Brigden's Operating Department Practice

For Churchill Livingstone:

Commissioning editor: Inta Ozols
Project manager: Valerie Burgess
Project controller: Derek Robertson
Design direction: Judith Wright
Page layout: Gerard Heyburn
Copy editor: Jennifer Bew
Indexer: Janine Fearon
Promotions manager: Hilary Brown

Brigden's Operating Department Practice

Edited by

Philip Clarke RGN
formerly Theatre Manager, Guy's Hospital, Director of Nursing, Lewisham Hospitals, Guy's and Lewisham NHS Trust, London

Josephine Jones RGN
Surgical Services Manager, Mount Vernon and Watford Hospitals NHS Trust, Northwood

Foreword by

Raymond J. Brigden PhD SRN
formerly Nursing Officer, Department of Health, London

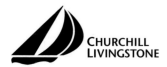
CHURCHILL
LIVINGSTONE

EDINBURGH LONDON NEW YORK PHILADELPHIA SAN FRANCISCO SYDNEY TORONTO 1998

CHURCHILL LIVINGSTONE
A Division of Harcourt Brace and Company Limited

Churchill Livingstone, Robert Stevenson House, 1–3
Baxter's Place, Leith Walk, Edinburgh EH1 3AF, UK

First published 1998

ISBN 0 443 05188 7

British Library Cataloguing in Publication Data
A catalogue record for this book is available from the British
Library.

Library of Congress Cataloging in Publication Data
A catalog record for this book is available from the Library
of Congress.

Medical knowledge is constantly changing. As new
information becomes available, changes in treatment,
procedures, equipment and the use of drugs become
necessary. The editors, contributors and publishers have, as
far as it is possible, taken care to ensure that the information
given in this text is accurate and up to date. However,
readers are strongly advised to confirm that information,
especially with regard to drug usage, complies with current
legislation and standards of practice.

Printed and bound in Great Britain by
The Bath Press, Bath

The
publisher's
policy is to use
**paper manufactured
from sustainable forests**

Contents

Contributors

Brenda Baxter RGN MRM
Business Manager, Anaesthetic Directorate,
Northwick Park and St Marks NHS Trust,
Harrow

*The National Health Service contracting process,
Quality in the operating department and Day-care
surgery in Ch. 1 Organization and Management*

Claire Campbell RGN ONC DipN
Senior Clinical Nurse – Theatres, Royal
Lancaster Infirmary, Lancaster

Ch. 5 Surgical preparation
Ch. 6 Surgical practice

Philip E Clarke RGN
formerly Theatre Manager, Guy's Hospital,
Director of Nursing, Lewisham Hospitals (Guy's
and Lewisham NHS Trust), London

*The operating department: management and
organization in Ch. 1 Organization and
management*

Bridget Dimond MA LLB DSA AHSM
Barrister-at-Law
Emeritus Professor, University of Glamorgan

Ch. 2 Legal aspects of operating theatre practice

Jennifer D East MSc RN
Director, Infection Management Ltd,
Harpenden

Ch. 3 Risk management

Christine Greenhaugh
Director, GCL Healthcare Management
Consultants, Macclesfield

*Information technology in theatres in Ch. 1
Organization and management*

Rachel Hodson RGN DN
Nurse Practitioner, Endoscopy,
Castle Hill Hospital, Hull

Endoscopy in Ch. 5 Surgical preparation

Josephine Jones RGN
Surgical Services Manager,
Mount Vernon and Watford Hospitals NHS Trust

*The operating department: management and
organization in Ch. 1 Organization and management*

Roger King BA FIOT Cert Ed
Senior Lecturer,
Thames Valley University

Ch. 4 Anaesthetic practice

Jane Sharp RGN
Recovery Room Sister,
Ashstead Hospital, Surrey

Ch. 7 Recovery practice

Marion Taylor BEd(Hons) DipN
Senior Lecturer, Middlesex University

Ch. 5 Surgical preparation
Ch. 6 Surgical practice

Sinclair Webster MA DipArch (Cantab.) RIBA FIHSE
Websters Architects, Woking

Ch. 8 Design considerations

Paul Wicker BSc RGN RMN CCNS
Eduction Co-ordinator, Theatres,
Royal Infirmary of Edinburgh NHS Trust,
Edinburgh
Editor, British Journal of Theatre Nursing

Principles, uses and hazards of electrosurgery in Ch. 5 Surgical preparation

Mike Mason Williams BA (Hons) FCA
Healthcare, KPMG, Birmingham

Business planning for theatres in Ch. 1 Organization and management

Foreword

The first edition of *Operating Theatre Technique* set out to provide a comprehensive reference book for operating theatre personnel. At that time there was no other all embracing document which covered the multitude of subjects of interest to theatre nurses. Two-thirds of the book comprised operating theatre procedures, the remainder dealt with theatre practice including basic design and the role of the theatre nurse.

Over the next two decades, evolution in the organization of the operating theatre as well as developments in surgical procedures resulted in a change of emphasis. Although surgical procedures still formed an important proportion of the content, more information was included in each subsequent edition on such aspects as theatre design, management and patient care. The last 10 years in particular has seen a rapid escalation not only in the range and extent of surgery undertaken, but also in the very wide range of information required by the operating department manager. The extension of day surgery and the use of non-invasive procedures are some of the aspects changing the approach to the provision of operating department services.

The primary consideration is, of course, maintaining a high standard of patient care but to achieve this, in addition to technical expertise, the theatre practitioner must be cognisant of many other aspects such as business planning, quality control, information technology, and legal implications such as health and safety legislation, etc.

The Editors of this new edition have reiterated the original objectives of 1962, namely to bring together a multitude of subject matter relevant to the theatre practitioner. This does not of course obviate the need to refer in depth to other specialized publications when appropriate. It is right that the majority of space in this book is devoted to theatre practice, although the reader will still find a good deal included on procedures, for example, in anaesthetic and recovery practice. I have no doubt that *Operating Department Practice* will continue to form a valuable source of reference to all operating department personnel.

RJB
Reading 1997

Preface

Raymond Brigden first published *Operating Theatre Technique* in 1962; he revised and updated subsequent editions to reflect the many changes affecting operating department practice. When asked to review and consider a new edition of the textbook we decided that the main focus should be directed towards the care of the patient and the preparation of the operating department team. The reader may be disappointed that there is little reference to operating procedures and more emphasis on organizational issues relating to practice. This is no reflection on the style and content of Bridgen's original textbooks but is an attempt to emphasise the need for a knowledge and research-based practice in the operating department.

Throughout the text reference is made to the practitioner. This definition includes nurses, operating department practitioners and assistants and those preparing for these roles.

We are extremely grateful to our contributors and would like to thank them for their help, patience and understanding during what has been a lengthy process. In addition we would like to thank Carrie Bonsey, Linda Carr, Kate Nightingale and Paul Wicker for their critical appraisal and professional help.

Our thanks also go to those who assisted by providing additional material, these include Merril Revill, Henri Choo, Kath Fullerton and Ruth Buxbaum. We are grateful for the help and advice given by the staff at Churchill Livingstone.

We are indebted to our colleagues from industry for allowing us to use their product information and illustrations. Among those we would especially thank are Johnson and Johnson, Ethicon Ltd, Codman, 3M Manufacturing Co., Rimmer Bros., Davis and Geck, Key Med, Valley Lab, Sims Medical Systems.

PEC and JJ
London 1997

1

Organization and management

The operating department: management and organization

P. Clarke   J. Jones

This chapter gives details of some of the systems used to ensure organizational efficiency.

The operating department is no different from any other service-providing facility in a hospital: it pulls together a complex range of organizational activities and is a major user of financial and other resources. Management challenges are presented in isolation from, but as part of, the whole hospital organization.

It must be recognized that organizational management has many facets. If the full potential of an operating department is not realized, the outcomes may lead to a form of crisis management. Failure to meet contractual requirements and service agreements could result in closure of theatre sessions, failure to fulfil patients' needs and a loss of jobs.

In this chapter the reader will find information on some of the processes relating to organizational management. A list of references is given at the end of each section.

The 1989 changes in the law governing healthcare to the nation have changed the way in which this care is provided.[1] The split between the purchasing of healthcare and the providing has resulted in a more businesslike approach and provided challenges to managers at all levels of service. The practitioner must have an understanding of the systems that need to be employed to maximize the use of resources, in order to achieve the quality of service deserved by the patient. The Health Service's Patient's Charter affects everybody working in healthcare delivery and charges each individual with accountability to ensure that the highest standards of care are achieved.

No one facet of organizational management can be taken in isolation. It will be seen in this section how each tool is dependent on the others, providing a thread to management objectives.

Data collection needs information technology (IT) but cannot be done in isolation without an understanding of organizational and personnel management, quality, educational needs and the contractual arrangements with the purchaser. Planning – not only day-to-day events but also long-term strategy – is dependent on recognition by both managers and personnel of the benefits of using these systems.

Resources, in terms of both staff skill mix and financial limitations, have to be considered innovatively to enable the operating department to provide an efficient and cost-effective service.

A whole new vocabulary of jargon has reached the operating department. However, the basis of good management remains, that is, getting things done. Objectives can only be achieved by the people and with the people that form the operating department team.

Human resources management is fundamental to the efficient organization of the department. Performance review of individuals within the team is paramount in promoting standards of skill and staff motivation, which will in turn provide a high level of morale, contributing to a well ordered team.

Performance review is insufficient in itself: it must be clearly planned, with skilled assessors and both parties understanding the function and objectives of the system in order to make the process dynamic. Individual action plans, which match the overall business objectives of the organization and the department, should be agreed. Coupled with this is the need to recognize the individual's ability to achieve outcomes and how additional help can be given in the form of coaching, education or training, the final step being an agreed plan of monitoring and review.[2]

The assessor must, of course, have skills in listening and the ability to be objective and honest with the individual. It is essential that the appointed 'grandparent' be supportive to both parties and aware of the objectives.

EDUCATION AND TRAINING

The operating department team will be made up of a variety of people with different skills, training and education, varying from the qualified nurse to the department assistant or practitioner, who form the cohort of the non-medical professional team. In addition there will be ancillary workers providing assistance to the professional team or carrying out specific tasks, including portering or housekeeping duties. Managers must have an understanding of the educational and training needs of all team members, which will be identified and reinforced by the performance review. It must always be borne in mind that individual requirements must be balanced with the overall objectives of the department.

COMMUNICATION STRATEGY AND TEAM BRIEFING

The need for effective communication, both verbal and written, should not be underestimated. This is a subject that cannot be ignored when considering organizational management. The operating list is an example of how effective communication is with all disciplines: medical staff, wards, clinical departments and support services. If this one basic element of a day's work is not well planned, the repercussions, not least for the patient, are endless.

The rate of change in organizational management and service delivery has been accelerating, and if we are to be sufficiently responsive and keep up with the changes we need better ways of keeping in touch. Systems that rely heavily upon formal meetings and written reports, and which span six or seven hierarchical layers, prevent rapid communication. As a result, those in higher management are seen to be out of touch. Recent trends have resulted in a flatter management structure, reducing hierarchies and enabling decisions to be made nearer to the point of service. The excellent organizations recognize that the people who know what is happening and can sense the way the world is moving are not exclusively at the top. It is those who work with the patients who know most about their changing needs. Everyday communication can be repetitive or ritualistic, but is necessary and needs particular attention and therefore requires a structured approach.

The process of information sharing begins by identifying the channels to be used in organizational communications: both downward and upward as well as lateral communication will be used. The choice of method depends on the direction and the specific nature of the message to be communicated. At the same time, for organizational communication to be effective it has to be carried out often and be of short duration for better memory retention.

One method of communication which is practised in the United Kingdom is team briefing. This can strengthen and reinforce the manager's role by sharing information about the organization at all levels of the service, demonstrating his responsibility for team performance and enhancing his reputation as a coach, a support and a provider of information. Building of trust will follow through working with the staff.

Good communication can help eliminate wastage, improve employee attitudes and increase their involvement at work, leading to an increase in job satisfaction.

Behavioural influence depends on the leadership climate within the operating department. The result of staff leadership is only effective if the climate is sympathetic to the adoption of more people-centred attitudes. Credibility is obtained by being able to demonstrate techniques and coaching staff into getting things right. The manager must be interested in what the workforce does and thinks about their work. One way of doing this is to walk the floor to listen and to value opinion.

The need for communication cannot be overemphasized: it is the central purpose of every individual working within any organization. The responsibility of every team member is to communicate and to ensure feedback from meetings, both educational and informational.

Communications within the organization as a whole will follow a framework, and clearly this will affect networking within the operating department. The manager must have a clear strategy for ensuring that staff are both informed and have the opportunity to express their views. This will engender *esprit de corps* and participative decision making. Team briefing is one approach that may be used to ensure that staff at all levels are aware of changes, developments and trends in service delivery.

In 1970, the Lewin Report on the Organization and Staffing of Operating Departments[3] recommended the establishment of a Theatre Users' Committee, a multidisciplinary forum whose objective was the efficient use of theatre services. Although the principles remain, many organizations have restructured this forum into a Theatre Management Committee, which reports to the Hospital Board and provides support to the theatre manager.

MANPOWER

Manpower planning identifies the systems best suited to an organization to enable the desired service to be provided. It also ensures that staff are deployed in a manner that is both efficient and cost-effective.

It is inappropriate to lay down guidelines on staffing levels and skill mix requirements because local needs vary. Staffing must be calculated taking into account workload and specialist needs and commitment to educational programmes.

With good manpower control it is possible to eliminate inefficient areas and at the same time maintain agreed standards of quality.

REFERENCES

1. Department of Health 1989 Working for patients. HMSO, London
2.. Stewart A 1982 Performance appraisal. In: Mumford A (ed) Handbook of management and development. McGraw Hill, Maidenhead
3. Department of Health and Social Security 1970 The organization and staffing of operating departments. HMSO, London

Business planning for theatres

M. Mason Williams

Put very simply, the process of planning is 'managing change'. This involves thinking ahead; looking at the wider picture; monitoring the progress of the theatre; and being in control rather than being overcome by events.

Business planning is not just a one-off exercise and it is not just the production of a business plan, which is typically used by the department as a resource bidding exercise to the Unit Board, but it is a 'culture' which should be adopted by the department. It is a fundamental part of the changing market for healthcare.

Everybody plans, either as an individual, as part of a group (for example a family) or as an organization. The term 'planning' can cover a whole range of formal or informal ways of agreeing where the department is at the moment, of deciding where it wants to go (its destination or goal) and how it is going to get there; and being able to monitor how successful it has been in achieving its goal. This process will result in change, both as a consequence of the process itself and because of external influences, for example a change in government. There is no mystery in planning: it is simply a discipline for defining and taking key decisions and for 'managing' the changes.

WHY BOTHER WITH PLANNING?

This is a question very often asked by staff connected with healthcare, particularly because healthcare is an area of great uncertainty where prediction and planning is very difficult. Therefore, why not wait for events to make actions urgent?

Does a doctor wait for a patient with abdominal pain to develop appendicitis before acting? Is there no chance that early diagnosis will make the patient's survival more likely and the treatment less painful? By acting early does the doctor not keep her options open, giving herself room for manoeuvre and choice? In waiting for a crisis the doctor has effectively removed any choice.

A department should try and plan, but it should accept that it cannot plan for all eventualities.

Changes in departmental organization

There have been major changes in the ways in which hospital departments, including theatres, are managed. These include, for example, the devolvement of budgets and accountability to departments and specialties; and a move towards competitive tendering and market testing. Business planning will enable the department to cope more effectively with these changes. This is just one of its benefits.

Benefits of planning

• The theatre is more likely to achieve its overall goal – to achieve health gain.

• An effective planning process leads to better management control and monitoring of results.

• The department will be better prepared to meet external changes and can take advantage of new opportunities, to the benefit of the patients. The absence of a plan guarantees confusion in changing circumstances.

• The department can actively maximize its assets, both quantitatively and qualitatively.

• The department will have a clearer awareness of its weaknesses and be better placed to overcome them.

• The department will be better placed to understand its priorities.

• Collective ownership of the department's goals can be achieved by communicating those goals and objectives effectively to the staff.

- In the modern environment of cash-limited funds, a department which provides detailed business cases/plans for future development will stand a better chance of obtaining the money it needs.

THE PLANNING PROCESS

The standard elements of the planning process[1] are outlined in Table 1.1. The important thing to remember is that the department should **plan to achieve results** and the planning process is about how this happens. This boils down to four basic questions:[2]

- Where are we now?
- Where do we want to get to?
- How do we get there?
- How far have we got?

Table 1.1 The standard elements of the planning process

Terms	Definition	Personal Example
Mission ↓	Overriding premise in line with the values of the department	Be healthy and look good
Goal ↓	General statement of aim or purpose	Lose weight
Objectives ↓	Quantification (if possible) or more precise statement of the goal	Lose 10 lb by 1 September
Strategies ↓	Broad categories or types of action to achieve objectives	Diet and exercise
Actions/tasks ↓	Individual steps to implement strategies	Eliminate desserts, snacks and butter. Limit alcohol to 1 drink/day and swim every day
Control ↓	The monitoring of action steps to reinforce objectives and hopefully leading to: assess the effectiveness of strategies and actions; modify strategies and/or actions as necessary	Weigh first thing every morning; if satisfactory progress, do nothing; if not, consider other strategies and actions
Rewards	A payoff for reaching the objective	Buy a new suit

STAGES OF BUSINESS PLANNING

Preparation for business planning

This is a key stage in the business planning process and one that, in practice, is commonly omitted. However, its successful completion is vital to the ultimate success of the planning process as a whole. There are three elements to this stage:

- appointing a project manager
- identifying the participants and agreeing their roles
- compiling a profile of the department's current services.

A department's profile should answer the following questions:

- Who are the users/customers of the services? For example, the various surgical specialties.
- What services are provided? For example, use of the theatre facilities.
- How are they provided and by whom? For example, by the theatre nurses.
- When are the services provided? For example, the availability of theatre time.

Quite often a department will benefit from doing this stage on its own as, having done so, many a department manager has remarked: 'I did not realize we did that and why are we doing it that way? It would be much better like...'.

Defining the department's purpose

This involves setting the department's mission and agreeing its core values and goals.

The mission statement is an expression of the ideal purpose for the department and what the services eventually hope to achieve. It defines the business the department is in and where it is going. It can be thought of as an expression of its *raison d'être*.

The value statements define the department's core values, in such areas as:

- availability of the service
- quality of the service
- care of the staff (training, staff development)
- innovation (new services, new methods)
- accessibility of the service.

The purpose of value statements is to help develop a service which is based on shared beliefs and to identify a need for change.

Goals are a general statement of direction for the department. Quite often they are qualitative in manner. They should be related to the mission and expressed in terms of outcomes or results. An example of a goal is 'to provide effective and flexible support to meet the changing needs of the theatre's customers'.

To achieve these goals it will be necessary for the department to have a greater number of more detailed objectives (see below).

Analysing the department's strengths, weaknesses, opportunities and threats (SWOT analysis)

SWOT analysis is simply an evaluation of how well the department is doing and what are the opportunities and threats facing it.

Strengths and weaknesses are areas which are **internal** to the department, and over which the department has direct control. Opportunities and threats are **external** factors, and so the department can only influence them. The purpose of this stage is to identify all the strengths, weaknesses, opportunities and threats of the department in the light of its mission statement, with the aim of:

- maximizing/exploiting the strengths
- taking corrective action to minimize the weaknesses
- being in a position to take advantage of opportunities
- being aware of, and prepared for, all known threats.

An example of a theatre SWOT analysis is as follows:

Strengths:
- trained and committed staff
- availability of the services
- utilization of the facilities
- quality of the service.

Weaknesses:
- poor standard of the facilities – lack of day theatres

- overreliance on key individual staff
- lack of management and organizational skills.

Opportunities:
- ability to provide services for other units/hospitals
- new technology (IT and clinical).

Threats:
- 'knock-on' effect of main specialties' problems
- market testing and competitive tendering.

Agreeing the department's objectives

Objectives are a quantification or more precise statement of a goal. They are the department's targets for the forthcoming year.

Ideally the department should focus its objectives on its **outputs** and/or **results**, that is, what its services aim to achieve, as opposed to purely the inputs, for example staff costs.

Objectives should be:

- specific (clear and unambiguous)
- measurable (not only quantity but also quality)
- agreed (must be 'owned')
- realistic (practical and achievable)
- time related (not 'open ended').

Examples of a theatre's objectives are as follows:

- all staff to meet their individual training development plans by the end of the financial year
- approval for the development plan for a day theatre to be achieved by 31 December
- agreed working practices/protocols to be documented and adopted by the department by 30 June
- establish a regular communication process with other departments and the specialties by 31 March.

Agreeing the department's strategies

Strategies are broad statements of intent which show the types of action required to achieve the objectives.

Areas of strategy include:

- staff (skill mix, training, development and review)
- facilities (space, equipment)
- processes (quality)
- services provided
- financial.

Determining the department's action plans

Action plans should be designed to implement all the strategies of the department, taking into account their relative priorities and the resources available.

Successful action plans have the following characteristics:

- Each task must be 'owned' by department staff.
- Plans should be communicated to all involved.
- Time limits should be set for each task.
- Plans should include a monitoring mechanism.
- Contingency plans should be prepared.
- Overall the plans should be flexible.

Monitoring and reviewing the department's results

This is the sometimes painful process of determining whether or not the department is succeeding. The monitoring and reviewing process can be referred to in one word: **audit**.

The monitoring and reviewing stage is very important to the success of the business planning process. It performs three loops back to earlier stages in the process:

- to allow corrective action to be taken
- to help identify new strategies and/or plans
- to make changes to existing strategies for future years.

Most departments will need to monitor:

- financial performance
- Service Level Agreement (SLA) performance (if applicable)
- overall activity/service levels
- quality
- key performance indicators (to be set by the department)
- progress with objectives.

REFERENCES

1. Johnson G, Scholes K 1993 Exploring corporate strategy. Prentice Hall International, Hemel Hempstead
2. Glynn- Williams WI 1992 Managing for results. Glaxo Pharmaceuticals UK Limited. NHS Relations Address at NAHAT Conference, Harrogate

The National Health Service contracting process

B. Baxter

The changes contained in the government's 1989 White Paper[1] introduced the market economy into the health service, separating the purchasing of healthcare from its providers. Prior to these reforms district health authorities were allocated funding to pay for healthcare provision and managed hospitals and community services providing care.

Following the introduction of the changes health authorities were designated as purchasing authorities. In addition, the concept of general practitioner fundholders was introduced, which allowed GPs to purchase independently some aspects of healthcare for their patients.

Hospitals and community services became provider units. Some were afforded self-governance through trust status, whereas others remained directly managed by the health authority.

PURCHASER'S ROLE

It is the role of the purchasing authority to identify service requirements in terms of the type of care needed, the volume and the location for care delivery. Information available to them to make these decisions comes from the study of historical activity, epidemiological studies and the views of local practitioners and their patients. The constraints on purchasing authorities are cash limits and the need for them to provide core services, such as:

- accident and emergency (A and E)
- immediate admission via A and E
- other immediate admissions
- services in support of the above.

GP fundholding practices can purchase healthcare for their patients from an agreed number of procedures. They do not purchase emergency or urgent admissions.

The providers are:

- NHS trust hospitals
- NHS community trusts
- private hospitals
- private community services
- directly managed units.

PROVIDER'S ROLE

Provider units produce a catalogue of services which they are able to offer to purchasers. The provider needs to inform the purchasers of the capacity available and the price of services.

TYPES OF CONTRACT

Block contract

These contracts are negotiated to a fixed sum, defining the service and a fixed volume of work.

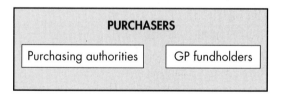

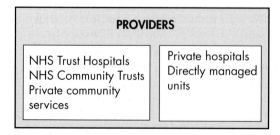

Figure 1.1 The relationship between purchasers and providers.

The contract will also include explicit quality standards and is expressed in finished consultant episodes, for example 6000 general surgery, 7000 general medical, 4000 orthopaedic, 4000 gynaecology, and so on. Block contracts do not normally distinguish between emergency, urgent and routine episodes.

Cost and volume

Such contracts define a service requirement and a base-level volume of provision. An initial fixed sum is agreed, with scope to increase the volume if this is agreed between the purchaser and provider at a later date. Quality standards are explicit in the contract.

Cost per case

This type of contract defines the service and is charged on a cost-per-case basis. The volume remains flexible and there are explicit standards included.

During negotiations the purchasers agree with the providers what percentage of the contract they expect to be completed as day care for each specialty.

IMPLICATIONS FOR THEATRE MANAGEMENT

Before contracting with purchasers was established, the allocation of theatre space depended on the number of operating sessions noted in consultant surgeons' contracts. These sessions may not have been linked to waiting-list numbers or adjusted for session over- or underutilization.

Contracting now means that once a contract is let, the total number of episodes for each surgical specialty has to be considered, using historical data. The percentage of admissions for each specialty which does not come to theatre then has to be extracted from the total. For example, in orthopaedic surgery a patient may be admitted with acute back pain, treated by bed rest and traction only and discharged. This is a finished consultant episode against the orthopaedic contract, but the patient did not come to theatre.

A percentage then has to be deducted for emergency and urgent surgery performed out of session time, again using historical data. There may be some scope in certain specialties to move urgent work into session time: trauma which has to be operated on within 48 hours could be moved into planned sessions.

Once the estimated number of cases in the contract that will occur in session time has been calculated, then for each specialty the total is divided into a 48-week operating year. This provides the total number of cases to be achieved for each specialty in one week.

The weekly number is then divided again by the average number of operations achieved by a specialty in a session, which provides the total number of sessions by specialty each week (Box 1.1).

Block contracts, and in some cases cost and volume contracts, do not currently distinguish between major, minor and intermediate operations. Banding of episodes of surgical intervention is being explored, and will help in the refinement of contracting.

Increases in cost and volume contracts or cost-per-case contracts will mean that additional theatre sessions may be required for given periods throughout the year. It therefore follows that flexibility in work patterns and in the use of temporary contracts, bank staff and gain share schemes requires to be implemented to cover peaks in theatre workload.

Purchasing authorities may provide funding for waiting-list initiatives at some stage during the year, over and above episodes agreed in the contract. These initiatives may only involve a certain specialty, for example orthopaedics to reduce the overall waiting time for routine hip replacement, and may encompass all surgical

---

Box 1.1   Formula for contracting

Annual contracted number for surgical specialty

Minus % that do not come to theatre
Minus % operated on out of hours
Divided by 48-week operating year
Divided by average number of cases per list
= Total number of lists per week for specialty

specialties to reduce the length of waiting time for all routine surgery. Similar calculations can be made to estimate the increase in operating lists required to accomplish the additional workload, as used to assess the main contract.

REFERENCE AND FURTHER READING

1. Department of Health 1989 Working for patients. HMSO, London
2. Mills I 1989 Caring for the 1990s. Resource management initiative information package – acute hospitals. Post progress and future plans. NHS Management Executive, London
3. Department of Health 1989 Contracting for health services: operational principles. NHS Management Executive, London

Quality in the operating department

B. Baxter

Within both service and manufacturing industries, greater emphasis is increasingly being placed on quality assurance. Consumer expectations are continually being raised, and within the health service this has been reinforced by the Patient's Charter, which sets targets for waiting times, waiting lists and other broad measurement targets, and this has resulted in the development of systems to measure and ensure that outcomes are achieved.

Purchasers of healthcare expect quality service which is relevant, timely and cost-effective. This will be reflected when contracts are negotiated and agreed. Employees expect standards which ensure a safe environment, good conditions of employment and effective communications.

In order to ensure that patients' and their carers' expectations are met, quality assurance strategies must be in place. This section outlines some of the methods which may be used to achieve high standards of care.

Quality can be defined as a level of excellence – freedom from doubt. In 1988 Dr C. Wilson stated that quality assurance was 'A management system by means of which we assure ourselves and others of the quality of work for which we have responsibility'.

TOTAL QUALITY MANAGEMENT

Total quality management (TQM) is a management process which has quality as an integral part, which is comprehensive, coherent, systematic and continuous throughout the whole of the organization.

All staff working within the organization, from the Chief Executive downwards, must be committed to ensuring that procedures carried out are right first time. Such a philosophy practised by all employees will save time on investigating complaints, reduce concern, anger and suffering for patients and their relatives, and reduce compensation claims.

John S. Oakland[1] states: 'To be successful in promoting business efficiency and effectiveness, TQM must be truly company-wide and it must start at the top with the Chief Executive, or equivalent, the most senior directors and management, who must demonstrate that they are serious about quality. The middle management have a particularly important role to play: they must not only grasp the principles of TQM, they must go on to explain them to the people for whom they are responsible, and ensure that their own commitment is communicated. Only then will TQM spread effectively throughout the organization. This level of management must also ensure that the efforts and achievements of their subordinates obtain the recognition, attention and reward that they deserve.'

Each member of staff must understand that their failure to perform effectively will have implications for other members of the team caring for the patient, and may adversely affect the outcome of treatment.

The involvement of all staff in understanding TQM will not only reduce errors, but also increase the consistency of staff performance and improve the function of the organization.

COST – VOLUME – QUALITY

Purchasers include in their contracts with providers the three elements of cost, volume and quality:

- cost = resources, input
- volume = output, total numbers achieved
- quality = outcomes of treatment.

Purchasers require to be assured that the contracts they agree with providers guarantee:[2]

- the appropriateness of treatment and care
- the achievement of optimum clinical outcome
- that all clinically recognized procedures to minimize complications and similar preventable events are followed
- an attitude which treats patients with dignity as individuals
- an environment conducive to patient safety, reassurance and contentment
- speed of response to patients' needs and minimum inconvenience to them (and their relatives and friends)
- the involvement of patients in their own care.

Specific standards will be explicit in the contracts which the providers must demonstrate. Systems must be in place to ensure that the right things are done in the right way and at the right time to ensure that agreed standards are met.

PROCESS

The National Health Service introduced Performance Indicators 1982–84,[3] which measured input and output for clinical activity,

finance, manpower and estates management. No measurement was made of outcomes.

There were two obvious defects in extrapolating the data from performance indicators: one is that it is uncertain whether they compare like with like; for instance, the minimum dataset for operating theatres asks for information on the number of lists held and the number of cases for each specialty carried out in those lists: it does not ask for information on the length of lists. In some hospitals a list session is 4 hours, in others it is 3.5 hours and in some it is 3 hours. The other defect is that the measure of activity does not prove the quality of the work, i.e. there is no outcome measure.

MEDICAL AUDIT

This is a system which looks at the outcomes of medical practice as providing peer review to investigate best practice and ensure that the treatment given to patients will provide the best outcomes. The development of treatment protocols based on current research is beginning, although some clinicians are concerned that this will erode their clinical freedom.

Medical audit occurs locally, whereby clinicians review patients treated and the outcomes achieved. There is also a national review of treatment and outcomes.

In 1982 a National Confidential Enquiry into Perioperative Deaths (CEPOD)[5] was initiated as a joint venture between the Association of Anaesthetists and the Association of Surgeons, funded by the Nuffield Provincial Hospital Trust and the King Edward's Hospital Fund for London. Three NHS regions were involved in a review of surgical and anaesthetic practice over 1 year. Funding was made available by the government in 1988–89 to enable a wider study covering all of the regions in England to continue the work of this group. The work of CEPOD continues, allowing doctors to examine their own practice and performance with the objective of reducing perioperative mortality.

CLINICAL AUDIT

Doctors do not work in isolation: they depend on nurses, paramedical and technical personnel as well as secretarial and hotel services staff. Clinical audit in a multidisciplinary setting is a way of developing standards that provide a good-quality service for the patient.

The shared values of the organization must be clearly defined in the objectives and goals of each group and department in the hospital, and used to set standards in all areas. Trust and a willingness to share information about performance reviews between professional and other groups must be built up, and the patient must be placed at the centre of all functions carried out within the institution.

STANDARD SETTING

'Standards are a mechanism for giving voice to concerns and empowering people to make changes in the light of these concerns.'

'Standard setting gives nurses and other healthcare professionals the power to put the patient back at the centre of the NHS.'

These statements were made by Christine Hancock[6] in July 1991 and demonstrate that setting and monitoring standards provides tools to demonstrate the need for change to improve care.

Achievable realistic standards must be developed from the philosophy and shared values of the organization. These must be set locally within each area using the bottom-up approach: the staff must feel ownership of the standards to ensure commitment. Standards must be relevant to the care given, based on current research and important for the quality of care. They must have measurable criteria to assist in the evaluation of care, help to identify problems and achievable solutions, and improve the quality of care.

The institution's infection control policies and relevant local and national policies must be included in the agreed standards. COSHH (Control of Substances Hazardous to Health) and health and safety legislation should also be reviewed when setting standards to ensure that requirements are noted.

The standard is the statement of the agreed level of service that should be achieved. The criteria are the measurable performance required to achieve the standard, and can be grouped into structure, process and outcome:

- structure = the resources that must be available to achieve the standard
- process = the actions carers take to achieve the standard
- outcome = the effect that the available resources and the carers' actions have on the achievement of the standard.

Audit of standards must be completed on a regular basis, the results evaluated and discussed with staff, and actions agreed and implemented when standards are not being met. Once action has been taken, the process of audit and evaluation must begin again to measure the effect this has had on improving care. Figure 1.2 illustrates a systematic approach to standard setting.

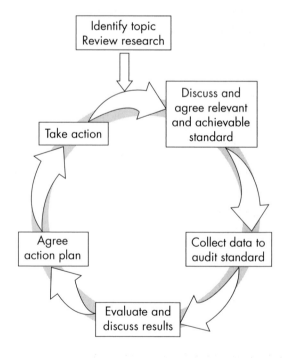

Figure 1.2 A systematic approach to standard setting.

QUALITY ASSURANCE

This is a system to ensure the quality of work for which management is accountable and to enable it to be demonstrated to others. Quality means different things to different people: the professional carer's view may differ from that of the patient receiving the care.

Methods of obtaining patients' views can be used: for example, the Audit Commission's Patient Satisfaction questionnaires on surgical day care for adults and children is a useful tool and can be compared with a national database.

There is a quality assurance package available from the National Association of Theatre Nurses which reviews:

- preparation of personnel
- preoperative care
- operating room care
- recovery care
- departmental organization.

The package gives standards and measurable criteria, and is currently in its third edition.

In 1994 the Association reviewed the package and felt there was a need to provide a more patient-focused tool which considered care at all stages of the operative process.

The tool is designed to follow the patient through the ward/department interface, through the theatre and recovery, and back to the ward. In addition there are aspects of the audit which consider management, and the whole is reinforced by a patient satisfaction questionnaire. The NATN tool document is in four distinct parts:

1. Patient care
2. Departmental management
3. Patient questionnaire
4. Action plan.

Part 1: Patient care

This part is split into five sections covering the patient's episode of care within the operating department.

Part 2: Departmental management

This part covers the following issues in departmental management:

- environment
- information
- manpower issues
- quality.

Part 3: Patient questionnaire

This part contains a questionnaire which is designed to obtain feedback from the patient about their experience within the operating department.

Part 4: Action plan

This part contains a template for constructing action plans following the quality assessment.

King's Fund Organizational Audit

Standards for acute hospitals have been developed by the King's Fund centre;[8] these were first published in 1989, with the second edition produced in October 1990. The definition of this Organizational Audit (Accreditation UK) is:

'1. A framework of organizational standards which relates to the systems and processes which must be in place to provide an efficient and effective service to patients and a good working environment to staff.
2. Evaluation of a hospital's progress towards meeting these standards by means of a survey conducted by a team of external senior healthcare professionals.'

This audit reviews management and support services, professional management and departmental management. Operating theatre service audit is included in the section on departmental management. Self-assessment forms are completed in each department, and are reviewed by the hospital project team to provide them with information on the progress made to achieve the standards. Copies are forwarded to the King's Fund at least 6 weeks prior to the survey. At the visit from the survey team the forms are completed based on the evidence produced by each department to support the various standards.

BRITISH STANDARDS

Healthcare service organizations are increasingly applying the British Standards Institute quality tool BS5750. This was developed by the Institute following consultation with representatives from the major manufacturing and service industries. The system audits all parts of the organization, including management, organizational, financial, personnel and safety functions, and is aimed at delivering a quality product for the consumer. BS5750 certification is awarded following the successful completion of an extensive audit process conducted by approved assessors.

Benefits

The patient should receive treatment which satisfies their expectations for an improved quality of life or, when this is not possible, to have a comfortable and dignified death. Treatment should be timely and in pleasant surroundings, with staff responsive to patients' individual needs, hopes and fears.

The staff understand the goals and objectives and have shared values with the organization. They receive training and support to assist them in meeting the standards set. They are involved in setting those standards, their views are sought, and they feel they are involved in the decision-making process.

The organization gains a stable and committed workforce. Money is saved on the recruitment, selection and orientation of new staff. Complaints are reduced and time is saved on the investigation of complaints. The reputation of the organisation is thereby enhanced.

The purchasers will receive documentary evidence, which they require as part of their contract, that quality care has been given with beneficial outcomes.

BENCHMARKING

Benchmarking is a system which has been used in industrial and commercial settings and is now being used in healthcare. It is a systematic, continuous process which identifies, observes and implements best practice. In this process a facilitating group decides what to measure and agrees the scope of the study. Data are then collected and analysed, goals are developed and action plans agreed. The changes and the processes are monitored and, if necessary, the benchmark recalibrated, with best practice being integrated into the existing system to improve the function of the organization.

All systems which are used to ensure quality must address whether the treatment was safe, accessible, equitable and legal. They must place the patient at the centre of the process and review all the layers of the service which affect the quality of clinical care given by doctors, nurses and technicians; the workload and deployment of staff to provide safe and timely care; systems for personnel management; organizational arrangements; the environment in which care is given; and the support services the professional team requires to function effectively, for example supplies and hotel services.

Target 31 from the World Health Organization states that 'By 1990, all member states should have built in effective mechanisms for ensuring quality of patient care within their health systems'. This was endorsed in 1994.

All managers must utilize quality assurance methods to monitor the provision of healthcare. This is an expectation of both patients and their carers and is a requirement embodied in the health service.

REFERENCES

1. Oakland J S 1989 Total Quality Management. Butterworth-Heinemann, Oxford
2. NHS Management Executive 1989 Contracting for health services: operational principles. HMSO, London
3. Department of Health Korner Reports 1982–1984 1: Hospital facilities and diagnostic services; 2: Patient transport; 3: Manpower; 4: Paramedical services; 5: Community services; 6: Finance. HMSO, London
4. Department of Health 1989 Working for patients. HMSO, London
5. Campling EA, Devlin HB, Lunn JN 1990 The Report of the National Confidential Enquiry into Perioperative Deaths. London
6. Hancock C July 1991 Quality Conference. London
7. Benchmarking Tenzer I, Stodd K, Spies MB 1994 Association of Operating Room Nurses Conference
8. King's Fund Centre 1990 Organizational Audit (Accreditation UK): Standards for acute hospital, 2nd edn. King's Fund Centre, London
9. National Association of Theatre Nurses. QUAD. July 1994 Harrowgate

Information technology in theatres

C. Greenhalgh

Information technology (IT) plays an increasing role in the management and delivery of healthcare. Without technology to rapidly collate, analyse and present enormous amounts of complex data we would have to rely on simple manual indicators of performance, and spend an inordinate amount of valuable time collecting and manually analysing data.

Theatres account for a large amount of an acute hospital budget, second only to that of nursing. Many patients require some form of operative procedure. The pressure for IT to help assimilate information for both operational and clinical management, as well as to understand resource utilization, is therefore a high priority.

In 1991 the Department of Health Resource Management Initiative, recognizing this as a key area for resource management, provided money towards the purchase of theatre IT systems. Before this time there were only one or two commercially available systems for specific use in theatres. Because of this opportunity a number of new systems were developed: these tended to focus on the need for information to manage the resources.

The current emphasis on clinical effectiveness as well as efficiency has redirected the trend towards systems that provide day-to-day operational and clinical benefits as well as management information. The majority of operating departments now have IT systems capable of providing information for both operational and management use. It is expected that all will eventually have such systems as the demand for better and more timely information continues to increase.

THE NEED FOR INFORMATION

Information technology should not be seen as simply a tool for management, although this is one very important use of IT in theatres.

Using IT to record patient details not only allows fast retrieval of patient data but also provides information required for legal and data protection purposes, and analysis of information for contracting and for clinical research.

Information is also needed to help in the day-to-day work of running the department. IT can speed up some of the more routine operational processes by reducing the amount of duplication of recording. In-patient clerks are able to provisionally book patients into theatre sessions, which saves time and effort and avoids duplication in the operating department. Systems can rapidly produce theatre lists, and reproduce such lists when changes are necessary. Systems may control the purchase and use of stocks to a given budget, automatically reordering when stocks are low, and keep up-to-date staff timesheets, plan rotas and maintain annual leave and absence records.

It is often used to assist in operational decision-making processes, such as the preparation of theatre schedules, by calculating estimated session lengths with different mixes of patients and procedures, producing lists that make the most efficient use of theatre time. Some even incorporate into this the availability of equipment and specialist staff before finalizing schedules, producing job sheets and equipment booking lists and staff rosters as well as theatre schedules.

Information is needed to provide management with an understanding of the effectiveness and efficiency of the operating department. Aggregated data from different sources, such as patient records, theatre lists and stock control systems, can provide this information. Examples include:

- theatre utilization
- staff workload
- comparative costs of procedures/patients

- extent of and reasons for late starts, early finishes and cancelled sessions
- statutory returns.

The advantage of IT in analysis is that it can compute vast amounts of data quickly, to produce comparative statistical data, over time periods, between theatres and specialties, or even between different firms or surgeons. The big bonus over manual systems is the ease with which slightly different analyses can be repeated.

FUNCTIONALITY IN CURRENT SYSTEMS

The functionality of the currently available systems differs widely, not just in the areas they address, but also in their approach and in the detail of how functions work. For example, not all systems offer stock control or personnel management functions. Some are highly sophisticated, designed over many years to provide a wealth of different types of function. Others have been designed more simply and address rather fewer functional areas, or with less detail.

It is not possible to discuss all the functions and differences in any great detail here. For those who wish to read more about the different systems there is a guide called *Operating theatre systems – a guide to existing and potential products.*[1] In this chapter, five key functions are described which give an indication of the programs available and their key differences:

- scheduling resources
- personnel management
- stock control
- patient and clinical information
- management information.

Scheduling resources

The principle of scheduling systems is that the computer assists the user to plan an operating list that makes the best use of theatre time and resources. There is a wide variety of ways in which different systems achieve this. Some allow the entry of planned procedures, using historical data on how long is needed and the resources required to plan an ideal schedule; some simply allow the user to enter a possible schedule; and some calculate the estimated session length based on average times for procedures, to demonstrate potential spare capacity/overruns, and allow the user to consider a change in the schedule.

Some systems will provide a facility for admissions clerks to find spaces in theatre schedules based on predetermined criteria. Others add patients to a theatre waiting list, the precise session and time to be worked out by the theatre manager at a later time. More sophisticated programs will schedule patients, equipment, prostheses and materials to a session. Using information about surgeons' preferences by type of procedure, the system provides information about availability and allows the users to 'book' what is needed, thereby preventing two surgeons/anaesthetists wanting the same equipment at the same time.

Systems can produce 'pick lists' detailing equipment and supplies needed, waiting lists, scheduled session lists, pre-booking lists and the checklist cards for admission to and discharge from theatre.

Personnel management

Not all systems provide a personnel or rostering function: some use other hospital-wide personnel systems or input theatre nursing staff on specific personnel/rostering systems.

Those that do provide staff allocation functions are very different from each other. Some use the planned theatre schedules to derive 'workload', which is translated into nurse hours required; these are then used to automatically produce planned duty rosters. Others simply allow the straightforward entry of planned rosters. Most then allow for changes to these to reflect actual hours worked.

There are systems that provide immediate access to the estimated costs of planned rosters. In this way users can see the impact that changing the staff skill mix has on costs/budgets in specific periods.

There are systems that collate personnel data

for the day-to-day management of staff. These provide information such as budgeted staffing versus in-post and establishments; vacant post analysis; sickness and absence analyses of individuals or groups of staff; turnover analyses; and, for each member of staff, hours worked, in sufficient detail for payroll input.

Stock control

Not all systems include facilities for stock control, although most record sufficient detail about usage to arrive at an indicative cost per patient.

Details may be stored listing surgeons' preferences, including lists of equipment trays and supplies used by individuals for specific procedures, which can be updated with changes as they occur.

Recording the use of consumables varies between systems. Some do not record what is actually used, and consequently any cost information produced is related to planned stocks/supplies use. Others not only record actual use of stocks and supplies but relate use directly to an inventory, enabling remaining stock levels to be monitored.

One particular system uses a handheld barcoding facility to easily upload data from inventories into the theatre system. There are systems that automatically reorder stocks by producing requisitions. In effect, such systems are mini stock-control systems interfaced with the theatre functions. The drawbacks of any theatre stock-control system in the past have included problems with multiple sites for storage and different ordering procedures for different types of stock; these are now being addressed.

Patient and clinical information

The extent of patient and clinical data held also varies between systems. All now provide information about the theatre episode by patient, using the patient administration system (PAS) number. Data will include:

- patient number
- date and time of operation
- theatre number/name

- surgeon, anaesthetist and nurses involved
- procedures.

Selected systems may provide additional data, including:

- complications
- details of anaesthetic used
- clinical progress in recovery/anaesthesia
- results of laboratory tests.

Reports can show comparative information about interventions between patients who have the same procedures and information about differences between surgical teams. Combined with other information, such as rates of recovery, dates of discharge and subsequent wound infections, theatre systems can provide considerable information for the audit of effectiveness.

Management information

It is perhaps in the area of theatre management that IT is recognized as being most useful. All systems provide information about theatre and session utilization. There will be data on overruns and poor use of theatre time, by session, by theatre and by day. Statistics may be produced numerically or graphically, and all systems can produce information for statutory returns. Additional information may include patient times in various areas, including preoperative, theatre and recovery.

Efficient management of theatre resources can be achieved using IT. Workload information may include utilization by surgeon, firm, specialty or procedure. Reasons, impact and timing of cancellations will provide comparative data to enable efficient rostering and deployment of staff. The provision of cost information by patient as well as operation is necessary to understand the range of times for the same procedures, in order to derive costs and prices for the contractual process.

Staff costs

The basis for the calculation of staff costs varies between systems. Ranges may include:

- actual staff time involved with specific patients
- estimated times of procedure and staff involved

- averages based on historical data
- reconciliation of average expected times with actual times available.

Stock costs

The basis for costing stock – trays, prostheses, implants, disposables and other supplies – also varies considerably. Some theatre systems do not provide costings but send details to case-mix systems. These tend to use predetermined weightings for type of procedure and likely use of consumables. Some, however, do attempt to record when items are used by each individual patient, and provide cost per patient to the case-mix systems and to the business management process.

The important thing to note is that to track accurately everything used by an individual patient costs money, time and resources. This needs to be weighed against the benefits of really accurate costing. Some units will consider the added accuracy to be not worth the added cost of collection.

The management information potential of the systems is considerable, but it is not always functionality that influences the usefulness of the data. There are other factors that may influence data usage.

DATA ENTRY METHODS

Systems also differ in their means of data entry, and each has its own advantages and disadvantages.

Many require data entry in what is called batch mode, which means collecting data manually for later entry in batches. Data entry may be at the end of each session, at the end of each patient episode in theatre, or at the end of the week. The speed of data entry obviously affects the usage and value of the information.

Optical mark readers (OMRs) may be used; these require information to be collected manually by 'ticks' on a specially designed form, which is then read electronically; this converts the markings into data for direct transfer to the computer system. This reduces the time spent on data entry but requires staff training and is more expensive.

There are also real-time data entry systems, which require data to be entered as events happen. This means terminals must be sited in all preoperative, theatre and recovery areas. Obviously this is expensive, but it has the advantage of greater accuracy as transcription errors from paper to computer are thereby obviated. Facilities may also be available for access to other clinical/operational systems which are useful during the patient's time in theatre.

FLEXIBILITY/CUSTOMIZATION

Some systems are flexible in functionality, providing customization according to information needs; for example, flexible operation could allow changes in rostering rules for different sessions or changes to data collection for specific specialties.

In others, customization is restricted to using the standard framework to set up local data, such as the names and times of sessions and the names and grades of doctors.

Systems also vary by virtue of the amount of coded and text data required, with some allowing non textual clinical entries. All systems use coded data to record procedures that have taken place and allow users to choose the coding system they wish to use. Some have provided facilities that allow the user to 'find the correct code' through direct interrogation, but most rely on codes being found manually and input directly into the system.

REPORTING FACILITIES

Programs vary in their ability to analyse and report on the data input. Some have a wide selection of standard reports designed specifically for management use, and some have facilities that allow interrogation of a whole range of different data collected, through the provision of report generators and/or spreadsheets. This interrogation might be limited to the data collected in a designated theatre system; however, in some hospitals theatres are not 'standalone' systems, but are part of what is known as the hospital information support system (HISS). In HISS environments there is a single clinical record for each patient. Data collected in theatres can be interchanged together with data from, say, pathology, or from the wards, allowing for information such as type of operation, theatre and surgeon to be linked with wound infection or length of stay.

Coupled with differences in reporting capabilities are the differences in the abilities of systems to present data. Many systems have now the ability to produce not only numerical tables, but also graphical presentations of data showing trends of expenditure on consumables, for example, or changing utilization of theatres. Graphics and modelling capabilities need not be part of the

theatre system, but may be bought separately and linked.

INTERFACES

Theatre systems are just one of many hospital-based patient systems that relate to each other. If we are going to see a reduction in effort and a maximization of data use, then interfaces must be developed. Figure 1.3 shows how the Information Management and Technology Strategy for the NHS in England and Wales views theatre information in relation to other information.

Most current theatre systems interface with other systems to avoid the duplication of data collection. In most this involves the uploading (transfer to the theatre system) or download-

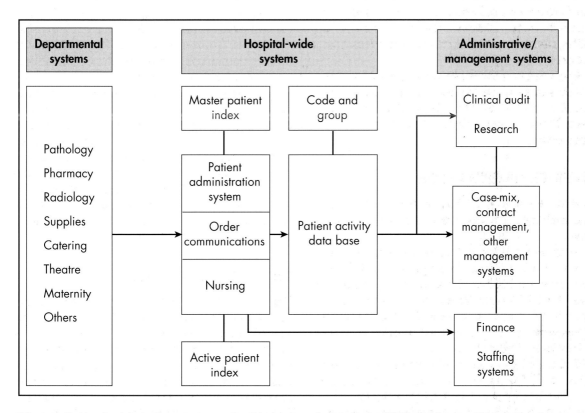

Figure 1.3 How the information management and technology strategy for the NHS in England and Wales views theatre information in relation to other information.

ing (transfer from the theatre system) between two different systems. Systems interfaced with theatres include:

- PAS/master patient index (usually to upload patient details to theatre system)
- PAS/waiting list (to book patients to theatre, or simply to transfer waiting-list details of individual patients)
- case-mix management (usually to download data on case-mix activity from the theatre system)
- contract monitoring system (usually to download patient cost information for contracts)
- personnel systems (usually to upload staff details to theatre systems, but sometimes to download roster information destined eventually for payroll)
- payroll systems (to download staff timesheet information)
- audit systems (to download patient-specific details).

These links may be made by batch transfer of data, for example all relevant records at the end of the day, or in real time (as things happen), such as when PAS is accessed and the user uploads specific patient details to the theatre system.

Other links may provide the ability to access other systems but do not allow data transfer, for example accessing other systems from the terminals in theatre to order pathological tests or items from the hospital stores.

All systems are different in the interfaces they have developed. In environments where theatre functions are part of the whole hospital system built around the single patient record, this tends to be referred to as integrated seamless data, rather than interfaced, as the data are transferred between different application functions.

DATA SECURITY

Many clinical staff express concern about the security of confidential information in computer systems. In fact, such information is, if anything, more protected than paper records could ever be.

To access any system requires some form of identification code for the system to recognize the user. Access to a different range of functions depends upon the status of the user and is defined by a unique allocated code. For example, some people may be able to look at data but not change them; some might not be able to access staff personnel data; some might not be able to schedule patients to theatre.

Many systems have an audit trail of transactions, which means they can discover (through the code) who made changes, what the changes were, and when. This knowledge can be used to investigate suspected system abuse or to recreate data after a system problem.

Obviously staff do get concerned that others might know their password, and sometimes staff watch others entering data. Not all security codes come up on the screen when entered, but it is possible that someone might watch where fingers are placed, which is why systems are set up to allow users to change their password as often as they like should they consider that others might have become aware of it.

People who are determined to 'hack the system' to obtain data might of course succeed, but anyone that interested could easily have extracted information from filing cabinets.

INTRODUCING NEW SYSTEMS

The introduction of a computer system into an operating theatre environment is a major project requiring many skills on the part of those involved. Changes are needed in:

- staff skills
- the culture of the working environment
- staff responsibilities
- staff working practices
- the physical environment
- the amount of data collected
- the use of the data and information.

There are a number of activities involved in introducing a new system; these fall broadly under the headings of preparation, selection, implementation and evaluation.

There is an excellent guidance document for the introduction of theatre systems, called *Operating theatre systems guidelines for selection and implementation*,[2] which gives a number of criteria that are necessary to secure a successful outcome:

- sufficient time for all stages
- structured approach
- the involvement of specialist staff
- clearly defined objectives and scope for both the project (selection and implementation) and the system functions
- a preimplementation assessment of the benefits expected from the introduction of the system and an assessment of the actual benefits realized postimplementation
- validation of outputs from the system, to check for software faults and to control the quality of data input
- ownership of, enthusiasm for and commitment to the system on the part of both direct and indirect users (including general managers)
- realization of the operational benefits before the strategic benefits
- evaluation of the system and identification of areas for improvement.

Information about the functionality of different systems can be found in *Operating theatre systems: a guide to existing and potential products*.[1]

It is not possible to cover all aspects of systems introduction here, but a number of important points are made below.

Planning

It cannot be stressed enough that this is the stage where future problems should be anticipated so that they can be avoided. Failure of systems to achieve what was expected is frequently due to inadequate preparation.

Activities to be included in planning are:

- establishment of the project management team
- production of a procurement plan
- seeking agreement to funding
- seeking commitment to processes for procurement, implementation and evaluation
- early preparation for change
- researching and understanding the available products

- development of risk analysis and containment plans.

Project management of major IT implementations will frequently use methodologies such as PRINCE (Projects in Controlled Environments), in which formal stages, processes and procedures will be defined, such as the production of a project initiation document and sign-off procedures at each stage and for each type of internal project, deliverable.

Preparation

The activities of preparation should include:

- baseline assessment of the current situation
- preparation of the statement of need
- production of EU advertisement
- production of the contract framework.

Any hospital thinking about buying a theatre system must advertise in the *European Journal* if the cost is likely to exceed prescribed levels (100 000 ECUs as at 1997) (goods and services). Suppliers will then respond if they are interested in tendering. An outline statement of need is often sent out at this stage, so that suppliers can decide if they wish to be considered.

The statement of need, which specifies the local operational requirement, describes what the users want the system to do. It is frequently issued with an invitation to tender to suppliers, and includes such information as:

- background information about the hospital
- a description of theatre information in the context of the rest of the hospital
- the broad functionality required
- detailed functionality, including information requirements, links to other systems, data items, reports
- system-wide requirements, including security, flexibility, archiving, transactions/usage, response times
- an indication of the hardware required, e.g. number of terminals, communications network
- requests for information from the supplier needed to evaluate responses, for example customer sites, size of company, ability to support product, etc.

Purchasing

The business case preparation activities involved in procurement include:

- selecting capable suppliers from responses to adverts
- shortlisting
- evaluating shortlisted suppliers
- preparation of detailed statement of need
- invite, confirm and expand tenders
- production/negotiation of draft contract
- evaluate offers and award contract
- debrief unsuccessful suppliers.

Evaluating shortlisted suppliers will include seeing demonstrations of the system as well as visiting other sites using it. A demonstration script is often used to ensure that all suppliers demonstrate the same functions, so that potential users can objectively value the nearness of fit to their particular priorities and requirements.

Once the shortlist has narrowed down to one (or sometimes two) suppliers detailed confirmation of how requirements are to be achieved is prepared. This provides more detail of what is required and how the particular system must meet these requirements, and is important as it is the basis of the contract with the supplier. Not preparing this, or getting it wrong, can lead to bitter disputes over what the system should have done. Note that at this stage the involvement of staff with experience of legal contracting is essential.

Guidelines for the procurement process can be found in *Procurement of information systems effectively (POISE)*, which is available from the NHS and provides a step-by-step framework for the procurement process, in conjunction with the Standards Enforcement in Procurement (STEP) documentation.[3,4]

Performing

Provided planning and preparation have been done well, this stage is not as onerous as it might be. If a system is not considered useful it is usually due to inadequate staff training. Training needs to cover awareness of IT, an awareness of why information is needed and why computers are useful in providing it. Specific system training, training in support processes to ensure that the information is accurate and complete, and training in the use of the information is necessary. It is frequently the latter that is inappropriately covered.

Points to note are that:

- training is ongoing: new staff have to be fully trained, not grasp what they can from whoever is around
- system training takes longer for staff unfamiliar with computers
- all staff will need some training
- training may not just be for nursing staff
- system training is only one small part of training
- the processes of information audit should inform training plans
- people who hardly know the system themselves do not make good trainers
- cascade training is not always appropriate.

EVALUATION OF BENEFITS

All purchases of any magnitude should be evaluated in terms of value for money. These approaches are variously called evaluations, cost–benefit studies or benefits assessment studies. All are based on the principle of demonstrating, as objectively as possible, the benefits accruing from buying the system. Approaches therefore rely on demonstrating change, which requires before-and-after studies, hence the earlier reference to a baseline review, which is a statement of where you are now and should be repeated after the system has been in operation for some time, to measure the extent of change.

Benefits should be considered from the viewpoints of patients, staff and the organization. The latter two will indirectly affect the patient as they will include cash and care benefits. They will also include both tangible and intangible benefits, for example savings in staff costs and improved morale. Cash values might also be accorded to different benefits, allowing comparisons of relative values. A guide to assessing benefits from nursing systems[4] provides some insights as to what might be necessary for this in theatres.

There has been some criticism of systems in

terms of benefits, although it needs to be noted that the same system might be criticized by one site while being lauded by another. This may be due to expectation: some sites appear to be clearer in their definition of requirements than others; or it may be a function of implementation – we still hear reports of systems that are inadequately funded, where insufficient training was given, or where local data support procedures are not adhered to. In some cases the systems themselves have in the past been less than perfect, and some were still being developed and 'site tested' during implementation.

THE FUTURE OF IT IN THEATRES

The future is likely to see the operational processes of whole hospitals dictating the need for systems, rather than for systems to be developed for discrete management functions related to specific service delivery areas. This will reflect a number of strategic intentions:

- for management data to be derived from operational systems
- for data to be patient centred (or person based), not service specific
- to provide appropriate data for questions about effectiveness
- to reduce duplication of effort
- to maximize the use of data collected.

We should therefore expect to see a movement away from theatre systems that are bought separately towards patient-focused integrated hospital systems, where theatre functionality is simply another function of the whole hospital and where there is a single, hospital-wide patient clinical record.

Not every hospital, however, will be in a position to change from the modular approach favoured to date, where patient data are extracted from separate service department systems and uploaded for analysis as needed.

Which systems survive will depend upon their ability to provide the information needed in the new business environment. This will depend largely upon their ability to interface, providing service-specific quality management information without too much duplication of effort.

The short to medium term will therefore see:

- more integration of functions, for example:
  — booking theatre time at the time of in-patient appointment
  — using the theatre lists to derive staff rosters
  — linking roster information to personnel and payroll systems
  — linking the use of stock items to stock control systems
- more flexibility in environment, for example:
  — choices of environment to fit the preferred IT strategy
  — theatre functions accessed where needed around the hospital
  — other hospital systems accessed from theatres, for example order/communications systems to, say, pathology
  — greater use of real-time data entry
  — more systems that have proven value for money, such as greater use of objective benefits assessment methods.

In the longer term we will also see changes in the type of IT used. Character readers – machines capable of reading handwritten textual information and translating it into code for computer analysis – are already developing, although not yet sophisticated enough to cope with all the different handwriting styles. We should also expect to see advances in the use of voice recognition systems, not just to allow access (they are often used for door security) but to intercept data as spoken for transfer to computer systems. Underpinning all of these developments will be a sensitivity to patient and staff confidentiality of the system contents.

REFERENCES

1. Operating theatre systems: a guide to existing and potential products 1993 GCL, Macclesfield
2. Operating theatre systems: guidelines for selection and implementation 1993 GCL, Macclesfield
3. Department of Health 1997 POISE: Procurement of information systems effectively, 2nd edn. HMSO, London
4. NHS Executive 1997 NHS IT standards in procurement (V4, March 1997) JMG E5226. NHS Executive, London
5. Benefits assessment studies: a practical guide 1992 Welsh Office, Cardiff

Day-case surgery

B. Baxter

In 1992 the Royal College of Surgeons published its Report of the Working Party on Guidelines for Day-Case Surgery, in which it is stated 'Day surgery is now considered the best option for 50% of all patients undergoing elective surgical procedures, though the proportion will vary between specialties'.[1]

The NHS Management Executive and the Day Surgery Task Force have made the strategic assumption that 50% of elective surgery can be carried out as day cases and that this is achievable within this decade.[2] Healthcare purchasers are negotiating with providers the percentage of day care that they require within each surgical specialty as part of contract agreements.

With the further development of minimally invasive procedures, laser surgical techniques and the development of hotel beds in acute hospitals, it should be possible to increase day-case surgery above 50% for all elective procedures.

ADVANTAGES

Patients

• Patients admitted for day-case surgical procedures will have to spend less time away from their home and family.
• With well planned postoperative analgesia and clear information as part of their discharge protocol, on average patients have a better postoperative recovery phase, earlier ambulation and a quicker return to work.

• Cancellations of operations for patients scheduled for day-case surgery should not occur at short notice because of emergency admissions. Beds and theatre time are designated for day-case surgery, therefore the patient can make the necessary plans both at home and at work.
• The risk of cross-infection is reduced as patients are separated from inpatients, spend only a few hours in hospital and recover in their own home.
• Spending only a short time in hospital is less traumatic for the patient – the length of stay is an important psychological factor. This is especially important when treating children and elderly patients.
• Day-case procedures are usually carried out by consultants or more experienced medical staff, which contributes to the overall higher quality of care and improved outcome for the patient.

Purchaser and provider

• Day-case surgery lowers the unit cost of an episode because of the reduction in the hotel element of treatment.
• A reduction in premedication, less invasive surgery and new anaesthetic drugs reduce recovery time and shorten the need for specialist post-anaesthetic care.
• Day-case surgery can reduce long waiting times and provide the ability to meet Patient's Charter standards.

• As day-case units have a planned workload, not affected by emergency admissions, they are usually more efficient in meeting value-for-money objectives.

• Savings made in lowering the unit cost of procedures and efficiency can be released to provide resources to expand and develop other services.

ACCOMMODATION

Day-case units which are self-contained, with their own admission facilities, beds, theatre and recovery area, have been purpose-built in many acute general hospitals. In some instances the day-case surgical facilities may be adjacent to the main theatre complex, using dedicated operating suites in that area to maximize the use of existing operating rooms and equipment.

Some hospitals may have a day-case ward, with patients operated on in the main theatres and recovering in the general recovery area. Some operating lists may be mixed, with both day and inpatient surgery.

Day-case beds may be allocated on inpatient wards, but this can create difficulties if such beds are filled by unplanned emergency admissions.

Whatever system a hospital adopts for accommodating day-case surgical patients, the ethos of preplanning admissions and ensuring that there are allocated beds and theatre time to undertake the procedures must not be compromised.

Admission of patients should take place in a reception area adjacent to the ward, where there should be sufficient comfortable waiting space for both the patients and their escorts. There should be an interview room for doctors and nurses to use while taking the patients' personal histories, to ensure confidentiality.

Office space for clerical staff booking admissions, preparing letters to patients, information to general practitioners and producing operating lists is required. Safe storage for patients' medical notes must be available.

Day-case surgical wards should be planned to provide easy supervision of patients by staff, but privacy for the patient must not be jeopardized. Separate changing facilities for male and female patients, with lockable cupboards for their clothing and valuables, are required.

Patient trolleys are available that can be used for both the surgical procedure in some specialties and for the recovery of the patient. These reduce the need for movement of the patient. A mixture of beds and trolleys can be used to provide for the individual needs of patients. All beds and trolleys must provide the head-down tilt necessary for the safe recovery of patients.

Bedhead facilities must include a nurse call system and power points; some spaces should be supplied with piped oxygen and vacuum outlets.

The provision of a sitting recovery area is required for patients undergoing surgical procedures using local anaesthetics and for the secondary phase of recovery for those who have had a general anaesthetic. Comfortable armchairs and reclining chairs can be used to furnish this area. The usual ancillary rooms are required:

• patients' toilets, with mirrors
• clean utility
• sluice
• beverage bay
• staff base
• safe storage for drugs and medicines
• storage space
• offices.

Operating theatre suite provision for day-case surgery must be comparable to that provided for inpatient care. The hazards of general anaesthetics are the same for day-case patients as they are for inpatients, therefore the anaesthetic room must be equipped with the same facilities, anaesthetic machine and patient monitoring apparatus as those provided in a main theatre complex.

Accommodation and equipment provided in the operating room should be of the same standard as that for inpatient surgery, including patient monitoring equipment, piped medical gases, vacuum and compressed medical air. Image intensification, lasers and equipment required for minimally invasive surgery could all be used in the day-case theatres. Policies, procedures and standards to ensure the safety of the patients and staff will be exactly the same as for inpatient surgery. Ventilation systems, lighting and other services must be comparable to those provided in an inpatient theatre suite. Scrub-up facilities, a preparation room and disposal area are required.

Primary recovery of day-case patients must take place in an area equipped and staffed to manage the high-dependency post-anaesthetic phase of their care. The full range of monitoring and resuscitation equipment must be available, as must piped medical gases, vacuum and ventilation apparatus.

Adequate storage for equipment such as video screens, microscopes, lasers, image intensifiers and table accessories is required and storage for all consumable items must be provided. Space for storing sterile packs and pharmacy goods is also necessary.

Staff changing areas, toilets, rest room, office and beverage bay will be needed in the day-case unit.

The design of any unit must consider the patient flow: it should be welcoming to both the patient and their escorts.

Short-term parking space is required for patients to be delivered and collected by their carers; such space should be used only for this purpose.

SELECTION OF PATIENTS

Selection of patients is dependent on three factors:

- procedure required
- general health of the patient
- social circumstances.

Procedures

The Audit Commission,[3] with advice from clinicians, identified a basic 20 operations ('basket of twenty') that could be carried out as day-case procedures. Table 1.2 shows a list of procedures, compiled by the Department of Health's Day Surgery Task Force, which is broader than the original 'basket of twenty'. The Task Force feels that none of the procedures listed can be performed on an outpatient basis, so any confusion between day surgery and outpatient is avoided. The procedures in Table 1.2 are divided into spe-

cialities and include the OPCS codes, the percentage of Finished Consultant Episodes (FCEs) carried out in 1990/91 on a day case basis in the NHS, and the equivalent upper quartile figures from the Audit Commission's 1992 report *All in a Day's Work*, in age bands. The OPCS codes included are the principal codes and are not comprehensive.

The Audit Commission took account of combinations of procedures and care should be taken to exclude combinations which are not suitable for day surgery.

Operations requiring general anaesthetic should not last longer than 60 minutes, and procedures where severe postoperative pain is likely should be excluded. Procedures where significant disability is likely – for example bilateral Keller's operation or bilateral carpal tunnel release – should not be undertaken as day cases.

General health

Patients with severe systemic disease, such as diabetes, heart disease, hypertension, pulmonary insufficiency and gross obesity, are not suitable for day surgery. Patients suffering from psychiatric illnesses are also not considered suitable.

The very elderly and infirm patient may also be excluded, but exclusion should be based on the biological condition of the patient rather than their chronological age. Elderly patients having procedures carried out under local anaesthetic can be considered for day surgery if a suitable carer is available to stay with them following discharge.

Normally patients will be selected who fall into the category of the American Society of Anesthesiologists Classification of Physical Status Class I (ASA I) or Class II (ASA II):

ASA I: a normally healthy individual; the surgery to be performed should be localized and not cause any systemic disturbance.

ASA II: a patient with mild systemic disease which does not interfere with normal life, including mild medical conditions which are well controlled with treatment.

Table 1.2 Operations which can be carried out as day-case procedures.

	OPCS code	NHS percentages for 1990/91	Audit Commission 'Basket of Twenty'		
			Age group 0–15	Age group 16–64	Age group 64+
General Surgery					
Repair inguinal hernia	T20 T21 except T21.4	6.0%	47%	6%	2%
Repair of femoral hernia	T22 T23 except T23.4				
Umbilical, paraumbilical and epigastric hernias	T24 T25 T24.4 T26 T26.4 T27 except T27.4	10.6%			
Varicose vein surgery	L85 L87	15.5%		22%	10%
Excision breast lumps & segmental resection of breast	B28	25.2%		50%	20%
Operations on duct of breast	B34	15.5%			
Anal stretch	H54 and H53.2	43.9%		75%	82%
Haemorrhoidectomy	H51 H52.1	4.1%			
Paediatric surgery					
Circumcision	N30.3	34.7%	68%		
Hydrocoele operation		33.7%			
Inguinal herniotomy	T19	27.4%	47%		
Repair umbilical hernia	T24	12.0%			
Repair epigastric hernia	T27 repair of other hernia of abdominal wall	10.6%			
Orchidopexy	NO8 Bilateral NO9 Other	18.1%	39%		
Anal stretch	H54 Dilation of anal stretch	43.9%			
Correction squint	All of C31 & C35 operations	9.1%	12%		
Myringotomy & insertion of grommets	D15.1	39.1%	84%		
Correction of bat ears	Pinnaplasty D03.3	19.8%	8%		

Table 1.2 Operations which can be carried out as day-case procedures (cont'd).

	OPCS code	NHS percentages for 1990/91	Audit Commission 'Basket of Twenty' Age group 0–15	Age group 16–64	Age group 64+
Orthopaedic surgery					
Carpal tunnel release	A65.1	57.1%		87%	90%
Dupuytren's contracture	T52.1 T52.2 T54.1	11.1%		25%	16%
Diagnostic arthroscopy	W87 of knee W88 of other joint	38.8%	54%	63%	37%
Removal of internal fixation of bone	W28.3	22.8%			
Amputation of finger	X08.3 X08.4 X21.6	9%			
Amputation of toe	X11 X27.3	11.1%			
Release of constriction of sheath of tendon including release of trigger finger	T27.3	55.7%			
Gynaecological surgery					
D & C	Q10.3	40.1%		69%	20% UQ
Termination of pregnancy	ICD9 CODE 635	55.7%		80%	
Laparoscopy	Q37, Q38, Q39, Q49, Q50	20.4%		48%	
Laparoscopic sterilization	Q35 and Q36.1	27.4%		48%	
Ophthalmic surgery					
Cataract surgery	All of C71 & C75	7.5%		4%	7% UQP
Squint surgery	All of C31 to C35	9.1%	12%		
Urological surgery					
Circumcision	N30.3	34.7%	68%	48%	
Excision epididymal lesion	N15.3	16.9%			
Hydrocoele surgery	N11	18.2%			
Orchidopexy	N08 Bilateral N09 Other		38%		
Orchidectomy	N05 Bilateral N06 Other	2.0%			
Reversal of vasectomy	N18.1	18.1%			

Table 1.2 Operations which can be carried out as day-case procedures (cont'd).

	OPCS code	NHS percentages for 1990/91	Audit Commission 'Basket of Twenty'		
			Age group 0–15	Age group 16–64	Age group 64+
Plastic Surgery					
Correction of bat ears	Pinnaplasty D03.3	18.8%	8%	45%	
Blepharoplasty	C13	30.4%			
Nipple and areola reconstruction	B29.8 B35.4	10.0%			
Breast augmentation	B31.2	2.7%			
Removal of breast implants	B30.3	4.0%			
Insertion tissue expanders	S48	2.1%			
ENT surgery					
Myringotomy & insertion of grommets	D15.1	39.1%	84%	77%	
Direct laryngoscopy & pharyngoscopy	E24, E25.2, E34, E35,E36	9.2%			
Submucosal diathermy turbinates	E04.1	12.2%			
Nasal polypectomy	E08.1	5.5%			
Turbinectomy	E04.2	1.2%			
Submucous resection	E03.1	0.8%	50%	11%	

Social circumstances

In the selection process it is important to ensure that the patient's home circumstances are adequate to provide conditions for their recovery in comfort, with suitable lavatory and bathroom facilities. There must also be access to a telephone in case additional help or advice is required following discharge.

Patients should live within 15 miles or 1 hour's drive from the hospital. They must not go home on public transport, they must not drive themselves home and they must have a responsible, fit adult to escort them home. For the first 24 hours following discharge the patient must have a fit, responsible adult available to stay with them.

At the outpatient appointment the surgeon will assess the suitability of the condition for day-case surgery. The surgeon should explain the operation and management to the patient and get the consent form signed. All preoperative investigations must be arranged prior to admission. In some centres the patient may attend an anaesthetic assessment clinic, or they may attend a nurse assessment clinic in the day-case unit.

It is particularly useful for children to visit the day-case unit with their parents prior to admission, to meet the staff, as this helps to allay anxiety.

Nurse-led preadmission clinics, at which the patient's general health and social circumstances and anaesthetic assessment following preagreed criteria can be reviewed, are becoming more routine because of the reduction of doctors' hours. At these clinics the nursing staff will ensure that all relevant information is given to the patient, both verbally and in writing, about their admission and preanaesthetic instructions, and their discharge plan can be agreed (see Appendix 1).

Nurses can undertake ECG recordings and take blood if required. This provides a 'one-stop' clinic for the patient and prevents them having to visit a number of departments in the hospital. Simple training and assessment programmes can be set up for the nurses to extend their role and undertake these tasks. The nursing staff in the day-case unit can complete the relevant clerking details for the patient.

If a problem which would preclude day-case treatment is discovered at the assessment clinic the nursing staff will contact the surgeon and anaesthetist. If this is in the general health status of the patient then an inpatient admission may have to be arranged.

If there is a change in the patient's social circumstances it may be possible to arrange an overnight stay in a 'hotel' bed if these are available in the hospital.

A date for admission should be agreed with the patient and information forwarded to their general practitioner about this date, the operation to be performed and that it will be day care, not an inpatient stay.

ADMISSION

Where possible, staggered admission times should be arranged. The patient will be required to reach the day-case unit in good time. Routine admissions procedures will be carried out by the nursing staff, who will also advise the patient's escort of the time to contact the unit for information on their progress. Preparation for surgery will be completed.

The surgeon will confirm the patient's understanding of the operation and the consent given. The anaesthetist will carry out the normal examination and explanation prior to commencing anaesthesia. Surgery is performed and the patient is then returned to the recovery area.

In the secondary phase of recovery the patient may be placed in the sitting recovery area and given a drink and a piece of toast, a sandwich or a biscuit.

DISCHARGE

The surgeon is responsible for discharging the patient, but may delegate this to the nursing staff, who will follow an agreed protocol. This should include the following:

- The patient's vital signs must have been stable for at least 1 hour prior to arrangements for discharge being made.
- The patient must have no signs of respiratory depression.
- The patient must be orientated to person, place and time.
- The patient must be able to retain oral fluids.
- The patient must be able to void urine.
- The patient must be able to dress themselves and walk without assistance.
- The patient must not have excessive pain, bleeding, nausea or vomiting.

If the nursing staff have any concerns they must inform the surgeon or anaesthetist and ensure that the patient is seen prior to discharge.

When the patient fits all the discharge criteria, arrangements can be made with their escort to come to the unit and collect them. The nurse completing the discharge should ensure that both verbal and written instructions are given to the patient about post-anaesthetic care and the postoperative instructions for the specific surgery that has been performed.

It must be reiterated that the patient should not operate any mechanical device, undertake domestic cooking or drink alcohol for 24 hours following discharge. Only prescribed drugs should be taken and the patient should be told to refrain from driving for at least 48 hours after a general anaesthetic.

Written information in the form of a discharge summary should be given to the patient with the request that this be retained for 24 hours in case assistance is required from a GP. After 24 hours the patient's carer should be requested to deliver the discharge summary to the GP's surgery. Written information on what to do if problems occur should also be given to the patient, and this should be explained verbally.

It must be made clear to both the patient and their escort that recovery is taking place at home rather than in hospital; when reaching home the patient should rest in bed and have a light diet. All postoperative instructions must be followed and resumption of normal activity will be gradual.

A contact number for advice should also be provided and an outpatient follow-up appointment date should be given to the patient prior to discharge. The surgeon will forward a discharge letter to the patient's GP.

POSTOPERATIVE PAIN CONTROL

It is extremely important to ensure control of postoperative pain for day-case patients. Local or regional blocks using a long-acting local anaesthetic can be inserted in theatre. Analgesics can be given in the form of suppositories or in sublingual form to prevent the need for injections. A small supply of suitable analgesics must be given to the patient to take home, with clear instructions and explanation for use.

AUDIT

Some centres have a system whereby the nursing staff telephone all patients discharged following intermediate surgery on the day after operation. They ascertain whether pain relief has been adequate, whether there have been any problems necessitating assistance from the patient's GP,

and whether the patient has any particular concerns. Records are kept and reviewed on a regular basis with surgeons and anaesthetists.

Locally devised questionnaires to patients on specific issues such as pain control or wound healing can be used to obtain feedback and, when necessary, to revise practice.

General practitioners can be requested to inform the day-case unit of any problems they have had to deal with when patients have been discharged.

An audit package is available from the Audit Commission[4] which contains 250 adult questionnaires and 100 children's questionnaires, plus a systems disk for a computer program. The results are compared with a national database.

The questions review the age groups treated as day cases, the procedures performed, the facilities at the hospital and the information the patients were given. Questions are also included to assess the postoperative discharge care, whether patients had to contact their GP, practice or community nurse, and what hospital facilities they have used since discharge. Patients are also asked to assess their perceived outcome of the operation, changes in symptoms, changes in day-to-day living and speed of recovery. These questionnaires are completed by the patient 3 weeks after discharge.

CONCLUSIONS

Day-case surgery is not a second-class 'cheap' option: to be successful it must be carefully planned and controlled. It must be consultant-led and regular audit is required to review practice and ensure quality care.

REFERENCES

1. Royal College of Surgeons of England 1992 Commission on the Provision of Surgical Services. Report of the Working Party on Guidelines for Day Case Surgery, Revised edn, March 1992. Royal College of Surgeons, London
2. NHS Management Executive 1993 Day Surgery. Report by the Day Surgery Task Force. Department of Health, Leeds
3. Audit Commission. Patients' Experiences of Surgery (Day Care) Adult and Children Package. Publications Section, Audit Section, Nicholson House, Lime Kiln Close, Stock Gilford, Bristol BS12 6SU
4. Audit Commission 1990 A short cut to better services. Day surgery in England and Wales. HMSO, London

2

Legal aspects of operating theatre practice

B. Dimond

The aim of this chapter is to consider those areas of the law which are of particular relevance to the professional who works in theatre. It is addressed not just to the operating theatre nurse but to all professionals and technicians other than medical staff, i.e.:

- theatre nurses
- anaesthetic nurses
- operating department practitioners
- recovery room nurses
- coronary care unit nurses
- intensive care nurses
- special care nurses
- perfusionists.

The term practitioner will be used to cover all these different staff.

It is assumed that the reader will have access to texts covering the more general topics that affect all health professionals (see Further Reading); even so, space permits only the briefest discussion of the specialist areas. The areas to be covered are listed below. For the most part they have been culled from seminars with theatre staff, both day and inpatient surgery, and represent those topics that cause the greatest concern.

- accountability
- patients' rights
- health and safety laws and consumer protection
- law relating to medicinal products
- employment law
- the internal market
- record keeping

- day-case surgery
- specialist operations, e.g.
  - termination of pregnancy
  - sterilization
  - transplants: removal of organs and donations of bone marrow

- Section 57 Mental Health Act 1983
- in vitro fertilization
- obstetrics and the safety of the baby
- circumcision.

Knowing the law

Why can law not be left to the lawyers? Why should the professional in theatre have any legal knowledge? Legal knowledge is important because:

- The legal framework is important.
- There may be insufficient time to obtain a lawyer's advice.
- Patients' rights must be known and observed.
- The nurse is accountable to the UKCC (United Kingdom Central Council for Nurses, Midwives and Health Visitors) and must know the significance of the Codes of Conduct and other UKCC advice.
- Nurse managers take decisions which have legal significance.
- Nurses need to know their rights as employees.
- The police/press/relatives and others make demands and professionals need to know the appropriate response. What are they obliged to do in law?
- Evidence may be required in a court of law. The principles of good record keeping and statements must be followed.
- Practitioners need to know when to seek legal advice.
- Practitioners may wish to press for reforms.

Legal framework is important

Nurses work within the context of the law. As a minimum they must know if an operation is lawful:

- When can they refuse to take part in an abortion?
- When would an abortion be unlawful?
- Is female circumcision lawful?
- Is male circumcision lawful?

Insufficient time to contact lawyer

There is not always time for an operation to be halted and a lawyer's opinion summoned. A knowledge of the basic principles of accountability and patients' rights is essential for all nursing work. Speedy decisions must often be made, and an understanding of the law is essential.

Patients' rights

The patient is unconscious. What is meant by a valid consent to treatment? Can medical students conduct a gynaecological examination? When can nurses oppose a surgeon's orders because they are protecting the rights of the patient?

Code of conduct and statutory authority guidance

The UKCC has issued extremely helpful guidelines to registered practitioners. What if the employer ignores these guidelines and, for example, expects employees to work in unsuitable accommodation with inadequate staffing; can they refuse? What is the legal significance of the Scope of Professional Practice? How do nurses prove their competence to carry out an expanded role if they do not have a certificate?

Nurse managers must understand the law

The theatre manager may have to stand up to senior consultant surgeons or to senior Trust managers. He or she needs to know the legal situation, as will be illustrated later in some specific situations.

Rights of employees important

What are the rights of staff when an NHS Trust is formed? What are the duties of an employer in relation to the health and safety of employees? Can an employee insist on attending a refresher training course? Can the employer be compelled to reimburse the employee's costs?

Police/press/relatives make demands: should they be met?

What duties exist in relation to confidential information relating to the patient? Can theatre nurses refuse to answer police questions after a death in theatre on the grounds that they would be incriminated or would incriminate someone else?

Evidence may be required from the nurse: record keeping/statements/ court witness

How should records be kept to ensure that they are of the utmost value to patient care and to any possible subsequent proceedings? What principles exist in the preparation of statements and the giving of evidence?

Need to know when to seek expert advice

There will be times when expert legal advice must be sought. However, only a good understanding of the law will enable someone to know when it is essential to bring in a lawyer, and what action should be taken and what should not be taken before that time.

Understanding leads to reform

The law is imperfect: changes are constantly being made. Theatre staff may be aware of abuses of patients' rights, where added legal protection is required. Unless there is a basic understanding they cannot press for reforms. There are many legal areas of which the theatre nurse should have an understanding. These will be considered in this chapter.

Accountability

To whom is the nurse accountable? If a patient dies on the operating table, what potential legal actions does the practitioner face?

Every such death must be reported to the coroner, who will decide whether to order a post-mortem and hold an inquest. The practitioner should have assistance in preparing the statement which the coroner is likely to request, and to have instruction in how to give evidence before the court. The circumstances will then determine if there are also to be civil and criminal or other proceedings.

First the nurse would have to give evidence at the coroner's inquest. The coroner's task is to ascertain the identity of the deceased and the cause of death. Secondly, in cases of gross recklessness and negligence there could be a criminal prosecution, and even if the practitioner is not the defendant he or she might well be a witness in the Magistrates' Court at the committal proceedings, and before the jury in the Crown Court.

Thirdly, relatives may wish to claim compensation for the death, and again the practitioner might be a witness in the civil courts, trying to establish that there was no negligence and that the employers were not vicariously liable. Fourthly, if the practitioner is a nurse he or she is accountable to the Professional Conduct Committee of the UKCC, to whom they must answer for any alleged misconduct. Other practitioners, if registered, will be accountable to their own registration body.

Finally, practitioners have a contract with their employers and must obey reasonable orders and act with reasonable care and skill. If they have failed to do this they could be disciplined or even dismissed. The remedy then is an application to an industrial tribunal for unfair dismissal.

Practitioners are also accountable to themselves. This principle is at the heart of the personal and professional accountability of the UKCC Code of Professional Conduct.

There are many cases of negligence brought in relation to actions in theatre and the recovery room, and there is no doubt that litigation is increasing. There may be a temptation, since the patient is unconscious, not to inform the patient and to attempt to conceal the facts. Practitioners should not assist in changing the account of what happened. They must have the professional courage to withstand any pressures to conceal and to ensure that the records state comprehensively and clearly exactly what took place. It is not for individual nurse practitioners to tell the patient what went wrong, but they should ensure that the senior manager is aware of the full facts and that these are notified to the patient. The patient is entitled to have access to his or her health records under the Access to Health Records Act 1990, and therefore openness in explaining matters is best. There is a chance that if the full details are made known at the earliest opportunity, the patient may be less likely to consider litigation than if they fear that there has been a cover-up.

Another example of negligence could be an anaesthetic nurse misreading the medication and administering the wrong drug. In such situations openness and a frank admission of the error is the essential and only policy. It may be necessary to seek the advice of pharmacy or of a poisons centre on whether an antidote is necessary. The nurse may well have to face disciplinary proceedings, but should have the opportunity to put his or her case and, if there are faults in the system, for these to be rectified so that there is no repetition.

CIVIL PROCEEDINGS

If civil proceedings were to be brought by a patient or relatives following an untoward occurrence, what would the person bringing the action have to show to obtain compensation in the civil courts? The elements to be established in an action for negligence are that:

• a duty was owed by the defendant

- this duty has been breached
- as a reasonably foreseeable result of this breach, harm has occurred.

A duty of care is owed to all patients to ensure that reasonable care is taken of them while they are in the care of the theatre staff. Where there has been a breach of this duty of care this would be tested against what the patient could have expected in relation to the reasonable standard of care exercised by a professional having those special skills following the accepted approved standard of care. This is known as the Bolam Test,[1] and was laid down in 1957:

When you get a situation which involved the use of some special skill or competence, then the test as to whether there has been negligence or not is … the standard of the ordinary skilled man exercising and professing to have that special skill. A man need not possess the highest expert skill; it is well-established that it is sufficient if he exercises the ordinary skill of an ordinary competent man exercising that particular art … He is not guilty of negligence if he has acted in accordance with a practice accepted as proper by a reasonable body of medical men skilled in that particular art.

Failure to follow the reasonable standard expected is not necessarily evidence of negligence if the practitioner's actions would be supported by a group of competent professionals. In a case where a patient challenged her doctor's decision to recommend a mediastinoscopy and her expert witness claimed that she was clearly suffering from TB, the doctor's suggestion that her illness could be Hodgkin's disease was therefore evidence of negligence. The House of Lords held that 'It was not sufficient to establish negligence for the plaintiff to show that there was a body of competent professional opinion that considered the decision was wrong, if there was also a body of equally competent professional opinion that supported the decision as having been reasonable in the circumstances'.[2] She therefore lost the case.

Causation

It is not sufficient for the plaintiff to establish negligence to obtain compensation: he must also prove that the harm that resulted arose from the reasonably foreseeable consequence of the breach of duty. Many patients who are operated upon are critically ill. There may be negligent acts, but it may be established that the patient would have died anyway. In a case involving a premature baby who was on oxygen therapy, the parents, in their case against the hospital,[3] failed to show that it was negligence in monitoring the baby's oxygen intake (the catheter was inserted in a vein rather than in an artery) that caused the retrolental fibroplasia. There must be factual causation[4] and the harm that resulted from the breach of duty must have been reasonably foreseeable.[5]

The thing speaks for itself

Sometimes it happens that harm occurs which should not if reasonable care is taken. If, in such circumstances, the plaintiff can show that the elements shown below existed, then the plaintiff can rely upon a legal device known as *res ipsa loquitur*, i.e. 'the thing speaks for itself':

- Harm should not occur if reasonable care is taken.
- Events were under the control of the defendants, their servants or their agents.
- The defendants are offering no explanation as to how that harm occurred.

The doctrine of *res ipsa loquitur* is frequently used in litigation following theatre incidents such as:

- a swab being left in the patient
- the wrong limb/organ etc. being amputated or removed
- the patient suffering from insufficient oxygen.

The effect of this doctrine is that defendants are responsible for showing on a balance of probabilities that there was no negligence on their part. This may be quite difficult to do, as the examples show.

Scope of professional practice

Where does the practitioner stand who is asked to take on the role of first assistant, having no experience or training in this work, and who burns a patient? A very helpful booklet has been prepared by the National Association of Theatre Nurses.[6] The basic principle is, of course, clear and is enshrined in the UKCC Code of Conduct and the Scope of Professional Practice: always work within your competence and refuse to practise outside it. The answer to the question, therefore, is that the nurse will face disciplinary proceedings by his or her employer, a professional conduct committee hearing, and possibly a claim for compensation in the civil courts, where the employer will be sued for vicarious liability for the nurse's negligence. A theatre sister in Cornwall was disciplined by her NHS Trust when she performed an appendectomy under the supervision of the surgical registrar.

Managerial control of theatre

Where does the manager stand if the surgeon insists that the list order be changed? Where does the manager stand if the consultant is not present in hospital when the registrar is about to commence the list? Both of these situations relate to the control of the theatre by the theatre manager. There are dangers in changing the order of the list: this is where mistakes can be made concerning the identity of patients and their operations. The theatre manager has the right to ensure that the theatre functions in such a way that no harm occurs. It is up to him or her to assess the risks and dangers from any request made by a surgeon and to balance the reasons why the request was made against any dangers that would result from the change. If the change is agreed to then the manager must take every precaution to ensure that the patients will be safe.

Each operation should be supervised by a consultant. If there are fears that junior staff are left unsupervised and there is no consultant on call within the hospital, the theatre manager is entitled to refuse to let the operation commence unless it is an emergency.

DEFENCES TO AN ACTION FOR NEGLIGENCE

The main defences against negligence are:

- denial of the allegations

- one of the elements of negligence was not established
- contributory negligence
- voluntary assumption of risk
- limitation of time
- exclusion of liability.

For further details reference should be made to the author's more comprehensive work.[7]

CRIMINAL LIABILITY

A death in theatre or the recovery room could lead to criminal proceedings if the Crown Prosecution Service considers that the events justify a charge of causing the death of the patient through gross recklessness and negligence, a crime known as involuntary manslaughter.

Involuntary manslaughter

This is where death results where there is no intention to kill. There will not be a charge of murder. Such cases may be prosecuted or there may be no prosecution at all. This can cause some confusion.

It was reported[8] that the police used to be reluctant to prosecute medical professionals following an unexpected death, but since it was set up in 1985 the Crown Prosecution Service has been less wary about such litigation. The Director of Public Prosecutions denied this assertion.

Box 2.1

Example 2.1
In 1991 two junior doctors were given a 9-month suspended prison sentence for the manslaughter of a 16-year-old with leukaemia. He died after being wrongly injected in the spine with a cytotoxic drug which should have been administered intravenously. The conviction for manslaughter was quashed by the Court of Appeal on the grounds that the jury should have been directed to decide whether the defendants were guilty of 'gross negligence' and not 'recklessness'.

cont'd

> **Box 2.1** (Cont'd)
>
> **Example 2.2**
> In this case the person charged was the anaesthetist in charge of the patient during the latter part of an operation. At approximately 11.05 a.m. a disconnection occurred at the endotracheal tube connection. The supply of oxygen to the patient ceased and led to a cardiac arrest at 11.14 a.m. During that period the defendant failed to notice or remedy the disconnection. He first became aware that something was amiss when an alarm sounded on the Dinamap machine, which monitored the patient's blood pressure. From the evidence it appeared that some 4.5 minutes would have elapsed between the disconnection and the sounding of the alarm.
>
> When the alarm sounded the defendant responded in various ways by checking the equipment and by administering atropine to raise the patient's pulse, but at no stage before the cardiac arrest did he check the integrity of the endotracheal tube connection. The disconnection was not discovered until after resuscitation measures had been commenced.
>
> The defendant accepted at his trial that he had been negligent: the issue was whether his conduct was criminal. He was convicted of involuntary manslaughter but appealed against his conviction. He lost in the Court of Appeal and then appealed to the House of Lords.

Subsequent to the case outlined in Example 2.2 in Box 2.1, the House of Lords have clarified the legal situation.[9] The stages they suggested were as follows:

• The ordinary principles of the law of negligence should be applied to ascertain whether or not the defendant had been in breach of a duty of care towards the victim who had died.
• If such a breach of duty was established, the next question was whether that breach of duty caused the death of the victim.
• If so, the jury had to go on to consider whether that breach of duty should be characterized as gross negligence, and therefore as a crime. This would depend on the seriousness of the breach of duty in all the circumstances in which the defendant was placed when it occurred.
• The jury would have to consider whether the extent to which the defendant's conduct departed from the proper standard of care incumbent upon him, involving as it must have done a risk of death to the patient, was such that it should be judged criminal.

The judge was required to give the jury a direction on the meaning of gross negligence, as had been given in the present case by the Court of Appeal:

The jury might properly find gross negligence on proof of (a) indifference to an obvious risk of injury to health; or of (b) actual foresight of the risk, coupled either with a determination nevertheless to run it; or with an intention to avoid it but involving such a high degree of negligence in the attempted avoidance as the jury considered justified conviction; or (c) of inattention or failure to advert to a serious risk going beyond mere inadvertence in respect of an obvious and important matter which the defendant's duty demanded he should address.

The House of Lords held that the Court of Appeal had applied the correct test and the appeal was dismissed. (An amended test is used in the case of a charge of involuntary death in motor accidents.)

The judge has full discretion over the sentencing in a case of a conviction for involuntary manslaughter.

A charge of involuntary manslaughter could be laid against any of the staff working in the operating theatre and its associated departments, since an error in carrying out their duties, whether it be the cleaning of the theatre, general maintenance or the connection of the equipment, could cause the death of a patient.

Patients' rights

The main rights of a patient recognized by law are:

- to receive a reasonable standard of care
- to give or withhold consent
- to receive information
- to confidentiality
- to have access to records
- to complain.

A REASONABLE STANDARD OF CARE

The right to receive a reasonable standard of care is considered part of the accountability of the professional whose duty it is to provide that care and to ensure that the standard is met.

THE RIGHT TO GIVE OR WITHHOLD CONSENT

The civil wrong of trespass is the unlawful touching of another person without his consent. If it can be shown that a person has apprehended or received direct interference with his person then he can claim compensation, even though he may have suffered no harm. The motive of the person undertaking the alleged trespass will not necessarily be an effective defence. The consent of the patient, in writing, by word of mouth or implied, is one of the most important defences to an action of trespass.

The following legal issues arising in consent will be considered here:

- the mentally competent adult
- the mentally incompetent adult
- the minor of 16 and 17 years
- the minor under 16 years.

The mentally competent adult

Imagine the situation where a patient is brought to theatre and it is established that he has been given premedication but the consent form has not been signed. There are perhaps three options:

- to obtain the signature even though the patient is now under sedation
- to carry on with the operation without a consent form
- to send the patient back to the ward to recover from the premedication, and then start all over again.

Signing the consent form after premedication would probably not result in an effective consent. To be legally valid, consent must be given freely, without coercion, by a competent person. It could be argued that a patient who is under premedication is not capable of making a reasonable decision. If the operation proceeded on the basis of a consent form signed at this stage the patient might well be able to challenge its validity. This is therefore not an acceptable option, but it will depend upon the patient's clinical condition.

If there is no actual consent given, those carrying out the operation risk an action for trespass to the person. It may be that one of the surgeons has already seen the patient and knows that he or she wants this particular operation to proceed, and in fact that the patient has already given consent by word of mouth. If this is the situation, and if the surgeon is prepared to substantiate it, then the operation could proceed on this basis. Otherwise there is the potential for a civil action for battery by the patient. Where possible, details of any witness who heard consent being given should be available before the operation proceeds.

There may, however, be clinical reasons why the operation should not be delayed, in which case it could proceed on the basis of necessity.[10] Here the professional must be acting in the best interests of the patient following the Bolam Test. The surgeon should be absolutely clear what necessity justifies acting in the absence of the consent of the patient.

It is not sufficient to act out of good motives. It is reported that a surgeon was carrying out a hernia repair when he noticed that the patient had an ingrowing toenail. So, while the patient was under the general anaesthetic the surgeon repaired the ingrowing toenail. On recovery the patient was surprised to see a bandage round his toe as well as a dressing on his abdomen, and made inquiries. He was then prepared to take legal action for a trespass to his person. The doctor's defence union was prepared to make an offer of compensation, since the claim was indefensible. In this case the patient had signed a consent form, but the words 'and any other procedure deemed necessary' was not sufficient to cover such a totally unrelated procedure to which the patient had not given consent.

If consent by word of mouth cannot be established then the preferred practice would be for the patient to return to the ward to recover from the premedication and then to give written consent. However, this would have to be balanced against the nature of the operation. Is it an emergency? What would be the effect of delay on the patient? A recent case where a surgeon was carrying out a hysterectomy when he discovered that there was a fetus present illustrates the problems. The surgeon was acquitted of a criminal offence under the Offences against the Persons Act. The mother later received £10 000 in respect of her civil claim for negligence.

The advantage of returning the patient to the ward would be an improvement in ward procedures, so that the consent would always be checked before the patient was given premedication. The disadvantage is that the patient might naturally be very exasperated, and make a formal complaint.

It follows that where the mentally competent adult refuses treatment or certain procedures, e.g. blood transfusion, even though this is contrary to his best interests, his refusal cannot be overruled.[11] The professional must establish the validity of the refusal. There are specific forms for Jehovah's Witnesses to sign whereby they give consent to the operation on the understanding that no blood or blood products will be given. It is a matter of trust that the theatre professionals accept this limitation on their work. Should they ignore the prohibition and the patient survives because of the transfusion, they could still face an action for trespass to the person.[12]

The mentally incompetent adult

At present the law does not recognize any system of proxy decision making for adults whereby one adult can give consent on behalf of a mentally incompetent adult. The situation is under review by the Law Commission, which has made recommendations for reform.[13] Until their proposals are implemented, professionals have, out of necessity, to act in the best interests of the adult, obtaining the approval of the court where necessary in the light of the seriousness of the operation.

In the case of Re F[10] the House of Lords issued a declaration that to carry out an operation for sterilization on a female patient with learning disabilities who lacked the capacity to consent would not be unlawful provided the doctors were acting in her best interests following the Bolam Test. They requested that in future such cases should come before the courts, and a practice note has been issued to this effect. According to this principle, professionals are protected by the powers given to them by the common law to act out of necessity in the patient's interests.

This principle also applies to the situation where a patient is unconscious following a road accident and needs life-saving treatment. In the absence of any information to the contrary (e.g. a card indicating that certain procedures or treatments were unacceptable) the patient can be treated.

It does not follow that because a patient is detained in a special hospital he or she cannot therefore give a valid refusal, as the following case shows.[14] The patient was a 68-year-old man who suffered from paranoid schizophrenia and was detained in Broadmoor Hospital. He developed gangrene in his foot and was removed to a general hospital, where the consultant surgeon said that he was likely to die unless his leg was amputated below the knee. He refused to give consent and was treated with antibiotics and conservative surgery. The hospital refused to give an undertaking that it would not in future carry out an amputation operation. The patient therefore sought an injunction to restrain the hospital from amputating his leg without his express written consent. He succeeded in his application. The court held that the evidence failed to show that he lacked sufficient understanding of the nature, purpose and effects of the proposed treatment, but instead showed that he had understood and retained the relevant treatment information, believed it and had arrived at a clear choice.

The minor of 16 and 17 years

The minor of 16 and 17 has a statutory right under the Family Law Reform Act 1969 Section 8(1) to give consent to medical, surgical or dental treatment. Treatment is defined to include all the ancillary and diagnostic procedures necessary, including the giving of an anaesthetic. Where the minor is mentally competent this consent will be an effective defence against an action for trespass to the person, even if the parents had disagreed with the operation proceeding.

Under the Act the parents' right to give consent is preserved (Section 8(3)), and so where the minor is himself incapable of giving consent the professionals can obtain consent from the parents. Where there is a clash the professional can determine the issue on the clinical necessity, but only in exceptional circumstances would the refusal of the child be overruled. This occurred in the case of Re W[15]: the patient was 16, under a care order, and suffered from anorexia nervosa. She refused to be treated and the Court of Appeal made an emergency order permitting her to be taken, without her consent, to the unit for eating disorders and to be treated there.

The minor under 16 years

It was held by the House of Lords in the Gillick case[16] that a minor under 16 years old could give a valid consent to treatment without the involvement of the parents if he or she had sufficient maturity to understand the implications. The context of the decision was family planning advice and treatment, but the same principles apply to other treatments. This principle of the participation of the child depending on his or her maturity and understanding in decisions affecting his or her care and treatment is set out in the Children Act 1989.

The capacity to consent must relate to the nature of the treatment taking place. A minor may, for example, be able to give consent to stitches being inserted but would be incompetent to give consent to brain surgery.

Where possible, it is recommended that parental consent should be obtained for surgery on the minor under 16 years. In February 1997 the Court of Appeal upheld the parents who refused to give consent to a life-saving liver transplant on their 18-month-old son, on the grounds that they were acting in the child's best interests.

TO RECEIVE INFORMATION

The duty of care includes the duty to provide information before consent is given. Should significant harm occur as a result of substantial risks which have not been explained to the patient, and the patient would not have consented to the treatment had these risks been explained, then the patient may bring an action for negligence.[17]

The Patient's Charter and local charters also set out the duty of providers to give information to patients, but this is not enforceable in a court of law, except under the principle considered above.

CONFIDENTIALITY

All theatre practitioners are bound by the duty to maintain the confidentiality of information relating to the patient. There may be exceptional circumstances where disclosure is justified, e.g. to the court, or in the public interest, but the guidelines laid down in 1996 by the UKCC in its Guidelines for Professional Practice which includes a section on confidentiality should be followed.[18]

ACCESS TO RECORDS

Under the Data Protection Act 1984 and the subject access provisions, the patient has a right to access to his health records kept in computerized form. The right of access to manually held records was given by the Access to Health Records Act 1990 for those records kept since 1 November 1991.

The right of access is not absolute, but for both manually held and computerized records is subject to certain exceptions, including the right to prevent access where serious harm would be caused to the physical or mental health of the patient or another person, or where a third person would be identified by the records and had not given consent to the access.

THE RIGHT TO COMPLAIN

There is a duty under the Hospital Complaints Procedure Act 1985 for a complaints procedure to be established. This duty is extended under the Patient's Charter.

Health and safety laws and consumer protection

The same areas of law cover liability in the field of health and safety as apply in the general care of the patient. These are: criminal laws under the Health and Safety at Work Act 1974 and its regulations; the contractual duty of employer and employee in relation to health and safety; civil duty of care in the tort of negligence, and under the Occupiers' Liability Act 1957 and the Consumer Protection Act.

PROFESSIONAL CODES OF CONDUCT
Health and Safety at Work Act 1974 and the Regulations

The Health and Safety at Work Act 1974 places a duty of care upon each and every employer 'to ensure so far as is reasonably practicable, the health, safety and welfare at work of all his employees' (Section 2(1)). In practice this covers every possible scenario, but the Act also sets out specific examples without reducing the scope of the general duty. Subsequently the duty has been detailed by regulations passed as a result of the European Directives, which set out specific duties in the following areas:

- Health and Safety (General Provisions) Regulations
- Provision and Use of Work Equipment Regulations
- Manual Handling Operations Regulations

- Workplace (Health, Safety and Welfare) Regulations
- Personal Protective Equipment at Work Regulations
- Health and Safety (Display Screen Equipment) Regulations.

All theatre staff must be aware of the contents of these regulations and ensure that they are implemented in the workplace. The individual employee owes a duty under the Health and Safety at Work Regulations:

To take such care for the health and safety of himself and of others who may be affected by his acts and omissions at work and as regards any duty or requirement imposed on his employer or other persons by or under any of the relevant statutory provisions to cooperate with him in so far as is necessary to enable that duty or requirement to be performed or complied with.

Enforcement of the Health and Safety provisions is through the cooperation of employers and employees in the workplace; by the appointment of trade unions of safety representatives who work with the employer on safety committees; and by the work of the health and safety inspectors, who visit and inspect, can issue enforcement or prohibition notices, and can commence prosecutions of both employers and employees.

CONTRACT OF EMPLOYMENT

The duties set out by the Health and Safety at Work Act 1974 are mirrored in the contractual duties in relation to health and safety implied in the contract of employment and placed upon employer and employee. The employer has a duty to take all reasonable care of the health and safety of the employee by providing a safe system of work, competent staff and safe premises, plant and equipment. The employee has a duty to obey the reasonable instructions of the employer and to take all reasonable care and skill in the carrying out of his duties. If the employee is in breach of these duties it could lead to disciplinary proceedings and ultimately justify dismissal. If the employer is in breach the employee might be justified in regarding the contract as ended. If the employee is harmed, he may be able to sue the employer for compensation.

CIVIL LIABILITY

The duty of care in negligence is considered above. In addition, there are other statutes that place duties upon the employer, occupier, manufacturer and supplier to take reasonable care not to harm others. Two will be considered in brief: the Occupier's Liability Act 1957 and the Consumer Protection Act 1984.

The Occupier's Liability Act 1957

Under this Act a duty is placed upon occupiers to take such care as in all the circumstances of the case is reasonable to see that the visitor will be reasonably safe in using the premises for the purposes for which he or she is invited or permitted to be there. 'Visitor' includes staff, patients, maintenance workers and any others who are permitted to be there. (Separate legislation, the Occupier's Liability Act 1984, covers the situation of trespassers.)

There may be several occupiers, as when contractors come to decorate the premises, and it is a question of fact as to whose liability it is if harm arises from their activities. Under the 1957 Act the occupier, if he has acted reasonably in entrusting the work to the independent contractors and taken such steps as are necessary to satisfy himself that they are competent and that the work has been properly done, should not be liable for any harm their activities have caused (Section 2(4)(b)).

Consumer Protection Act 1987

This Act introduced into the health and safety laws a right of compensation against producers and suppliers of products if a defect in the product caused personal injury, death, loss or damage to property. It was passed in compliance with EEC Directive No 85/3741/EEC and came into force on 1 March 1988. The person claiming compensation must be able to show:

- that there was a defect in the product
- that loss or harm has occurred
- who was the producer or supplier of the product.

It is then up to the defendant to prove either that there was no defect or that he was not a producer or supplier of the product, or one of the defences given by Section 4(1) of the Act. The defendant can rely upon the fact that at the time the product was produced or supplied, the state of scientific knowledge was such that the defect could not have been discovered. This is also known as 'the state of the art defence'.

One important point for theatre staff to be aware of is that if the person harmed can be told who the original suppliers of the product were, then provided there has been no subsequent modification of the product, that person becomes the defendant. Records showing the source of supply are therefore extremely important, since if the original supplier cannot be traced then the theatre department, and hence the employers of that department, could be regarded as the supplier and would therefore become the defendant.

Theatre staff must also be aware that the supplier can say in defence that instructions on the use of the product have not been followed. This means that if the manufacturer makes it clear that certain products are for single use only, and this is ignored and the product is autoclaved and reused, it would be the responsibility of the hospital and not the manufacturers should harm result.

Since 1988 there have been very few cases under the Act. One reported in March 1993[19] led to Simon Garratt being awarded £1400 against the manufacturers of a pair of surgical scissors which broke during an operation on his knee; the blade was left embedded and a second operation was required to remove it. Had he relied upon the law of negligence to obtain compensation he would have had to show that the manufacturers were in breach of the duty of care that they owed to him. Under the Consumer Protection Act 1987 he had to show the harm, the defect and the fact that the scissors were produced by the defendant. A report by the National Consumer Council 1995 showed that the Act has been used very little and it offered recommendations on how the process of making civil claims in consumer cases could be improved.

It should be noted that the Consumer Protection Act also covers staff who are injured in course of employment. They also have the protection of the Employers' (Defective Equipment) Act 1969, which means that if they can show that they have been harmed while in course of employment as the result of negligence by a third party, they can obtain compensation directly from the employer, who then would have the task of obtaining the funds from the supplier or producer. The 1969 Act does not apply to harm where loss or damage to property is caused.[20]

Legal issues relating to AIDS/HIV infection

Exactly the same principles apply in relation to the care of a patient with HIV/AIDS and the protection of staff from cross-infection as apply in any other health and safety situation. The employer has a duty to ensure that all reasonable care is taken to prevent any harm arising to theatre staff. This probably does not permit a patient to be refused an operation, but all reasonable equipment should be provided and a safe system of work adopted.

What is the position of theatre staff if the patient is a drug addict and there is a high risk of AIDS/HIV? This is another question of patients' rights. Some surgeons would like to insist that all patients be tested for AIDS/HIV before surgery, but this is not lawful: an operation cannot depend upon the patient being prepared to consent to a test.

The professional has to carry out practice on the basis that everyone is potentially infected. This is, of course, the situation with hepatitis, which some say is a more dangerous concern to theatre staff. There can be false negatives, so a test is not conclusive and it would be unwise to rely upon it. However, the employee can expect the employer to provide the necessary equipment and protective clothing, and to ensure that there is a safe system of work to enable the employee to be reasonably safe from infection. Even if it were known that a patient was an AIDS sufferer this would not enable a registered nurse practitioner to refuse to care for the patient, as the UKCC has made clear.

What if a surgeon or other member of staff fails to use sound cross-infection techniques?

There may be surgeons whose practices do not accord with sound cross-infection techniques. Here it must be the theatre manager who will have to decide, in the light of the hazards to patients and staff, what action is required. He or she is bound by the professional duty of care not to endanger the health and safety of any patient and theatre staff should work through the manager.

If he or she fails to act appropriately then there would be justification for junior staff to report the dangers to other senior managers. Such 'whistle-blowing action' should be protected by the Department of Health's guidance for staff on relations with the public and media.[21] This makes it clear that no-one should be penalized for expressing their views about health service issues, and suggests the setting up of a local procedure for hearing about concerns. This should aim at resolving such concerns informally at a local level. Otherwise, they should be taken up through the management hierarchy, or a designated officer should be identified to hear and resolve them. Such internal measures should be taken before the issue is made public. The confidentiality of patient information should be respected and, if public interest justifies disclosure, this should only take place following advice from specialists.

What if one of the staff has hepatitis or is HIV positive?

The practitioner has a duty not to endanger the safety of other staff and patients. Recent guidance has been issued on the action that professional staff should take if they know themselves to be HIV positive. Exactly the same rules should apply to other dangerous infections. If an occupational health department exists the member of staff should be referred to that. It may be possible for them to be given non-invasive work while they are fit to work but still a carrier. In the case of Bliss v. SE Thames Regional Health Authority[22] it was held that there was no legal obligation on a consultant to submit to a medical examination when asked, unless the employer had reasonable grounds for believing that he or she might cause harm to patients or adversely affect the quality of their treatment. The situation does, however, depend upon the contract of employment: if it contains a clause requiring an employee to submit to medical examination if a specified cause occurred, the situation might be different. It should be noted that under Rule 39 of the Midwives Rules[23] a practising midwife shall, if the local supervising authority deem it necessary for preventing the spread of infection, undergo medical examination by a registered medical practitioner.[24] Failure of any registered practitioner to notify his or her employer of their HIV or hepatitis status and to continue to practice in a clinical situation could lead to a criminal conviction and loss of registered status.

Law relating to medicinal products

The legislation dealing with the safety of medicines cannot be discussed in detail here, but all theatre staff should be aware that there are laws that make it illegal for unauthorized staff to be involved in the administration or supply of drugs. Stringent rules apply to the storage and movement of controlled drugs, and all staff should ensure that the operational policy of the theatre on the use, storage and movement of drugs is obeyed.

Where does the nurse manager stand if an anaesthetic nurse becomes addicted to drugs? As with the hepatitis case above, it is recognized that the nurse manager has a professional duty to take appropriate action and, if harm occurs as a result of the anaesthetic nurse's condition, both the nurse and the manager could find themselves before the UKCC: the nurse possibly before the Health Committee; the manager before the Professional Conduct Committee.

Employment law

Each employee has a contract of employment with a health authority, an NHS Trust or private hospital employer. Nowadays, with the use of bank or agency nurses and others for crisis situations, it is a question of fact as to whether these persons are employed by the hospital or by the agency. Reference should be made to those books on employment law cited in the Further Reading section to obtain more details.

Within the NHS the Whitley Councils, through a system of collective bargaining, negotiated terms for each category of staff for the whole of the NHS. Now, with the establishment of Trusts, individual terms can be agreed with each employee or category of employee through local collective bargaining. The NHS Trust does not, however, have complete freedom over the contracts of consultant medical, surgical and dental staff. The transfer to Trusts has raised certain issues.

Where do practitioners stand if the directly managed unit becomes a NHS Trust and they are asked to accept less favourable terms?

The basic principle that applies to the change of contracts is that one party cannot change the terms unilaterally, i.e. without the agreement of the other party. The transfer of staff from one employer to another is protected by the EU rules on the Transfer of Undertakings and by Sections 6 and 7 of the NHS and Community Care Act 1990. Section 6(3) states:

... subject to Section 7 the contract of employment between a person to whom this section applies and the health authority by whom he is employed shall have effect from the operational date as if originally made between him and the NHS trust.

There have been cases on this subsection and the courts have interpreted it fairly tightly, so that where a person was transferred to a slightly different post after the Trust came into being she was held not to be protected by the Act. For the most part, however, staff are entitled to retain their existing terms and conditions. However, if they seek promotion or a different post, or if they move to a different Trust, then they lose that protection and can be asked to accept new terms, since there will be a new contract.

It was thought initially that there would be a strong move towards local collective bargaining, but this has not happened and for the most part Trusts are only slowly moving to develop terms and conditions outside the Whitley Council system.

Where do practitioners stand if their colleagues wish to work as an independent self-employed agency?

The development of the internal market has opened the way for new forms of delivering care. In some districts we have seen the formation of organizations of professions supplementary to medicine offering their services on a fee-for-service basis to Trusts and other providers, such as GP fundholding practices. For the present the arrangement of direct labour staff of each Trust is likely to remain, but it is possible that more of the services will be put out to tender and negotiated with the organizations of the professionals concerned. If nurses come under pressure to join such an organization they are entitled to stick to their contract of employment with the Trust. However, if the Trust were to decide to privatize the theatre services then the direct labour staff would be made redundant, as has happened in the field of domestic work, portering and other ancillary services.

These changes are possible, and the best protection for staff is to ensure that they remain at the highest level of training and skill so that their services will be required whatever the contractual arrangements.

The internal market

Since the implementation of the NHS and Community Care Act 1990, health services for patients have been purchased by purchasers from providers. Where this agreement takes place between NHS health service bodies it is known as an NHS agreement, but it is not enforceable in a court of law. The NHS agreement sets out the quantity and quality of the services being purchased. More and more GPs are becoming members of group fundholding practices, which means that the purchasing budget is delegated from the health authority to them. Where the services that are required are covered neither by an NHS agreement nor through group fundholding purchasing plans, the patient may be referred to another organization, or to a person not necessarily within the NHS, as an extra-contractual referral.

What are the implications of these changes for theatre staff? First, it is essential that theatre staff should have a clear input into the negotiation of the NHS agreement in relation to theatre services to ensure that the quality of the service can be maintained. Secondly, they should be involved in the setting of the standards that are laid down in the NHS agreement. Thirdly, they should be involved in the monitoring of these standards, so that the lessons learnt can be used to vary or modify the next NHS agreement. This involvement should concern all theatre staff, and not necessarily just the senior surgical and nursing staff.

Record keeping

It should be understood from the section on accountability that theatre records are extremely important in the event of any untoward incident. Since it may take many years for a case to come to court it is essential that the principles set out in the UKCC document *Standards for records and record keeping* are closely followed and monitored. The UKCC is the registration body for nurse, midwife and health-visiting practitioners, and its advisory paper is of relevance to every-one working in theatre who keeps records, including the surgical staff. Where mistakes have been made in the writing of records it is important that they should not be blanked out but clearly crossed out, so that what was originally written can be seen and the reason for the change made clear. The person altering the record should sign and initial the change, and a record should be kept of those signatures and the staff on duty at any one time.

Day surgery

This form of care is increasing, with twice as many operations being performed on an outpatient basis over the last few years. For the most part the law is no different in its application to day surgery than to inpatient surgery: exactly the same principles of standard of care apply and the rights of the patient are no different. However, because there is no safety net for postoperative problems as there is for inpatients, the assessment of the patient as being suitable for day surgery becomes very important. Preoperative selection must take place:

- when the possibility of day surgery is first considered
- when the patient is sent an appointment for care
- when the patient arrives for the operation.

After the operation a similar assessment must be made to ensure that the patient is fit to return home. As far as possible information concerning contraindications for day surgery should be given to the patient in writing, supported by communication with GPs over information they have that makes day surgery an unacceptable risk.

Can the patient insist upon day surgery when there are contraindications? The answer is probably no, since it would not be acceptable professional practice to undertake a procedure where there are clear reasons why the risks are unacceptable.

Can the patient insist upon inpatient surgery when there are no justifications for a hospital stay? The answer is probably not, but it is likely that there will be some bargaining with the patient along the lines that day surgery could be carried out much sooner than inpatient surgery. In addition, it is important to find out why day surgery is not acceptable to the patient, as this might show that it is inadvisable anyway: for example, the patient may have no support at home for the postoperative period.

Special requirements in certain operations

The following are types of operation where specialist laws apply:

- termination of pregnancy
- sterilization
- transplants: removal of organs and donations of bone marrow
- Section 57 of the Mental Health Act 1983
- in vitro fertilization
- obstetrics and the safety of the baby
- circumcision.

TERMINATION OF PREGNANCY

Before a termination of pregnancy takes place theatre staff should ensure that the requirements of the Abortion Act 1967, as amended by the Human Fertilization and Embryology Act 1990, are met. Clearly, once the patient has come to theatre it will be too late to check whether the necessary statutory conditions were present, but the theatre staff should check the documentation and ensure that the two certificates to be provided by the doctors are present and there is a consent form signed by the mother. The statutory requirements for a valid termination which would protect staff against the Offences Against the Person(s) Act (1861) are as follows:

1(1) Subject to the provisions of this Section, a person shall not be guilty of an offence under the law relating to abortion when a pregnancy is terminated by a registered medical practitioner, if two registered medical practitioners are of the opinion formed in good faith:

(a) that the pregnancy has not exceeded its 24th week and that the continuance of the pregnancy would involve risk, greater than if the pregnancy were terminated, of injury to the physical or mental health of the pregnant woman or any existing children of her family; or

(b) that the termination is necessary to prevent grave permanent injury to the physical or mental health of the pregnant woman; or

(c) that the continuance of the pregnancy would involve risk to the life of the pregnant woman, greater than if the pregnancy were terminated; or

(d) that there is substantial risk that if the child were born it would suffer from such physical or mental abnormalities as to be seriously handicapped.

1(2) In determining whether the continuance of a pregnancy would involve such risk of injury to health as is mentioned in paragraph (a) or (b) of subsection (1) of this section, account may be taken of the pregnant woman's actual or reasonably foreseeable environment.

1(3) Except as provided by subsection (4) of this Section, any treatment for the termination of pregnancy must be carried out in a hospital vested in the Minister of Health or the Secretary of State under the National Health Service Acts, or in a place for the time being approved for the purposes of this Section by the said Minister or the Secretary of State.

1(3A) The power under subsection (3) of this section to approve a place includes power, in relation to treatment consisting primarily in the use of such medicines as may be specified in the approval and carried out in such manner as may be so specified, to approve a class of places. (Abortion Act 1967 (as amended by the Human Fertilization and Embryology Act 1990))

The Act gives a right of conscientious objection to taking part in a termination of pregnancy, but this right does not exist in an emergency situation when the life of the mother is at risk.

Termination in an emergency

The statutory provisions set out above do not apply in an emergency. The relevant section of the Abortion Act 1967 is given below. In an emergency the hospital does not have to be one approved by the Secretary of State for carrying out terminations:

1(4) Subsection (3) of this Section, and so much of subsection (1) as relates to the opinion of two registered medical practitioners, shall not apply to the termination of a pregnancy by a registered medical practitioner in a case where he is of the opinion, formed in good faith, that the termination is immediately necessary to save the life or to prevent grave permanent injury to the physical or mental health of the pregnant woman.

STERILIZATION OPERATIONS

There is no legal requirement that the spouse should sign a consent form agreeing that the patient can have an operation for sterilization, although good practice should ensure that both partners are counselled before consent is obtained from the patient.

Sterilization of a minor

Where the operation is to be carried out on a minor the operating staff should ensure that consent forms are signed by the parents, and in the event of a non-therapeutic operation, i.e. one to be carried out on social grounds in the case of a person who is severely mentally impaired, there should be the authority of the court. Court approval would also be required in the case of a mentally impaired adult who could not give a valid consent herself.[25]

In the light of recent cases it is also good practice to ensure that the patient has a pregnancy test before the operation. What is the legal situation if during the sterilization it is found that the woman is pregnant? The surgeon would have to decide if clinically it were possible to stop the operation and allow the woman to recover and decide whether the pregnancy should continue, or whether the requirements of the Abortion Act were satisfied. If the surgeon were to continue and in effect terminate the pregnancy, this would probably not be an offence under the Act provided that the requirements shown above applied.

TRANSPLANT SURGERY

This can affect the operating staff in two ways: they might be involved in an operation to collect the organs which are to be donated, or they might be involved in an operation to transplant those organs into the recipient.

Collection of organs from the deceased

By the time the patient reaches theatre it is likely that the decision has already been made that they are brain dead and that doctors unconnected with the transplant team have certified death. Operating staff should, however, be aware from the documentation as to whether the patient was a donor card carrier or had given consent in the ways set out in the Human Tissue Act 1957 (see below), or whether the relatives had given consent (see also below). In a case where consent had been given by the deceased, there should also be an authority by the person in possession of the body (probably the unit manager) that the Act's requirements were satisfied.

Human Tissue Act 1957: prior consent
Section 1(1) If any person, either in writing at any time or orally in the presence of two or more witnesses during his last illness, had expressed a request that his body or any specified part of his body be used after his death for therapeutic purposes, or for purposes of medical education, or research, the person lawfully in possession of his body after his death may, unless he has reason to believe that the request was subsequently withdrawn, authorize the removal from the body of any part or, as the case may be, the specified part for use in accordance with the request.

Human Tissue Act 1957: no prior consent
Section 1(2) The person lawfully in charge of the body of a deceased may authorize the removal of any part from the body for use for therapeutic, medical education or research purposes, if having made such reasonable enquiries as may be practicable he has no reason to believe:
(a) that the deceased had expressed an objection to his body being so dealt with after his death;
(b) that the surviving spouse or any surviving relative of the deceased objects to the body being so dealt with.

At present, because of the shortage of donor organs and the growing waiting list of patients requiring transplants, discussions are taking place about changes to the law; some have suggested an opting-out system so that there is a presumption in favour of donation unless the person has actu-

ally made a declaration to the contrary. There is now a system of registration of potential donors through the licensing authority for drivers.[26]

Donation from living persons

Theatre staff should check that there is no breach of the Human Organ Transplants Act 1989, which restricts transplants between live patients of tissues that cannot be replicated. The Act does not therefore apply to bone marrow transplants. The Act makes it a criminal offence to sell organs (whether from dead or living persons) which are intended for transplantation (Section 1). Where transplants are to take place between live persons it is a criminal offence to remove an organ from a living person which is intended for transplantation to a recipient who is not genetically related to the donor, unless the approval of the Unrelated Live Transplant Regulatory Authority has been obtained. Theatre staff should ensure that the necessary documentation is present giving approval to the taking of organs.

Where it is alleged that the donor is genetically related to the recipient the nature of that genetic relationship should be identified in accordance with the Regulations.[27]

Under Section 4 the health bodies could be held responsible for any offences committed under the Act, and therefore they should establish procedures for compliance.

Operations implanting donated organs

Staff involved in these operations also have a duty to ensure that the legal requirements set out above in relation to the taking of organs are met, since they could also be involved in committing a criminal offence under the Act.

Donations of bone marrow

This does not come under the 1989 Act as it is regenerative tissue. However, since very young children could be donors it is essential that staff ensure that a valid consent form is present, and that the operation does not proceed unless it is. If there are any risks from the surgery, and it is not in the best interests of a donor who is a minor, the operation should also be stopped.

SECTION 57 OF THE MENTAL HEALTH ACT

In the case of treatment for mental disorder, a surgical operation for destroying brain tissue or for destroying the functioning of brain tissue and the surgical implantation of hormones for the purposes of reducing male sex drive[28] cannot be performed unless the requirements set out under Section 57 of the Mental Health Act 1983 are met. Operating staff should insist upon the production of Form 37. This sets out the following points:

A registered medical practitioner and two other persons appointed by the Mental Health Act Commission must certify that the patient…:
   (a) is capable of understanding the nature, purposes and likely effects of the treatment (the treatment must be described); and
   (b) has consented to that treatment.
The doctor must specify the names of the two persons he has consulted; one must be a nurse and the other professional neither nurse nor doctor who have both been professionally concerned with the medical treatment of the patient. The full name and status of each must be on the form.
The doctor must certify that having regard to the likelihood of the treatment specified alleviating or preventing a deterioration of the patient's conditions, the treatment should be given.

The theatre staff should ensure that there is also a valid consent form from the patient, since Section 57 requires the consent of the patient to be given before the operation can proceed. They must also check that the operation which is to be undertaken is that authorized on the form.

In an emergency Section 62 of the Mental Health Act 1983 enables any action to be taken for the treatment of mental disorder if it is necessary to save the life of the patient. This could apply to Section 57 treatment, in which case Form 37 would not have been completed, but staff should ensure that there is some documentary evidence that this is a situation to which Section 62 applies.

The sixth Biennial Report of the Mental Health Act Commission 1993–5 shows that there were 30 referrals under Section 57 in the period under review, and 24 certificates were issued authorizing the operation to proceed. Table 1 on page 181 of the Report shows the operating centres and types of operations performed:

> Brook Hospital – stereotactic subcaudate tractotomy;
> Pinderfields Hospital – stereotactic bifrontal tractotomy;
> Atkinson Morley's Hospita l– limbic leucotomy;
> University Hospital of Wales – bilateral capsulotomy.

IN VITRO FERTILIZATION

The Human Fertilization and Embryology Act 1990 regulates research and treatment for infertility that makes use of gametes (eggs and sperm) and embryos. The Act requires that a licence must be obtained from the Human Fertilization and Embryology Authority, which was established under the Act so that a person can bring about the creation of an embryo to keep or use an embryo. Theatre staff should therefore satisfy themselves, if they are involved in such work, that a valid licence has been obtained. Even with a licence there are certain activities which are illegal and would be criminal offences:

- placing a live embryo other than a human embryo in a woman, or live gametes other than human gametes
- keeping or using an embryo after the appearance of the primitive streak (i.e. over 14 days old)
- placing an embryo in an animal.

Other activities which cannot be authorized are set out in Section 3 of the Act. In January 1997 the Court of Appeal confirmed that written consent of a husband, now deceased, was required before his widow could be fertilized with his stored sperm. It was, however, possible for the widow to obtain treatment abroad, subject to the approval of the Human Fertilization and Embryology Authority.

OBSTETRICS AND THE PROTECTION OF THE CHILD

In Re S,[29] a case heard in 1992, a woman who made it clear that she was unwilling to have a caesarian operation on religious grounds, and who was supported in this by her husband, became the subject of a court hearing and the court declared that it would be lawful for the operation to proceed to save her life and that of the baby. Not surprisingly, the case led to considerable controversy. Subsequently, the ethics committee of the Royal College of Obstetricians and Gynaecologists has declared that this case should not be used as a precedent. Its recommendations include the following:

A doctor must respect the competent pregnant woman's right to choose or refuse any particular recommended course of action while optimizing care for both mother and fetus to the best of his or her ability. A doctor would not then be culpable if these endeavours were unsuccessful.

We conclude that it is inappropriate, and unlikely to be helpful or necessary, to invoke judicial intervention to overrule an informed and competent woman's refusal of a proposed medical treatment, even though her refusal might place her life and that of her fetus at risk.

There has been no legislation following the case of Re S. However, the basic principles relating to consent apply as described above and theatre staff should ensure that the documentation is in order.

In two cases in 1996 a judge ordered two women to have a compulsory caesarean section on the grounds of the women being incompetent to make a valid refusal. In a third case, a woman sectioned under the Mental Health Act 1983 and then compelled to undergo a caesarian section is at the time of writing challenging the validity of that decision through an application to the High Court for judicial review.

CIRCUMCISION

Male circumcision for religious reasons is legal and is often carried out by officials of a religion outside the hospital. It may also be indicated on clinical grounds.

Female circumcision, however, was made illegal by the Prohibition of Female Circumcision Act 1985, so whatever the religious views of the parents, the operation cannot be carried out lawfully in this country except in specific circumstances. The provisions of the Act are set out below:

Section 1 (Subject to Section 2) It shall be an offence for any person to:

- excise, infibulate or otherwise mutilate the whole or any part of the labia majora or labia minora or clitoris of another person; or
- to aid, abet, counsel or procure the performance by another person of any of those acts on that other person's own body.

Section 2 Section 1(a) shall not render unlawful the performance of a surgical operation if that operation:

(a) is necessary for the physical or mental health of the person on whom it is performed and is performed by a registered medical practitioner; or

(b) is performed on a person who is in any stage of labour or has just given birth and is so performed for purposes connected with that labour or birth by (i) a registered medical practitioner or a registered midwife; or (ii) a person undergoing a course of training with a view to becoming a registered medical practitioner or a registered midwife.

(2) In determining for the purposes of this Section whether an operation is necessary for the mental health of a person, no account shall be taken of the effect on that person of any belief on the part of that or any other person that the operation is required as a matter of custom or ritual.

REFERENCES

1. Bolam v. Friern Hospital Management Committee QBD 1957 2 All ER 118.
2. Maynard v. West Midlands Regional Health Authority HL 1985 1 All ER 635
3. Wilsher v. Essex Area Health Authority 1988 1 All ER 871
4. Barnett v. Chelsea HMC 1968 1 All ER 1068
5. Roe v. Minister of Health 1954 2 QB 66
6. National Association of Theatre Nurses 1993 The role of the nurse as first assistant in the operating department. NATN, London
7. Dimond BC 1995 Legal aspects of nursing, 2nd edn. Prentice Hall, Hemel Hempstead
8. Slapper G 1994 Shortcut to jail for surgeons. The Times 28 June 1994
9. R. v. Adomako House of Lords The Times Law Report, 4 July 1994

10. Re F. v. West Berkshire HA [1989] 2 All ER 545
11. Re T. (Adult refusal of medical treatment) [1992] 4 All ER 649
12. Malette v. Shulman (1988) 63 OR (2d) 243 Ontario High Court
13. Law Commission Consultation Papers 1991 No. 119, 1993 No. 129 and 1995 No 231
14. Re C. (adult refusal of medical treatment) [1994] 1 All ER 819
15. Re W. (a minor) (child in care: medical treatment) [1992] 3 WLR 758
16. Gillick v. West Norfolk and Wisbech AHA and the DHSS 1985 3 All ER 402
17. Chatterton v. Gerson [1981] 3 WLR 1003; Sidaway v Bethlem Royal Hospital governors and others 1985 1 All ER 643
18. Dimond BC 1993 Patients' rights, responsibilities and the nurse. Quay Publications, Lancaster
19. Dimond BC 1993 Protecting the consumer. Nursing Standard 7: 18–19
20. Dimond BC 1995 Legal aspects of nursing, 2nd edn. Prentice Hall, Hemel Hempstead
21. NHS Management Executive 1993 Executive letter EL (93)51
22. [1987] ICR 700
23. United Kingdom Central Council Midwives Rules 1993. UKCC, London
24. Kloss D 1994 Occupational health law, 2nd edn. Blackwell Scientific, Oxford
25. Re F. v. West Berkshire HA 1989 2 All ER 545.
26. Dimond BC 1993 Transplants and donor cards – the legal significance. Accident and Emergency Nursing 1: 49–52
27. Human Organ Transplants (Establishment of Relationship) Regulations 1989 2017
28. Mental Health (Hospital, Guardianship and Consent to Treatment) Regulations 1983 regulation 16
29. Re S. (Adult refusal of medical treatment) 4 All ER 671

USEFUL ADDRESSES

Abortion Law Reform Association
27–35 Mortimer Street
London W1N 7RJ
Tel 0171 637 7264

Action for Sick Children
Argyle House
29–31 Euston Road
London NW1 2SD
Tel 0171 833 2041
Fax 0171 837 2110

Action for the Victims of Medical Accidents
Bank Chambers
1 London Road
Forest Hill
London SE23 3TP
Tel 0181 291 2793

Association for Improvement in the Maternity Services
40 Kingswood Avenue
London NW6 6LS

Association of Community Health Councils
30 Drayton Park
London N5 1PB
Tel 0171 609 8405

Association of Supervisors of Midwives
Maternity Unit
James Paget Hospital
Lowestoft Road
Gorleston.
Great Yarmouth
Norfolk NR31 6LA
Tel 01493 452269
Fax 01493 452819

British Association of Operating Assistants
70a Crayfor High
Street
Dartford, Kent DA1 4EF

British Dental Association
10 Queen Anne Street
London W1M 0BD

British Homoeopathic Association
27a Devonshire Street
London W1N 1RJ
Tel 0171 935 2163

British Orthoptic Society
Tavistock House
North
Tavistock Square
London WC1N 9HX

British Paediatric Association
5 St Andrews Place
Regent's Park
London NW1 4LB
Tel 0171 486 6151
Fax 0171 486 6009

British Pregnancy Advisory Service
Austy Manor
Wooton Wawen
Solihull
West Midlands
B95 6BX
Tel 01564 793226

Carers National Association
20–25 Glasshouse
Yard
London EC1A 4JS
Tel 0171 490 8818
Carers line:
0171 490 8898

Child Accident Prevention Trust
4th Floor Clerk's
Court
18–20 Farringdon Lane
London EC1R 3AU
Tel 0171 608 3828
Fax 0171 608 3674

Community Hospitals Association
Shepherd Spring
Medical Centre
Cricketers Way
Andover,
Hants SP10 5DE
Tel 01264 361126
Fax 01264 350138

English National Board
Victory House
170 Tottenham
Court Road
London W1P 0HA
Tel 0171 388 3131
Fax 0171 383 4031

ENB Resource and Careers Department
as above

Equal Opportunities Commission
Overseas House
Quay Street
Manchester M3 3HN
Tel 0161 833 9244
Fax 0161 835 1657

General Medical Council
44 Hallam Street
London W1N 6AE

Independent Midwives Association
Nightingale Cottage
Shamblehurst Lane
Botley
Southampton

Medical Defence Union
3 Devonshire Place
London W1N 2EA

Medical Protection Society
50 Hallam Street
London W1N 6DE

National Association of Clinical Tutors
6 St Andrews Place
London NW1 4LB
Tel 0171 935 5556

National Association of Theatre Nurses
22 Mount Parade
Harrogate HG1 1BX
Tel 01423 508079
Fax 01423 531613

National Nursery Examination Board
8 Chequer Street
St Albans,
Herts AL1 3XZ
Tel 01727 847636
Fax 01727 867609

NHS Training Directorate
St Bartholomews
Court
18 Christmas Street
Bristol BS1 5BT

Patients Association
18 Victoria Park Square
Bethnal Green
London E2 9PF
Tel 0181 981
5676/5695
Fax 0181 981 6719

Royal College of General Practitioners
14 Princes Gate
Hyde Park
London SE7 1PU

Royal College of Midwives
15 Mansfield Street
London W1M 0BE
Tel 0171 580 6523/
0171 637 8823
Fax 0171 436 3951

Royal College of Nursing
20 Cavendish Square
London W1M 9AE
Tel 0171 409 3333

Royal College of Obstetricians and Gynaecologists
27 Sussex Place
Regent's Park
London NW1 4RG
Tel 0171 262 5425/
0171 402 2317
Fax 0171 723 0575

Royal College of Physicians
11 St Andrews Place
London NW1 4LE

Royal College of Surgeons of England
Lincoln's Inn Fields
London WC2A 3PN

Still Birth and Neonatal Death Society (SANDS)
28 Portland Place
London W1N 4DE
Tel 0171 436 5881
helpline
Tel 0171 436 7940
Fax 0171 436 3715

Society of Radiographers
14 Upper Wimpole
Street
London W1M 8BN

United Kingdom Central Council for Nursing Midwifery and Health Visiting
23 Portland Place
London W1A 1BA
Tel 0171 637 7181
Fax 0171 436 2924

Welsh National Board for Nursing Midwifery and Health Visiting
Floor 13
Pearl Assurance
House
Greyfriars Road
Cardiff CF1 3AG
Tel 01222 395535
Fax 01222 229366

Women's Nationwide Cancer
Suna House
128/130 Curtain Road
London EC2A 3AR
Tel 0171 729 4688/ 1735
Fax 0171 613 0771

FURTHER READING

Beddard R 1992 Human rights and Europe, 3rd edn. Grotius Publications, Cambridge

Brazier M (ed) 1988 Street on Torts, 8th edn. Butterworths, London

Brazier M 1992 Medicine, patients and the law. Penguin, Harmondsworth

Clarkson CMV, Keating HM 1990 Criminal law text and materials, 2nd edn. Sweet and Maxwell, London

Dale and Appelbe's Pharmacy law and ethics, 5th edn, 1993. Pharmaceutical Press, London

Dimond BC 1990 Legal aspects of nursing. Prentice Hall, London

Dimond BC 1993 Patients rights, responsibilities and the nurse. Central Health Studies, Quay Publishing, Lancaster

Ellis N 1994 Employing staff, 5th edn. BMJ, London

Finch J 1994 Speller's Law relating to hospitals, 7th edn. Chapman & Hall, London

Hunt G, Wainwright P (eds) 1994 Expanding the role of the nurse. Blackwell Scientific, Oxford

Kidner R 1993 Blackstone's Statutes on employment law, 3rd edn. Blackstone, London

Kloss D 1994 Occupational health law, 2nd edn. Blackwell Scientific, Oxford

Mason D, Edwards P 1993 Litigation: a risk management guide for midwives. Royal College of Midwives, London

Miers D, Page A 1990 Legislation, 2nd edn. Sweet and Maxwell, London

Morgan D, Lee RG 1991 Human Fertilization and Embryology Act 1990. Blackstone, London

Philips 1989 James, Introduction to English law. Butterworths, London

Pyne RH 1991 Professional discipline in nursing, midwifery and health visiting, 2nd edn. Blackwell Scientific, Oxford

Royal College of Midwives 1993 Examples of effective midwifery management. RCM, London

Rowson R 1990 An introduction to ethics for nurses. Scutari Press, London

Rumbold G 1993 Ethics in nursing practice, 2nd edn. Baillière Tindall, London

Salvage J 1988 Nurses at risk: guide to health and safety at work. Heinemann, Oxford

Salvage J, Rogers R 1988 Health and safety and the nurse. Heinemann, Oxford

Selwyn's Law of employment, 8th edn, 1993. Butterworths, London

Selwyn's Law of safety at work. Butterworths, London

Smith and Keenan English law, 10th edn, 1992. Pitman, London

Stanley, Loebetal 1992 Nurse's handbook of law and ethics Springhouse Corporation, Pennsylvania, USA

Steiner J 1992 Textbook on EC law, 3rd edn. Blackstone, London

Thompson R Thompson B 1993 Dismissal: a basic introduction to your legal rights; Equal pay; Health and safety at work; Injuries at work and work related illnesses; Women at work. All published by Robin Thompson and Partners and Brian Thompson and Partners

Tschudin V, Marks Maran D 1993 Ethics: a primer for nurses. Baillière Tindall, London

Young AP 1989 Legal problems in nursing practice. Harper Row, London

Young AP 1994 Law and professional conduct in nursing, 2nd edn. Scutari Press, London

Reference should also be made to the many articles on different legal aspects of nursing practice which can be found in *Nursing Times, Nursing Standard*, the *British Journal of Nursing*, and other journals for registered practitioners in general.

A bibliography of general and specialist books on midwifery, nursing and medical books is available from Meditec, Nursing Book Service, York House, 26 Bourne Road, Coldersworth, Lincs NG33 5JE.

Glossary

alleged   Put forward before it has been established.

civil   Used as distinct from criminal in relation to court proceedings which are brought in the civil courts of the country (i.e. County Court, High Court (Family Division, Queen's Bench Division and Chancery Division). See also torts.

common law   Judge-made law, i.e. law which is derived from principles established in cases heard before judges. A hierarchy of courts and a system of recording decisions enables judges to decide what previous decisions are binding upon them as precedents.

contract   A legally binding agreement between two parties based on an agreement and supported by consideration where there is an intention to create legal relations. Hence contract of employment. An NHS agreement between health services bodies for the purchase and provision of services within the NHS does not create a legal contract which is actionable in the civil courts. (See Section 4 NHS and Community Care Act 1990.)

contributory   Adding to: used in relation to negligence as a defence where the person seeking compensation is alleged to be partly responsible for the harm that occurred.

coroner   A person (in many cases qualified as both a doctor and a lawyer) appointed to inquire into a death which has arisen in specific circumstances, by means of an inquest.

criminal   Relating to proceedings brought in the criminal courts, i.e. Magistrates' and Crown Court, where offences are prosecuted against alleged offenders, usually by the Crown Prosecution Service or others such as the Health and Safety Inspectorate or NSPCC. Individuals can also bring private prosecutions. There is no clear distinction between whether an action or omission counts as a civil wrong or a criminal wrong and some may be both, e.g. assault, theft.

inquest   Proceedings held, in specified circumstances, to determine the identity of the deceased and the cause, place and time of death. Presided over by the coroner, who has inquisitorial powers to determine the answers to the set questions. He also has the power to order a postmortem.

litigation   Taking action through court procedures, usually to obtain compensation.

negligence   A civil action in the law of torts for breach of a duty of care which has caused harm.

plaintiff   A person commencing an action in the civil courts.

statute   An Act of Parliament which sets out the law. It may be supplemented by statutory instruments which are drawn up through powers delegated to a Minister or others, and which are placed before the Houses of Parliament. Statutory law contrasts with the common law.

torts   Civil wrongs (excluding breach of contract) which are actionable in the civil courts. They include trespass, negligence and defamation.

UKCC   United Kingdom Central Council for Nursing, Midwifery and Health Visiting, the registration body of such practitioners.

Vicarious liability   The liability of an employer for the tortious acts of an employee who was acting in the course of employment.

3

Risk management

J. East

Introduction

The concept of **risk** addresses the probability that an **untoward incident** will occur. An untoward incident results from a set of circumstances which may have harmful consequences; the likelihood of it happening is the **risk** associated with it. The degree of risk and the possible consequences can be increased or decreased by the impact of various risk factors. Some, such as toxins and infectious agents, are present in the physical environment; some, such as smoking, lack of effective hand-washing and driving without seatbelts, are behavioural; some, such as instability or socioeconomic deprivation, are part of the social environment; and some, such as predispositions to certain diseases, are hereditary. Often there is no clear relationship between a risk factor and a specific outcome. For example, devitalized tissue in a surgical wound is known to predispose it to infection. However, a surgeon who does not routinely tie off bleeding vessels or eliminate dead spaces does not always have patients with infected wounds; conversely, some superb surgeons may occasionally have patients who do. In the healthcare setting professionals have a responsibility to identify risks over which they have some control and to take appropriate measures to minimize those risks.[1] This process, when actively undertaken, is referred to as **risk management.**

Risk management:

… is a systematic process of risk identification, analysis, treatment and evaluation of potential and actual risks. The primary purpose is safeguarding the assets of the institution by identifying and controlling the risks before losses occur. Or by continuing to function in the event of a major loss without severe hardship to the financial stability of the organization.[2]

Risk management serves as the mechanism for risk reduction, elimination and avoidance of economic losses. It has to be a planned programme, requiring commitment from management, clinical staff and all employees, to prevent, control and monitor areas of risk exposure.

THE ORIGIN OF RISK MANAGEMENT

Risk management has emerged as an operational component of the healthcare industry as a result of:

- rising healthcare costs
- the government's need to contain costs
- the development of the division between the purchaser and the provider of healthcare
- increasing costs and numbers of claims against providers of healthcare
- escalating court settlements.

THE GOALS OF RISK MANAGEMENT

There are many reasons for implementing an effective risk management programme. These include:

- the continuing survival of the organization following a major loss:
  — ensuring sufficient assets to regain pre-loss stature
  — freedom from worry about a potential loss
- to enhance the quality and standard of care
- to minimize the risk of clinical or accidental injuries and losses
- to ensure the programme's effectiveness and efficiency through management direction and control
- to coordinate and integrate current policies, programmes, committees and all aspects of the risk management process
- to avoid adverse publicity as a result of litigation.

THE RISK MANAGEMENT PROCESS

To manage identified risks effectively it is neces-

sary to follow a formal cyclical process, which consists of five main steps:

1. Identification of the problem or risk
2. Analysis of the actual/potential risk
3. Identification of possible risk solutions
4. Implement the agreed corrective action
5. Evaluate the effectiveness of the action and monitor the risk reduction.

Step 1: Risk identification

Risk identification requires a systematic process to identify **actual** and **potential** losses, rather than relying on random identification, which may not identify risks before losses occur. It is the most important step because unless they are identified risks cannot be managed effectively. It is also important as it is the beginning of deciding the best solution to implement.

A prerequisite to risk identification is a thorough understanding of:

- the scope of the services provided in a particular environment:
  — general description of the services provided, diagnostic or therapeutic
  — the equipment and supplies used
- the legislation and regulations affecting the provision of care
- the potential liability exposures of providing those services:
  — the previous claims history
  — information gathered from incident/accident reporting, committee activity, local audits, etc.

When carrying out this process it is likely that a number of risks will be identified, and it is possible that the volume of information gathered can become overwhelming. It is necessary to prioritize the variety of risks that may be identified to ensure that the risk management process becomes more effective. The risk assessment process should identify:

- the probable or possible severity of the loss
- how often this risk is likely to occur
- whether there are trends or patterns
- how much it will cost to eliminate or reduce the risk
- whether the problem can wait.

Step 2: Analysis of actual or potential risks

The risk manager or local manager must determine which exposures are significant enough to treat and which can be safely ignored. There are a number of ways to approach this:

- Determine the probable/possible severity of the risk exposure by using past claims experience, incident/accident report data, local or external experience.
- Determine the effect of the potential loss on the organization, i.e. would there be adverse publicity, would there be a loss of patient revenue?
- Integrate subjective opinions and objective data from legal counsel, insurance company input, risk management, health and safety groups, etc.

Possible effects of the risk and the potential or actual loss may be financial loss, either through a legal claim or loss of revenue, or adverse publicity, either internally or externally.

Step 3: Identification of possible risk solutions

When deciding which resolution would be the most appropriate there are three stages that should be considered:

- avoidance or elimination: avoiding a type of procedure rather than accepting the risk
- prevention of the risk exposure: by introducing suitable controls that prevent exposure to the risk
- reduce the risk to those exposed: implement controls to reduce the potential severity of the risk.

The key to selecting the best alternative is identifying the best technique that contributes to the most cost-effective approach to managing the risk.

Step 4: Implementing the agreed risk solution

The solution should be agreed by those who are affected by the risk or who have a responsibility to ensure the safety of others, be they patients, staff, contractors or visitors.

It may be necessary to introduce new techniques, equipment or working practices. Where major changes are made to working practices then it may be necessary to devise and agree new policies and protocols. Suitable staff training programmes may also be required.

Step 5: Evaluation and monitoring

This step requires there to be an ongoing assessment of the effectiveness of the risk identification, analysis and treatment procedures implemented. Is the implemented change working? This can be evaluated by a decrease in or the elimination of the previously identified problem:

- a reduction in the number of incidents/accidents
- a reduction in the number of claims
- fewer patient complaints or injuries
- potential adverse events are identified early
- a decrease in the number of adverse patient outcomes, etc.

Part of this process must also include the ability to identify further action that needs to be taken, issues that might contribute to the prevention of risk reduction, and further changes in practice which will enhance the risk reduction process.

The rest of this chapter will address the major areas of risk within the operating theatre environment, including:

- health and safety
- environmental safety
- infection control
- control of substances hazardous to health (COSHH)
- electrical safety
- radiological protection and laser safety
- equipment management
- sterilization and disinfection
- latex sensitivity.

Health and safety in the operating theatre

The Health and Safety at Work Act 1974[3] places on employers a statutory duty to safeguard the safety and health of their employees at their place of work. Section 2(3) of the Act requires every employer to prepare, update and bring to the notice of employees a written statement covering two distinct aspects:

- general policy with respect to the health and safety at work of employees
- the organization and arrangements for carrying out that policy, including, where appropriate, reference to safety representatives and safety committees.

The policy should therefore outline the general policy and the organization and arrangements to carry it out. It should start with a statement outlining the employer's intent to provide a safe and healthy working environment. The principles contained within the policy should then be interpreted by local managers to make it relevant for their own work areas. Each layer of management has its own responsibility to ensure that the policy is carried out in each workplace.

The Chief Executive has the ultimate responsibility to ensure that there is an effective, up-to-date policy in place.

Senior managers devise the policy, ensure that it is ratified, and make sure it is regularly reviewed and kept up to date and that, where necessary, action is taken to maintain a safe environment.

Local managers have a responsibility to interpret the policy and ensure its implementation in their own work areas, including:

- Carrying out safety audits with safety representatives to identify local hazards and, where necessary, taking action to ensure that local policy is complied with.
- Ensuring that staff are trained in the requirements of the policy, safe working practices, maintaining a safe environment, reporting unsafe environments or practices.

- Identifying individuals who will be responsible for health and safety on a daily basis.
- Ensuring that new staff understand the policy and that all staff are informed if there are any changes in policy or working practices.

Individuals also have responsibilities, including carrying out the requirements of the policy by working safely and maintaining a safe environment. Everyone, of whatever grade, should have their individual responsibilities written into their job descriptions, which should be assessed annually as part of the individual performance review.

MANAGEMENT OF HEALTH AND SAFETY AT WORK REGULATION 1992[4]

On 1 January 1993, following the adoption of European Directives, the requirements of the Health and Safety at Work Act were more clearly defined in six new Regulations or Guidelines, which came into effect on that date. Of these documents the most important is the umbrella regulation, the Management of Health and Safety at Work Regulation 1992, which:

- applies to all areas of work activity
- places the responsibility for health and safety management on the employer
- sets out the general principles for instigating health and safety management
- requires the employer to designate competent personnel to take charge of health and safety
- places the responsibility to ensure that there are adequate emergency arrangements, including fire safety, first aid, etc.
- requires employers to provide information and training for all staff as necessary
- requires employees to take care of themselves and others.

WORKPLACE (HEALTH, SAFETY AND WELFARE) REGULATION 1992[5]

This second regulation places further responsibilities on the employer by requiring employers:

- and other managers to comply with health, safety and welfare requirements
- to ensure the maintenance of equipment and devices used for and in the course of work
- to provide basic facilities for staff toilet, washing, rest and changing facilities
- to provide and maintain adequate ventilation, temperature, lighting and cleanliness
- to provide safe workstations, traffic routes, etc.

THE PROVISION AND USE OF WORK EQUIPMENT REGULATION 1992[6]

This requires that:

- equipment must be suitable for its purpose and regularly maintained
- access be restricted to equipment used for specific hazards
- measures be taken to minimize risks
- control systems must be safe and allowances made for breakdowns
- there must also be regular maintenance of work equipment.

THE PERSONAL PROTECTIVE EQUIPMENT AT WORK REGULATION 1992[7]

This requires:

- the employer to ensure assessment of the risk of the task
- the selection of suitable protective equipment giving adequate protection, which fits correctly and is compatible with the work to be undertaken
- the provision of essential protective equipment free of charge and maintained in good order
- information, instruction and training in its use to be provided.

THE DISPLAY SCREEN EQUIPMENT REGULATION 1992[8]

This regulation states that:

- employers must assess workstations for risks, and where necessary correct them
- employers must ensure that workstations meet minimum standards
- managers should plan work activities to allow for periodic breaks and changes
- provision should be made for eye tests for employees who meet the criteria, if they need them
- information and training must be provided for display screen workers.

MANUAL HANDLING OPERATIONS REGULATION 1992[9]

This final regulation requires:

- an assessment to be made of **all** manual handling operations
- where possible, the avoidance of hazardous manual handling operations
- the reduction of the risk of injury where possible
- the appropriate training of all staff whose job involves manual handling, pushing, pulling or lifting goods.

To comply with the requirements of the Health and Safety at Work Act and the current regulations every working environment must be audited. The Act and Regulations must be translated into practical assessments of risk, analysis of that risk, the implementation of risk avoidance or reduction techniques, and regular evaluation of the effective implementation of safe working practices.

THE PROCESS

There must be a hospital-wide health and safety policy, which is interpreted locally where necessary. In the operating theatre there are many risks specific to that environment which will need to be addressed. This includes policies and guidelines identifying the risks, and safe practices associated with:

- environmental and ventilation systems
- scavenging of anaesthetic gases and maintenance of these systems (also required under Control of Substances Hazardous to Health Regulations, COSHH)[10]
- other COSHH assessments
- assessment of manual handling operations and risks
- possible assessment of VDU operations and risks
- infection control protocols related to general safe practice
- blood and body fluid exposure and appropriate controls, including vaccination cover for hepatitis B
- appropriate waste disposal
- decontamination of equipment before recycling, maintenance and repair, etc.

The next step is to devise an appropriate audit tool and carry out the audit. There are many examples available which can be reviewed and adapted to local needs. The majority of hospitals will already have an audit tool which will only require minor adaptation. One such tool is shown in Appendix 2. Others are available from organizations such as the National Association of Theatre Nurses.

When risks have been identified they must then be evaluated and prioritized, in particular:

- the frequency of risk
- the severity of the risk
- the possible cost of correction.

It must be remembered this is not a one-off process but will require regular assessment to ensure continuing safety improvement, both in identified risks and in identification and control where practices change and new activities are introduced. It is also essential as part of this process that action which is taken to minimize risk is monitored to ensure continuing improvement.

Essential elements for assessment are as follows:

- Appropriate training for managers and safety representatives to enable them to recognize what needs to be assessed and what procedures are needed to control and minimize the risks.

- Training for all staff in their responsibilities in identifying and maintaining a safe working environment, for both themselves and others.
- It will also be necessary to establish safe systems of work and to ensure that these are carried out.
- Is this environment a safe place of work?
- Environmental controls that will need to be assessed:
  — heating, lighting, ventilation
  — hygiene and cleanliness
  — waste storage and disposal
  — fire and electrical safety
  — noise, dust
  — toxic materials handling and disposal
  — first aid provision
  — staff protection and welfare, etc.

Controls which will be required

- Training for all staff, at induction and ongoing, to ensure that they are aware of potential risks and appropriate control measures: what are their responsibilities under the Health and Safety at Work Act to themselves, to colleagues and other staff; to the employer; to others who may use their working environment?
- Development of appropriate safety procedures.
- Changes in working practices, substitution of risk activities by safer practices, introduction of better controls.
- Improved ventilation and extraction if necessary.
- Review of housekeeping in its widest sense: improved storage, improved waste control, keeping corridors and traffic routes clear, etc.
- Provision of appropriate protective clothing and ensuring that staff use it when necessary.

Gowns

The primary purpose of wearing a gown around the operating table is to provide a barrier to contamination, which can pass from staff to patient as well as from patient to staff. It has been demonstrated that the bacterial penetration of a given material depends largely on the degree of stress placed on it. Impermeability to moisture is a basic necessity of barrier material because of the wicking effect, which tends to transmit bacteria in both directions. There is continuing research on both disposable and non-disposable materials. Consideration must also be given to the deteriorating effect of multiple laundering of the newer non-disposable materials.

Caps/hoods

Various types of hair covering are now available, and hoods have been shown to be more effective in reducing the risk of shedding of hair and bacteria than has been experienced with caps.

Gloves

In a number of studies it has been shown that up to 12% of gloves are perforated during surgery, and that this occurred in more than 30% of operations.[11] Traditionally gloves have been worn to protect the patient, but today, with the potential risk of transmission of bloodborne diseases to the healthcare worker, there is continuing interest in the quality of gloves and the possible decrease in risk by double-gloving and the need to change gloves frequently during an operation.

Masks

Everyone who enters the operating room during an operation is required to wear a high-efficiency mask to cover the mouth and nose. If the mask becomes soiled or wet during the procedure it should be changed. Orr, in 1981,[12] argued that the efficiency of the face mask in preventing wound infection has not been proven but that its efficiency in reducing bacterial contamination has. He noted no increase in wound infection in a general theatre when masks were not worn, and concluded 'that the wearing of a mask has very little relevance to the wellbeing of patients undergoing routine general surgery and it is a standard practice that could be abandoned'. However, the issue of staff protection is again raised, and so whenever there is a risk of splashing or contamination of the oral or nasal mucosa then masks should be worn.

Protecting the staff where the patient may be the risk

A great deal of emphasis is currently placed on protecting the employee from acquiring infectious diseases from an actively infected patient or carrier. The potential for exposure to bloodborne diseases such as hepatitis B virus (HBV), hepatitis C virus (HCV) and human immunodeficiency virus (HIV) is high in the operating room, since needle-sticks, sharps injuries and blood splashes to the skin or mucous membranes do frequently occur in this environment. The risks appear to be directly proportional to the length of time spent in the operating room, the type of operation performed and the local seroprevalence of the patient population. In a recent study of 1300 cases in San Francisco General Hospital accidental exposure to the patient's blood occurred in 84 procedures.[13] It was found that parenteral exposure occurred in 1.7% of cases and cutaneous exposure in the others. The risk of exposure is increased if the procedure lasts more than 3 hours, when the blood loss exceeds 300 ml and when major vascular or intra-abdominal gynaecological surgery is involved. The authors also conclude that preoperative HIV screening does not reduce the frequency of exposure. Universal precautions, including the limited and careful use of sharps, routine double-gloving, the use of face shields or safety glasses and the wearing of barrier gowns that prevent strikethrough, appear to offer the best protection against accidental exposure to blood. The role that the HIV-infected surgeon or operating room employee plays in patient seroconversion, and whether steps should be taken to curtail their work, still requires further research; however, the Department of Health has produced guidelines[14] which will assist in making these difficult decisions. There is now, however, substantial evidence that patients have acquired hepatitis B infection from their surgeons, and there has recently been guidance on screening and vaccination programmes for staff working in high-risk areas.[15] There is currently no evidence that hepatitis C infection has passed either from patient to staff or from staff to patient, but the possibility of this remains.

EVALUATION OF THE PROCESS

It is essential that audits are carried out regularly, that risks identified are addressed and that improved standards are maintained. Where identified risks cannot be resolved locally these must be notified to managers responsible for health and safety within the organization and, where necessary, remedial action should be taken. As part of the process it will also be useful to review relevant incident/accident reports, which may highlight particular areas of risk. As part of the continuing review these reports should also be monitored to ensure a reduction in numbers associated with a reduction in risk exposure.

Environmental safety in the operating theatre

There are many environmental issues within the operating theatre that need to be considered to ensure effective risk management within the department. These include:

- theatre design
- ventilation, heating, lighting, etc
- traffic routes
- hygiene and cleaning practices
- clinical storage and stock control
- waste collection, storage and disposal.

OPERATING THEATRE DESIGN

There are a number of considerations here, including the layout, design, building and equipping of the department. There are both national and professional guidelines available on the topic. There are certain features which are important to reduce the risks. These include:

- The department's location, with easy access to intensive care unit, Accident and Emergency, X-ray facilities, possibly the obstetric delivery suite and to the sterilizing and disinfecting unit.
- Whether the suite is divided into zones of increasing control and cleanliness, i.e. aseptic, clean, protective and disposal, which is consistent with the Medical Research Council recommendations.
- The number of corridors and the provision of a transfer zone.

There is unfortunately little research to show that this type of relatively expensive layout is justified, as there is no scientifically validated evidence to show that it contributes to the reduction of patient risk. Also, the discipline required of staff in maintaining clean and dirty areas is frequently breached by people taking the shortest route between two points. Moreover, in those suites being used almost as planned, no notable reduction in infection rates has been observed over previous rates or in suites designed with a single corridor. However, it may be justified to grade access to the department for security reasons:[16]

- general access: reception area, general store rooms, porters room
- limited access: staff rooms, offices, X-ray, endoscopy room, disposal areas
- restricted access: scrub-up area, anaesthetic room, clinical storage, preparation areas and the operating room.

The layout should focus attention on the importance of good discipline within the department as staff move towards the operating room and the operating field. Other important considerations should include easy-to-clean theatre walls, floors and fittings. The floors should be capable of withstanding heavy moving loads, frequent cleaning, heavy-duty cleaning with scrubbing machines, and be slip-resistant under wet conditions. Wherever possible built-in horizontal surfaces should be avoided. Adequate storage facilities are also essential, otherwise there is the added risk of cluttered and possibly dirty corridors. The provision of changing areas, rest rooms, toilets and emergency showers is also necessary.

The optimal size for most routine operating rooms is 20 × 20 ft with 10 ft ceilings, which allows for easy gowning, draping, circulation of personnel and the use of equipment without the risk of contact contamination. The door of each operating room should be kept closed except for the passage of equipment, staff and the patient. Intraoperative surveillance of the activity in the operating room and the levels of bacteria in the environment bears direct relation to the number of personnel, the degree of activity and whether or not the doors are kept closed.

Concern was recently expressed over the frequency of sternal wound infection following cardiac surgery (East 1990, personal communication). Each case was reviewed and it was found that no single organism was responsible, indicating that individual personnel were unlikely to be the source. On further investigation it was found that all the operations concerned were carried out on a day when only one instead of two operating rooms were in use, creating the need for a faster turnaround between patients than usual. Following discussion with the staff it was decided that it would be appropriate to establish the bacterial air counts during an operating list when only one theatre was in use. On reviewing the results it was clear that there were certain times during each operation when air counts increased to high levels (Fig. 3.1). These included placing the patient on the operating table; when

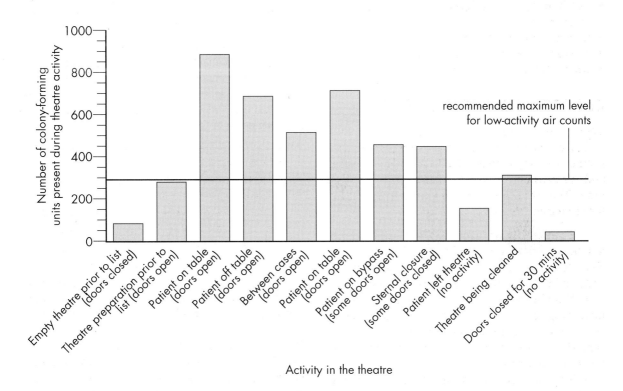

Figure 3.1   Microorganism air counts during different theatre activities.

cardiopulmonary bypass was being established; when coming off bypass; and at the end of the case when taking the patient off the table. Each increase was directly associated with a time of high activity in the operating room. Once the patient had left the area, the cleaning was completed and the doors were closed, the air counts dropped to zero. When this evidence was shared with the staff they reviewed their practices, in particular the handling of bedclothes, the numbers of staff and their activity during surgery, and the discipline of keeping the doors closed at all times. These practices are important for all types of surgery, not only cardiothoracic.

VENTILATION, TEMPERATURE AND HUMIDITY REQUIREMENTS

Conventional theatres

Almost all non-orthopaedic theatres are now plenum ventilated, with 20 air changes per hour without recirculation. In 1972 the Medical Research Council and the DHSS set out specific requirements for general, non-orthopaedic theatres, to ensure comfortable working conditions, to prevent the build-up of anaesthetic gases and to protect the wound from airborne bacterial contamination by dilution and transfer of the bacteria away from the cleanest areas (see Chapter 8 for further details).

Orthopaedic theatres

The risks to patients from the dispersal of low-grade pathogens in the theatre are much greater where there is a prosthesis to be introduced. Consequently, bacteriological standards must be much higher. In conventional theatres there is a degree of air turbulence because the air is introduced near the ceiling and is then deflected by the heat from the operating team and lights, the movement of personnel and the opening and closing of the doors. Research has shown that doubling the air flow increases the removal of airborne bacteria by up to 45%. Ultraclean air systems, together with body-exhaust suits and prophylactic antibiotics, significantly reduce the

incidence of deep sepsis following total hip or knee replacement.

The ultraclean systems provide clean filtered air in the operating zone by means of a unidirectional discharge of air from a filter bank or diffuser, positioned usually vertically over the sterile field (see Chapter 8 for further details).

LIGHTING REQUIREMENTS

Lighting should primarily assist the surgeon by providing adequate illumination with a broad beam of light, and, having regard to aerodynamic properties, also contribute to air quality. Cruciform or small multidomed shaped lights are preferable to single large lights, as the latter add to the air turbulence, particularly in theatres with ultraclean laminar air-flow systems.

TRAFFIC ROUTES

The number of corridors in the department, access to them and their layout should facilitate the efficient movement of staff, patients, equipment, supplies and waste disposal. A single corridor system is the simplest, and there is no evidence to show that this contributes to increased risk. It may be necessary to ensure that a single corridor in a large unit complies with fire regulations. It is essential that these corridors are wide enough to accommodate the passage of two patients in their beds and any additional equipment, without disruption or accident.

A transfer area may also be provided where patients can be received and handed over to the care of the theatre staff. Recent research has shown that the practice of transferring patients from a ward trolley to a theatre trolley is not necessary, since this does not reduce the carriage of general hospital flora into the operating room and may actually increase the risks of lifting injuries to staff and also distress to the patient. However, a transfer area may help to restrict access to the department to essential staff.

OPERATING ROOM CLEANING

Research over the years has shown that patients are at greatest risk from their own bacteria, and less so from members of the surgical team. In the early morning before people enter, the operating room environment is virtually sterile. Wet mopping of the floor between cases and wet scrubbing and vacuuming of the suite at night keeps the floor clean. The practice of closing operating rooms for 24–48 hours following 'dirty' cases makes no more difference to bacterial air counts than does closing the doors for 30 minutes following routine cleaning. Also, it is unnecessary to schedule 'dirty cases' at the end of the day or in a special theatre. In modern, well-managed operating suites the chance of environmentally- spread infection remains remote, primarily owing to the high degree of efficiency in sterilizing instruments and surgical devices, efficient ventilation systems that provide clean air, and adequate cleaning of the environment between cases. Cleaning of the walls in the relevant area must be done as soon as possible after direct contamination occurs. Also, all instruments should be covered and linen and waste bagged and labelled before they are removed from the operating room to the recycling or disposal areas. All gowns, gloves and masks should be disposed of prior to leaving the operating room.

CLINICAL STORAGE AND STOCK CONTROL

There is frequently not enough storage space available in operating theatres. Where a new department or refurbishment is planned, adequate space must also be planned. Where space is inadequate it often leads to cluttered and potentially dirty corridors and storage areas. There should also be extensive shelf storage for clinical supplies, within the department but not in the operating or preparation rooms. A system of strict stock control should be developed and the use of the department as a supplier of emergency stocks for the rest of the hospital must be discouraged. As part of the risk management programme particular attention must be paid to the storage of volatile and inflammable liquids and gases. All liquids must be stored in a fireproof cabinet and all gas cylinders must be stored in appropriate restraints.[10] As part of maintaining a safe environ-

ment it is also recommended that there is a regular planned review and removal programme of all unnecessary and obsolete equipment.

WASTE COLLECTION, STORAGE AND DISPOSAL

As a waste producer, both the department and individuals are bound by a 'duty of care'[17] to ensure that waste is disposed of safely. There are a number of pieces of legislation which require this care, including the Health and Safety at Work Act 1974, COSHH regulations 1988 and 1994, and the Environmental Protection Act 1990.[18] There are also a number of guidance documents which interpret the laws.[19] Hospital and local guidelines must be developed to ensure the safety of patients, staff and the general public, emphasizing the need for staff training in safe practices; segregation of types of waste; labelling of waste; provision of safe storage prior to collection.

Staff training

All staff who may be required to handle waste should understand the need to comply with the following:

- Fill all bags no more than two-thirds full.
- Check that all bags are effectively sealed.
- Ensure that the origin of the waste is clearly marked on each bag or box.
- Handle bags by the neck only.
- Understand the special problems associated with the disposal of sharps.
- Check that the seals on any waste container are unbroken when it is moved.
- Know the procedure in the case of accidental spillage, and report any accidents.

It is the manager's responsibility to ensure that all staff are trained and that the policy is complied with.

Segregation of waste and used laundry

Different waste materials will require different methods of disposal, and it is essential that all staff comply with these requirements. Segregation can be best achieved by the use of colour-coded bags and boxes. These include:

- yellow bags and boxes for any clinical waste and used sharps
- black bags for domestic waste
- glass, broken glass and crockery, aerosol cans and batteries must be disposed of separately
- items for return to central sterile services department, particularly if likely to be an infection risk, may be placed in sealed clear bags.

Labelling of waste

Under the requirements of the Environmental Protection Act each bag and box must be labelled as to its place of origin. In the operating theatre this should be each individual operating room. Both clinical and domestic waste should be identified.

Safe storage prior to collection

- This storage should allow for the separation of clinical and domestic waste.

- Surfaces in the storage area should be smooth, impermeable and easily cleaned.
- The area should not offer harbourage to insects and pests.
- The waste should be removed as frequently as circumstances demand. It is recommended that the minimum removal is once a day.

Laundry disposal

Again there should be a clear policy on the safe disposal of used linen. The policy must comply with the Health and Safety at Work Act 1974 and the NHSE Hospital Laundry Arrangements for used and infected linen HSG (95) 18.[20] As with waste disposal, staff training, segregation, labelling and safe storage must be addressed.

Segregation under a colour-coding system is essential, and allows priority laundry to be easily identified and rapidly processed. It is essential that only used linen is sent to the laundry and that no miscellaneous items are included.

Infection control in the operating theatre

There are two major areas to consider when reviewing infection control in the operating theatre. These are the risks to the patient and the risks to the staff. As each one can have an impact on the other, both are equally important. To ensure that the risk of acquiring an infection is kept to a minimum, the process of risk management can again be used:

- What are the risk exposures?
- What methods are suitable to control those risks?
- Which is the best control method?
- Implement suitable controls.
- Evaluate and monitor improvements in risk reduction.

INFECTION RISK MANAGEMENT FOR STAFF

What are the risks?

Is the working environment safe? Review the health and safety audit for possible areas of risk and suitable controls.

Are there patients who may pose a risk to staff? Because of the sometimes unpredictable nature of the work and the need to provide emergency care, it is frequently impossible to make an appropriate assessment of all patients. Therefore the approach should be to ensure minimal risk to staff from patients. It is much more appropriate to establish a routine, high standard of safe working practice rather than to suddenly introduce stringent measures for individual patients perceived to be a particular problem.

For example:

• Keep the operating room clear of equipment not required for the current operation.
• Keep the number of staff to a minimum to ensure safety in the operating room during surgery.
• Ensure that all equipment, instruments and extras are available at the start of a case to minimize movement in and out of the operating room.
• Ensure that all staff in direct contact with the patient wear the appropriate protective clothing:
   — gloves
   — face masks
   — impervious protective clothing
   — protective shoes.
• Train staff to identify the risks to themselves and others and the appropriate protective measures required.
• Routine nasopharyngeal and other microbiological cultures of personnel within the department are not necessary; however, screening of staff may be necessary in the presence of an outbreak of infection which can be traced to an infection acquired during surgery.
• Where possible visit the patient prior to surgery to identify any possible risks, which can then be prepared for.
• Ensure that staff are trained to behave in a manner that minimizes their risk exposure.
• Scrub staff must prepare themselves and behave in such a manner that they reduce the risk to themselves and others throughout the operation. In particular they should:
   — scrub up and don sterile clothing effectively
   — conduct themselves appropriately when scrubbed
   — wear sterile protective clothing when carrying out any invasive procedures
   — remove clothing at the end of operations carefully and discard safely.
• Train staff in the safe handling, labelling and transport of specimens.

• Provide circulating staff with appropriate protective clothing.
• Control the handling of soiled swabs, urine drainage, wound drainage, etc.
• Make the process of clearing the theatre simple:
   — ensure that all dirty instruments are safely handled from the operating room to ultimate recycling or disposal
   — ensure safe sharps and waste disposal, with closure of bags and boxes prior to removal from the operating room
   — provide appropriate cleaning materials and train staff in effective, safe methods of cleaning.
• Provide adequate first aid facilities and record all incidents and accidents; also follow up incidents to ensure that risks are minimized.
• Ensure that staff are adequately trained in the risks and risk prevention techniques.

INFECTION RISK MANAGEMENT FOR PATIENTS

Is the environment safe? Again, review the health and safety audit, in particular:

• effective ventilation systems appropriate to the type of surgery
• adequate heating and lighting to ensure that staff can work in optimum conditions
• high-quality hygiene and cleaning practices
• safe waste disposal
• high-level sterilization and disinfection practices
• equipment purchase, checking, cleaning, maintenance and repair protocols.

Despite the high standards set for professionals' performance and equipment, the controlled environment remains potentially hostile to both the patient and the surgical team.[21] The risks that the patients will be exposed to also need to be considered and minimized where possible. These include:

• Predisposing host factors, such as old age, obesity, malnutrition, the presence of underlying immunocompromising diseases such as diabetes mellitus or diseases requiring corticosteroid therapy, the duration of preoperative stay and the presence of infection at another site at the time of surgery.

• Surgery-related risk factors, for example the surgical wound class, emergency surgery, operative site, duration of surgery and levels of wound contamination at the time of surgery.

• Other factors which may contribute to increased infection risk, including the preparation of the patient both physically and psychologically, the use of perioperative antibiotics, methods of skin disinfection, timing of razor shaving, use of drains and methods of wound closure.

Recent research has shown that of all the above factors there are four major ones which are highly significant in the patient's predisposition to acquiring an infection perioperatively.[22] These are:

1. Surgical wound class:

• **Clean**: uninfected operation wounds in which no inflammation is encountered and in which the respiratory, alimentary, genital and urinary tracts are not entered.

• **Clean–contaminated**: those wounds in which the respiratory, alimentary, genital or urinary tract is entered under controlled conditions and without unusual contamination.

• **Contaminated**: these include open, fresh, accidental wounds, operations with major breaks in sterile technique or gross spillage from the gastrointestinal tract, and incisions in which acute non-purulent inflammation is encountered.

• **Dirty** or **infected**: these include old traumatic wounds with retained devitalized tissue and those that involve existing clinical infection or perforated viscera.

The wound infection in clean wounds is usually due to exogenous (from external sources) microorganisms such as *Staphylococcus aureus*, whereas the usual source of infection in all the other classes is generally the polymicrobial aerobic–anaerobic endogenous flora (the patient's own flora at the time of surgery). Infection rates for the different classes range from:

• clean: 1–5%
• clean – contaminated: 3–11%
• contaminated: 10–17%
• dirty: more than 27%.[23]

The greater the contamination the greater the risk of acquiring an infection, particularly when added to the other risk factors.

2. American Society of Anesthesiologists (ASA) classification:[24]

• I – normally healthy
• II – mild systemic disease which is not incapacitating
• II – severe systemic disease which may or may not be incapacitating
• IV – severe systemic disease which is a constant threat to life
• V – a moribund patient who is not expected to survive more than 24 hours without operation.

3. The duration of the surgery: the longer the operation the greater the risk, in particular if an operation is extended beyond the generally accepted norm for that type of surgery.

4. Intraoperative contamination: this has been shown to be highly predictive of an increased risk of infection.

The probability of infection in patients within a particular wound class is increased six-to eight-fold when patients in a high ASA group have a lengthy duration of surgery.

As part of the risk management process the patient's infection risk exposure during the perioperative phase should be assessed as part of the intraoperative care plan. It can be helpful to consider the potential risks by reviewing both the patient's and the surgical risks against previously identified criteria known to predispose a surgical patient to the risk of infection (Table 3.1).

Table 3.1 Infection risk assessment

Risk	1	2	3
Age	6–49	50–69	0–6 70+
Invasive procedure	None	Injections i.v. cannulation	Catheterization central lines, TPN surgery
Body fluid exposure	No contact with body fluids	Contact with vomit, sputum, urine, faeces, blood, etc.	Large skin lesions, pressure sores, burns, secondary closure of surgical wounds, etc.
Mobility	Mobile	Unable to move independently	Unconscious
Immunity	Normal response	Immunity compromised by diabetes, anaemia, smoking, alcoholism, psychological stress	Immunosuppression due to cytotoxic therapy, transplantation, dialysis, medical condition
Communication	Has a healthy concern for self-care. Understands healthcare communication	Needs some help and advice on hygiene, prevention of infection. Some language problems	Has little understanding of hygiene, prevention of infection. Requires translation

NB: The degree of risk increases with the addition of higher risk factors:
   1–7 low risk
   8–14 medium risk
   15–21 high risk; in this instance it will be essential to introduce effective risk management strategies, such as increased physiotherapy sessions, improved nutritional intake, antibiotic prophylaxis, etc.

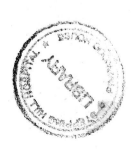

Control of Substances Hazardous to Health (COSHH) Regulations 1988[10] and 1995

The COSHH regulations came into force in October 1989. They require an employer to evaluate and control the risks to the health of employees posed by hazardous substances and to do everything reasonably practical to control those hazards. A hazardous substance is defined as a substance that creates a risk to the health of a person arising out of, or in connection with, his or her work. These are categorized as:

- very toxic, toxic, harmful, irritant or corrosive
- substances that have a maximum exposure limit or occupational exposure standard
- a microorganism hazardous to health
- dust of any kind when present in quantity.

Where possible, employers must ensure that employee exposure to such substances is prevented or adequately controlled. Controls may consist of:

- elimination of the substance
- changing practices so that the substance is no longer used
- substitution with a substance that is less hazardous
- controlling exposure by working in a closed environment
- improving local exhaust ventilation systems and general ventilation
- developing systems for safe handling of the substance
- ensuring that written work procedures are kept up to date
- educating and training staff.

Personal protective clothing should be the last control considered when other methods prove impractical. These may include respiratory protective equipment, appropriate protective clothing and gloves.

A COSHH assessment entails a number of objectives and procedures. It should:

- Involve a comprehensive assessment of all hazardous substances used in a particular area of work.
- Ensure that hazard data sheets are obtained from suppliers on all substances used in a work area.
- Establish whether the substance is controlled by a maximum exposure limit (MEL) or an occupational exposure limit (OEL).
- Identify any individuals within the organization who can give expert advice to staff.
- Establish whether there are any health effects to those exposed.
- Identify how the substance enters the body, for example through ingestion, inhalation, skin or eyes. Will it cause harm? Who is likely to be harmed?
- Facilitate the review and/or rewriting of workplace policies and procedures.
- Establish whether the substance is being used correctly by assessing work procedures; identifying how often, how much and for how long the substance is used; implementing safer procedures; monitoring usage, with updating if necessary; and monitoring staff health if necessary.

It is essential that all stages of the assessment are clearly documented, and a number of forms have been devised to facilitate this.[25]

PRACTICAL IMPLICATIONS FOR HEALTHCARE

All categories of hazardous substance need to be addressed in the healthcare setting.

Dust

The least likely to cause general problems is the production of dust, but dust in the fracture clinic or plaster theatre from the removal of plaster casts and splints should be controlled. If necessary, some form of dust extraction should be considered to protect staff. Also, the risk of dust created by building works will need to be assessed and, if necessary, appropriate control measures implemented.

Toxic, irritant, corrosive substances

Many substances used in hospitals fall into this category, and are generally found in laboratories and in patient care settings. The most notorious of these are the aldehyde preparations used in disinfection and sterilization procedures for heat-labile equipment. The first priority when assessing the risks associated with this type of chemical is to find out how it is used. A questionnaire has been developed (Fig. 3.2) to try to find out where, how and why aldehyde-type preparations such as glutaraldehyde are being used. The results of surveys carried out in a number of hospital settings using the questionnaire reveal several inappropriate uses, including the cleaning of work surfaces, disinfecting needles and sharp probes, which should be sterilized before use, and soaking contaminated equipment before cleaning. Glutaraldehyde is a fixative and so it is unlikely to be effective in the presence of organic material. The questionnaire also revealed the use of these substances in inadequately ventilated work areas without suitable exhaust ventilation systems. After evaluation of the survey results, control measures were introduced.

1. Do you use aldehyde-based products in your department? **Yes No**
   e.g. Cidex, Asep, Giagasept, formaldehyde, etc.

2. What are you using these products for?
   ....
   ....

3. Where are you using these products?
   ....
   ....

4. Are they stored in a covered container when not in use? **Yes No**

5. Are they used in a naturally ventilated area? **Yes No**

6. Is there an active local exhaust ventilation system? **Yes No**

7. Where do you activate the products before use?
   ....
   ....

8. Where are the products discarded when they are out of date or no longer required?
   ....
   ....

9. What protective clothing is available for staff?
   gloves, state type(s) .... **Yes No**
   glasses/goggles .... **Yes No**
   respiratory protective equipment .... **Yes No**

10. Have any of the staff complained of symptoms associated with sensitivity? **Yes No**

Figure 3.2 Use of glutaraldehyde questionnaire.

CONTROL MEASURES

1. Is the use of this chemical really necessary? In about 50% of cases it was not, and in most instances the sterile services department was able to provide a better service. Where it was necessary to use glutaraldehyde it was issued on a licensed basis, ensuring its use in a controlled environment.

2. Is it possible to use a less toxic chemical? Where glutaraldehyde is used appropriately there is no suitable alternative. However, there are a number of products undergoing research which may prove to be less toxic.

3. Is it possible to control exposure? The current Health and Safety Executive (HSE) Occupational Exposure Standard (OES)[26] is a 10-minute time-weighted average (TWA) value of 0.7 mg/m (HSE guidance on OELs), although recent experiments in the West Midlands have shown that individuals were still experiencing health problems at levels below the HSE standard.[27] Some measures that have been shown to be effective are decanting the chemical inside a fume cabinet; using an automatic endoscope washer/disinfector within a fume cabinet; using glutaraldehyde in an area with a local exhaust ventilation system, which is examined and tested once every 14 months to comply with COSHH Regulation 7; and ensuring that access to the working area is limited to staff undertaking the process.

4. Is it possible to ensure safe handling? This may not be possible in every circumstance, but all staff involved in the use of chemicals must be trained in the risks and be aware of their responsibilities. It is also necessary to provide personal protective equipment, such as long-sleeved latex gloves and nitrile gloves for extended exposure, and plastic aprons, face masks and goggles if splashing is likely. Respiratory protective equipment should also be provided, especially in units where large quantities of chemicals are used. Safe storage in a cool area away from direct sunlight is necessary, and great care must be taken if transporting, especially in immersion tanks. Splashes and spillage must be prepared for and all staff should be trained in the appropriate procedures and first aid practices.

5. Are staff well trained and do they work to written standards? Staff must be trained in safe practices and given written details of the agreed guidelines. Inexperienced employees should be adequately supervised until they reach an agreed level of competence.

Although glutaraldehyde has been considered, the same processes can be applied to other toxic, irritant or corrosive substances used in healthcare. Substances used in the operating theatre will include:

- glutaraldehyde, formaldehyde
- anaesthetic gases
- bone cement (methyl methacrylate)
- plaster of Paris and synthetic plasters
- control of legionellae
- disinfectants, in particular hypochlorite.

MICROORGANISMS HAZARDOUS TO HEALTH

It is the purpose of infection control to limit the acquisition and spread of pathogenic microorganisms. This can be achieved by appropriate policies and procedures to ensure the prevention of cross-infection, and by educating and training all healthcare staff. Many employees in healthcare are very concerned about their safety when working with patients, and their need for personal protection. Historically isolation practices have provided the backbone of infection prevention efforts. As in other areas of medical advancement, traditions have tended to become rituals.[28] In recent times many infection control teams have chosen to review their recommendations to staff to ensure a more rational approach to patient care. This change relies not on identifying specific diseases but on isolating body substances, such as faeces, blood, urine and wound drainage. These are the potential sources of pathogenic organisms, even in good health, and are usually transferred by the hands of staff. They can be eliminated primarily by wearing gloves and by effective hand-washing.

This system, usually called universal infection control precautions, eliminates many of the ritual practices while instituting protective measures against contact with all moist body substances, giving a uniform interaction of care with all patients from the time they enter hospital, regardless of diagnosis. These precautions have two purposes:

- to reduce cross-transmission of organisms among patients, primarily via the hands of healthcare staff
- to protect staff from unidentified organisms that may be carried by patients.

This practice is also a better way of protecting staff against bloodborne viruses than relying on testing patients, which can never be done in all cases and is impossible in an emergency. A guide to the implementation of universal precautions is given in Figure 3.3. Under this system, the only patients who will require single-room nursing and special precautions in theatre are those who have, or are suspected of having, an airborne communicable disease, or who are unable to prevent contamination of the environment. A successful infection control programme is one that is integrated into the individualized care planning process of each patient.[29] Infection risks should be assessed on admission and regularly thereafter, particularly prior to surgery.

MAINTAINING SAFETY: IMPLEMENTING THE COSHH REGULATIONS

The COSHH regulations have now been in place for more than 8 years. The following procedures must now have been implemented:

- A coordinator and COSHH team should be established.
- Inventories should have been carried out in every department.
- Hazard data sheets should be available in each work area.
- Assessments of high-risk areas should have been undertaken and checked by the COSHH team.
- Any necessary control measures should have been implemented, including improvement in ventilation systems.
- Systems for monitoring local exhaust ventilation systems should be in place; regular monitoring of environmental levels may be necessary.
- An appropriate health surveillance and immunization programme should be implemented.

---

1. **WASH** hands after every patient contact, and immediately if in direct contact with body fluids, even if wearing gloves.
2. **WEAR GLOVES** when you expect to have direct contct with blood and/or body fluids, mucous membranes or non-intact skin.
3. **WEAR SUITABLE PROTECTIVE CLOTHING** if your clothes are likely to become soiled. Plastic aprons provide an impervious barrier to moisture and are therefore better than cotton gowns.
4. **PROTECT YOUR EYES** and oral and nasal mucosa from splashing by wearing masks, safety glasses or goggles.
5. **DISPOSE OF SHARPS** (i.e. needles, razors, lancets, trocars, etc.) in a rigid, puncture-proof container that conforms to the current British Standard. This must be done by the individual who uses the sharps.
6. **LINEN AND WASTE** contaminated with body substances should be placed in appropriately coloured leakproof containers and stored securely before disposal.
7. **DISPOSAL** of fluid waste should be handled with care to ensure there is no splashing. Spillages should be dealt with as soon as they are discovered, using a locally recommended method and disinfectant. Domestic cleaning will then require no special precautions.
8. **COMMUNICATION** between staff is essential, in relation to both the assessed risks associated with each patient and the precautions necessary.

Figure 3.3   Guide to the implementation of universal precautions.

- Training of staff should have been carried out and all staff should be aware of their responsibilities, including reporting accidents and incidents.

It is the responsibility of everybody in healthcare to ensure that they are knowledgeable about the requirements of the Control of Substances Hazardous to Health Regulations, to ensure that they know what their personal risks are and the appropriate protective measures required to maintain their own and their colleagues' safety.

Electrical safety

The law governing the safe use and installation of electricity in the workplace is the Electricity at Work Regulations 1989,[30] which came into force on 1 April 1990 under the Health and Safety at Work Act 1974. The regulations outline the basic principles for safety, for good working practices and for objective means of meeting the standards.

Again, as with other regulations that have been recently introduced, there is a prime requirement to assess the risks, which requires both recognition and awareness of the possible dangers that may result from poor or deteriorating installations, unsafe work practices, unsuitable protective measures and wrongly selected equipment. To comply with these requirements it is necessary to establish a regular programme of inspection.

PROGRAMME OF INSPECTION

This must be carried out by a competent person, i.e. an electrician trained to make such assessments. However, this does not fully remove responsibility from managers and individuals working in a particular environment. With any inspection whatever you see should be assessed, and if it is felt that it looks incorrect or abnormal then further advice should be sought. The basic elements of an electrical inspection should include a general inspection of the installation:

- Are cables laid or run tidily?

- Are they terminated with no core or loose covering showing?
- Are conduits and trunking securely fixed?
- Is the installation and connected equipment assembled safely?
- Is the installation and equipment maintained adequately?
- How are the equipment and installation being used?

The rest of the regulations and guidance will need to be carried out by a trained and competent electrician, and will include:

- working with dead and live systems
- permits to work
- posting notices
- extra precautions when working with high voltages
- regular checking of portable electrical equipment.

It is the responsibility of the local manager to ensure that:

- all new electrical equipment is checked and added to the asset register prior to being used
- all electrical equipment is included in the planned preventive maintenance programme
- all staff using electrical equipment are trained to use it safely and are aware of the possible risks
- staff are aware of the procedure to follow if electrical equipment fails.

Radiological and laser safety

RADIOLOGICAL PROTECTION

The use of X-ray equipment in the operating theatre is subject to a number of regulations and guidelines, including the general requirements of the Ionizing Radiations Practice Regulations 1985 and 1988,[31] the Approved Code of Practice (ACOP) 1985,[32] and Health Service Use of Ionizing Radiations HC(89)18 1989.[33] The regulations and guidance documents require healthcare establishments to devise policies and protocols aimed at protecting patients and staff. These should include:

1. Identification of individuals with responsibility for ensuring safe practice, including:
   - the Chief Executive with overall responsibility
   - departmental manager responsible for ensuring safe practice within their unit
   - Radiation Protection Supervisor, a local expert with specialist knowledge
   - Radiation Protection Adviser, who can advise the employer on compliance with the regulations and other radiation protection matters. The name of this individual should be notified to the Health and Safety Executive. They must also have experience and expertise to the level of Principal Grade Physicist.
2. Control of radiation areas, including:
   - ensuring that appropriate warning signs are placed at the entrances to the operating room before X-ray equipment is switched on
   - ensuring that the controlled radiation area is identified when the X-ray equipment is in use.
3. Protocols on the protection of staff during X-ray use, including:
   - ensuring that only staff required for safe patient management remain in the controlled area

- the radiographer will warn non-essential staff to leave the controlled area
- ensuring that essential staff who remain wear protective clothing and a radiation monitor (monitors may not be necessary if only image intensifiers are used)
- pregnant staff must not remain in the operating room during procedures.
4. Control of direction of exposures, to include:
   - instructing the radiographer; this can only be undertaken by clinicians who meet the training requirements in Radiation Protection regulations or hold a certificate of training in the Core Knowledge of Radiation Protection
   - setting up and operating the X-ray equipment may only be carried out by a trained radiographer.
5. Emergency procedures, to include:
   - immediate reporting of equipment malfunction to the Radiation Protection Supervisor. Defective equipment must not be used on patients and must be isolated from the mains supply
   - where any person may have received an unplanned or excessive exposure this must be reported to both the Radiation Supervisor and the Adviser as soon as possible.
6. Radioactive sources: the use of radioactive sources in the operating theatre is subject to the same regulations and constraints as above. Senior theatre staff are responsible for placing warning notices and ensuring that the entire operating room and attached rooms are used as a controlled area.
7. Protection of staff in the controlled radiation area:
   - only essential staff and those undergoing training in the procedure should remain in the operating room
   - staff must wear radiation monitoring badges and stay as far away from the source as possible, consistent with their duties

• pregnant staff must be excluded when the radiation source is exposed
• radioactive sources should not be sent for or brought into the operating room until clinical preparations have been made, to ensure that the source is inserted immediately on exposure
• manipulations of the source must be carried out behind lead shielding as far as possible
• transfers and insertions must be carried out speedily and the source must be handled with appropriate forceps and tongs. Sources must **never** be touched by hand
• lead shields should be placed around patients undergoing treatment with radioactive sources, both in the recovery room and on return to the ward
• a record of each radioactive implant must be kept in a separate register as well as the operating register.

8. Clinical control:
• only clinicians holding a current Administration of Radioactive Substances Act 1978[34] (ARSAC) licence, which covers the relevant procedure, or a clinician acting in accordance with their direction, may apply radioactive sources to a patient for therapeutic purposes
• clinicians must also meet the Ionizing Radiations Regulations 1988 training requirements.

9. Control of radioactive sources:
• all radioactive sources brought into the operating room must be accounted for before the patient, dressings, instruments or bedding leave the room;
• in the event of the suspected loss of a source a search must be undertaken by a physicist until it is recovered.

10. Emergencies:
• damaged sources must not be used on a patient and must be placed behind a lead shield prior to speedy removal from the department by a physicist
• if there is any suspicion that a member of staff has received an excessive radiation dose the Radiation Protection Supervisor and Adviser must be informed as soon as possible.

LASER SAFETY[35]

Again, this type of equipment is hazardous unless used in carefully controlled circumstances. It is essential that local safety rules are devised and implemented. These should include:

• A Laser Safety Supervisor should be appointed within the operating theatre department to take responsibility for ensuring safe practice.
• No unauthorized person should use any laser equipment.
• The Laser Safety Supervisor should ensure that an up-to-date register exists of persons authorized to operate the laser, and of nominated personnel authorized to assist in its use and maintenance, also to assume overall control of the installation and its operation. The Laser Supervisor also has responsibility for notifying the Laser Protection Adviser of any changes in this register.
• The key to the equipment should be clearly labelled and kept securely when not required. A record should be kept when it is issued to authorized persons.
• It is the responsibility of those authorized to be present when the equipment is used, to be aware of the nature of the hazards involved and to ensure that the requirements for their own safety and the safety of the patients are met at all times.
• The operator of the laser must ensure that persons assisting in the procedures are fully trained in the safe performance of their duties and will be responsible for any visitors present.
• Calibration and verification of the laser power delivered by the attached accessory, usually a fibreoptic cable, will only be performed in accordance with the particular laser equipment operating manual.
• It is recommended that one particular theatre is designated for laser use and is designated a controlled area when the laser is energized. No other procedures should take

place in the controlled area, entry to which must be limited to essential personnel only.

- When a patient is undergoing treatment there must be at least two authorized personnel present at any time. Spectators must only be allowed in the area if required safety measures are taken.

- Laser light is dangerous: when improperly used it can damage the retina and skin and start fires. Therefore:
  — the laser beam must never be directed at or near the eye, even when protective goggles are worn (except for patients undergoing treatment on this area), nor at highly reflecting surfaces
  — highly reflecting objects must not be used in the vicinity of the beam. Persons working in the area must remove all personal accessories which have a reflecting surface
  — care must also be taken to prevent exposure of the skin to the beam, even at the lowest operating settings
  — all equipment not required in the operating room should be removed prior to the start of the session, and the laser beam must not be pointed towards any reflective furnishings or fittings
  — the laser beam must not be pointed towards any inflammable materials. Gauze and swabs should be moistened with water
  — inflammable anaesthetics or solvents must not be used in the laser control area when the laser is activated
  — the laser output must only be used when transmitted by an optical fibre correctly into the main unit
  — when a laser session is under way the beam must never be pointed towards doors, and the doors must remain closed when the laser is functioning. All windows, including those in the doors, must have closed blinds during the session.

- The laser emits an invisible operating beam and therefore it is essential that everyone present, including the patient, wears protective goggles. If the fibre is used in conjunction with an endoscope then an appropriate filter must be fitted over the eyepiece before the laser is armed. It must be remembered that even appropriate eyewear may not afford adequate protection if the beam or a reflection is directed at the eye.

- Switching on and off procedures must be clearly defined and followed exactly.

- The footswitch releasing the therapeutic beam must not be depressed until:
  — all personnel and the patient have been warned that the treatment is about to begin
  — all door interlocks and warning signs are set and window blinds closed
  — all personnel in the laser control area and the patient have their goggles correctly in place
  — goggles must not be removed by anybody, including the patient, at any time while tissue is being treated.

- All personnel except the operator and the assisting nurse must keep away from the operating area, in particular the direction of the operating beam.

- Whenever the laser is unattended by an authorized operator the control panel must be switched off and the key removed and kept in the safe custody of the authorized operator.

- If illumination falls on the unprotected eye, the individual must be examined by an ophthalmologist within 24 hours of exposure and an incident form completed. The Laser Protection Adviser must be notified of any such incidents as soon as possible by the Laser Protection Supervisor.

- Recent studies on the smoke plume emitted during laser use have suggested that there is a risk to staff working in close proximity to the patient. It is therefore recommended that appropriate face masks are also worn.

- The Laser Protection Supervisor must also review with the Laser Protection Adviser any safety implications of changes in operating procedure.

Equipment management

As with many other areas of healthcare there is increasing regulation of the quality and safety of equipment and medical devices. These include:

- Consumer Protection Act 1987, Part 1 Product Liability[36]
- Active Implantable Medical Devices Directive 1993[37]
- Medical Devices Directive 1993[38]
- Reporting adverse incidents, reactions and defective products, etc., guidelines MDA SN 9701[39]
- Management of Equipment, Health Equipment Information 1990[40]
- Decontamination of Equipment, Linen, etc. 1991[41]
- Good Manufacturing Practice 1989.[42]

PRODUCT LIABILITY

Part 1 of the Consumer Protection Act of 1987 covers the requirements of product liability. It is a popular belief that if things go wrong then the responsibility lies with the manufacturer, but this is not necessarily the case. The manufacturer has strict liability for defects in their products; however, the supplier, who may not be the manufacturer, is responsible for supplying a safe product. Any company or individual providing maintenance or repair services also has a responsibility to provide a safe product. Also, any individual who alters a product or recycles products not intended to be reused then takes on the responsibility for the provision of a safe product. The Consumer Protection Act 1987, s2(1) states that where damage is caused wholly or partly by a defect in a product the following persons may be liable for damages:

- the producer
- any person putting his name or trademark on the product
- any person importing the product.

The main target for liability is therefore the producer. The producer is defined as:

- the person who manufactures a product; or,
- in the case of a product which is not manufactured, but whose essential characteristics are attributable to an industrial process, the person who carries out that process.

Liability presupposes that there is a defect in the product. Defect is defined as the absence of safety in a product, which implies an entitlement to an expectation of safety on the part of the consumer. The risks to operating theatre staff become real when they reuse items which the manufacturer expressly states are for single use only. The possible cost savings in reuse may in the long term not be worth the risks, particularly in light of the changing medicolegal environment.

MEDICAL DEVICES DIRECTIVES

Medical devices are defined as instruments that are used in response to a variety of human conditions, for example for diagnosis, prevention, monitoring and the treatment of various diseases, injury or handicap; for the investigation, replacement or modification of the anatomy or of a physiological process; and for birth control. Pharmaceutical and chemical products are excluded.

Each country is responsible for ensuring that such devices are fit to be placed on the market and that the health and safety of patients, users and other persons are protected. In the UK this responsibility is undertaken by the Medical Devices Directorate of the Department of Health, which is responsible for medical devices and products used by the NHS and other healthcare sectors. They are concerned with ensuring the safety, quality and effectiveness of these items by:

- operating the Manufacturer Registration Scheme, which ensures manufacturing quality by monitoring supplying companies' manufacturing standards and practices and provides information to the NHS to assist in purchasing decisions

• coordinating adverse incident reports and investigating these via the National Reporting and Investigation Centre (NATRIC), which receives reports from the healthcare sector concerning accidents and incidents involving medical equipment, devices and materials

• undertaking equipment evaluations

• participating in the development of standards with the British Standards Institute and the European equivalents;

• playing a major role in the development and implementation of the EU Directives on medical devices. Member states must allow free movement of medical devices, which must bear the CE mark.

European standards are currently being developed and implemented to meet the safety requirements for most medical devices; these will then receive the CE mark. This includes standards in the areas of:

• biocompatibility
• sterilization methods and criteria
• quality systems
• labelling
• medical alarms and signals
• clinical investigations (trials)
• terminology
• symbols
• packaging.

REPORTING ADVERSE INCIDENTS

All staff working in the healthcare environment have a responsibility to report adverse incidents associated with medical devices and equipment to NATRIC. These incidents are an extremely useful source of information, enabling the Department of Health to advise users, on a national basis, concerning potential hazards and safety matters. MDA SN 9701 from the Medical Devices Agency details the guidelines for reporting adverse incidents.[39]

General managers and Chief Executives are responsible for ensuring the prompt reporting of adverse incidents, etc. and to ensure that prompt action is taken on receipt of hazard or other notification warnings. Managers should ensure that:

• adverse incidents, reactions and defective products are reported promptly

• procedures for reporting are followed

• for medical devices, a liaison officer is appointed at unit level to take responsibility for reporting

• products involved in an adverse incident should be kept until the department's officers have been given the option of investigating the incident

• healthcare staff are made aware of their responsibilities at induction and on a regular basis thereafter, in particular the procedures for reporting and isolation and retention of defective items

• warnings issued as a consequence of reports are circulated to all potential users and that prompt action is taken.

MANAGEMENT OF EQUIPMENT

To protect both patient and staff it is essential that all clinically related equipment is purchased through a controlled process. This usually consists of a committee of selected staff with relevant expertise. The process should include:

• committee review of all requests for new equipment, considering both the cost and the revenue consequences

• where necessary the committee will organize controlled, documented trials of equipment

• equipment should be purchased only from those companies registered by the Medical Devices Directorate

• the MLQ form is completed by the manufacturer, establishing conformity with the required safety standards

• the MLQ form is sent to the electronic and medical engineering department (EME) of the establishment for their approval

• the supplies department can then order the equipment

• when equipment is delivered it must be

checked by the EME department prior to use, whether it is freestanding or fixed *in situ* by the manufacturer

• where innovatory equipment is being trialled then the Local Ethics Committee approval should be sought and the EME department must check equipment prior to use

• as soon as equipment is delivered it should be identified in a preventive maintenance programme for regular servicing and calibration

• on delivery of a new piece of equipment, all staff must receive suitable training in its use.

It must also be remembered that individuals have a personal responsibility to ensure that they are providing a safe standard of care, including being knowledgeable about the equipment they will be required to use.

Management of contaminated equipment prior to maintenance

There has not been a recorded case in the UK where an employee of an NHS establishment, equipment manufacturer or supplier has contracted serious disease when undertaking maintenance of equipment. Nevertheless, on many occasions maintenance personnel are presented with equipment to work on that is in a foul condition; there are also occasions when equipment is handed over with a statement that it has been decontaminated, yet which remains visibly soiled. Consequently these staff face a potential risk, which health establishments and departmental staff have a duty to minimize. It is impractical to guarantee that any article is completely free from contamination, except possibly radioactivity, but good hygiene precautions should safeguard staff. Therefore a suitable safe system of work must be implemented, which should include:

• staff training at induction and whenever there are changes in practice
• a clear safety policy which is regularly reviewed
• provision of suitable equipment for decontamination purposes
• compliance with COSHH regulations and Health and Safety at Work Act

• a certificate of decontamination for equipment leaving the department for maintenance or repair.

The Health Notice HN(91)[41] and subsequent annual issues states the general legal requirements as they apply under the Health and Safety at Work Act and subsequent safety legislation. The major requirement is for each healthcare establishment to have a written safety policy to cover any person who undertakes maintenance, inspects/investigates, or is a third-party recipient of healthcare equipment which has been issued in a clinical environment. The policy should include:

• risk assessment
• user's responsibilities
• advice to staff on cleaning and decontamination
• safe areas of work within the department
• specialist advice available to staff
• completion of the decontamination certificate
• maintenance staff, manufacturer's safety
• sending equipment for inspection, maintenance or repair.

GOOD MANUFACTURING PRACTICE

All authorized manufacturers have to comply with strict quality and manufacturing practices. It is also necessary for all sterile services departments to comply with the same standards, as under the Consumer Protection Act they are also regarded as manufacturers. The Institute of Sterile Services Management produced a guide to the manufacturing process, from the collection of used materials, their progress through washing, drying, repacking and sterilization, to their redistribution to wards and departments. The document provides guidance on the standards to be achieved throughout the process, from the receipt of used equipment to its return to the user. The document provides guidance on:

• clean room facilities, packing room, etc.
• materials entry and exit
• raw materials storage
• sterilization area, work flow, batch numbering, autoclave and other methods of

sterilization, checking, sterile stock storage, etc.
- record keeping, including autoclave checking before use and cycle records, batch logs, etc.
- collection, delivery and transport of used and sterile materials
- linen preparation room
- cleaning and cleaning schedules, control of dust, pest control
- personnel training and hygiene
- quality assurance and control

- packaging, labelling, batch numbering and product recall procedures
- waste control, storage and disposal.

As a part of the overall risk management programme within the operating theatre it is essential that the sterile supplies also come from a controlled environment. The staff of the operating theatre have a responsibility to ensure that all materials supplied to the department are processed to the highest standards.

Sterilization and disinfection

The need for appropriate disinfection and sterilization has been shown by many reports documenting infection after the inadequate disinfection of patient-related equipment. Also, because it is not always necessary to sterilize all patient care items, hospitals must have clearly defined policies that identify whether cleaning, disinfection or sterilization is indicated on the basis of the items' intended use.

DEFINITIONS

Sterilization The complete elimination or destruction of all forms of microbial life. This can be achieved by either physical or chemical processes. Steam under pressure, dry heat, ethylene oxide gas, low-pressure steam and formaldehyde and liquid chemicals are the usual methods in a hospital.

Disinfection Describes a process that eliminates nearly all microorganisms on inanimate objects, with the exception of bacterial spores. This is generally accomplished using liquid chemicals or wet pasteurization (although this method has fallen into disrepute recently, as it is difficult to ensure adequate time for microbial destruction). The efficacy of disinfection may be affected by a number of factors, including:

- prior cleaning of the object
- the organic load on the object

- the type and level of microbial contamination
- the concentration of and exposure time to the disinfectant
- the physical shape of the object (e.g. crevices, hinges, lumina, etc.)
- the temperature and pH of the disinfection process.

Disinfection can be further divided: **high-level disinfection** can be expected to destroy all microorganisms, with the exception of high numbers of bacterial spores; **intermediate-level disinfection** inactivates *Mycobacterium tuberculosis*, vegetative bacteria, most viruses and fungi but not bacterial spores; **low-level disinfection** can kill most bacteria, some viruses and fungi, but cannot kill resistant bacteria such as tubercle bacilli or bacterial spores.

Cleaning The removal of all foreign material (e.g. soil, organic material) from objects. It is normally accomplished with water, mechanical action and detergents. Cleaning must precede disinfection and sterilization procedures.

Germicide An agent that destroys microorganisms, particularly pathogenic organisms. A disinfectant is a germicide that inactivates virtually all recognized pathogenic organisms, except bacterial spores, on inanimate objects.

Antiseptic A chemical germicide for use on the skin or tissue; it should not be used to decontaminate inanimate objects.

In 1968 E. H. Spaulding[43] devised a classification system designed to identify which type of object required sterilization or disinfection. These categories are based on the degree of risk of infection involved in the use of the items. The three categories of risk described were critical, semicritical and non-critical.

Critical items

Items in this category present a high risk of infection if contaminated by microorganisms or bacterial spores. These include all objects that enter sterile tissue or the vascular system. This category include surgical instruments, cardiac and urinary catheters, implants and needles. Where possible such items should be purchased sterile or sterilized by steam under pressure. If heat labile, the object may be treated by low-temperature steam, formaldehyde, ethylene oxide or, if other methods are unsuitable, then a chemical sterilant. It must be remembered that chemicals such as 2% glutaraldehyde-based solutions are only effective if adequate cleaning precedes treatment and if proper guidelines as to organic load, contact time, temperature and pH are met.

Semicritical items

Semicritical items are those which come into contact with mucous membranes or non-intact skin. These must be free of all microorganisms, with the exception of bacterial spores. Intact mucous membranes are generally resistant to common bacterial spores but are susceptible to other organisms, such as tubercle bacilli and viruses. Anaesthesia and respiratory therapy equipment and endoscopes are included in this category. Semicritical items generally require high-level disinfection by chemical germicides if they are not sterile. Glutaraldehyde, chlorine and chlorine compounds are dependable high-level disinfectants, provided the factors ensuring effective use, mentioned above, are followed.

Laparoscopes, arthroscopes and other scopes entering sterile tissue should ideally be sterilized. However, if high-level disinfection is used a thorough sterile water rinse after disinfection must be completed. If necessary, drying of these items should not recontaminate them (e.g. use filtered hot air).

Non-critical items

These items only come into contact with intact skin and not mucous membranes. Intact skin acts as an effective barrier to most microorganisms and sterility is not critical. Examples of these items include bedpans, patient trolleys and operating theatre furniture. Most non-critical reusable items may be cleaned with a neutral detergent. Disinfection is only required if items are soiled with blood or body fluids.

DISINFECTANTS

A large number of disinfectants are available for use in the healthcare setting, including alcohol, chlorine and chlorine compounds, formaldehyde, glutaraldehyde, hydrogen peroxide, iodophors, chlorhexidine, phenolics and quaternary ammonium compounds. These disinfectants are not necessarily interchangeable and the appropriate compound should be selected depending upon the task to be undertaken. All disinfectants are most effective in their recommended dilutions: increasing the level of disinfectant in solution does not increase its effectiveness but may well increase the costs and the risks associated with its use. Occupational skin diseases have been associated with the use of several disinfectants, such as formaldehyde, glutaraldehyde, chlorine and others, and appropriate precautions (e.g. gloves and proper ventilation, etc.) should be used to minimize exposure.

Alcohol

There are two alcohol preparations used in the healthcare setting, ethyl alcohol and isopropyl alcohol. These are rapidly bactericidal against vegetative forms of bacteria, fungicidal and virucidal, but do not destroy bacterial spores. The optimum bactericidal concentration is between 60% and 90% by volume. Alcohols are not recommended for the disinfection of surgical materials because of their inability to penetrate protein materials or bacterial spores. Alcohol can be useful to disinfect clean hard surfaces and skin, but in other circumstances has as many drawbacks as advantages. Alcohols are also inflammable and consequently must be stored in a cool, well ventilated area, and in a fire-proof cabinet if kept in large quantities.

Chlorine and chlorine compounds

Hypochlorites are the most widely used of the chlorine disinfectants and are available in liquid and solid forms. They have a broad spectrum of antimicrobial activity and are inexpensive and fast acting. Their use has to be restricted, however, because of their corrosiveness to metals, their inactivation by organic matter and their relative instability. In the operating theatre they are most useful for disinfecting surfaces contaminated with blood and body fluids. If there is a large volume of blood it should be mopped up with disposable wipes prior to disinfection. Hypochlorite preparations must not be mixed with volumes of urine as a chlorine gas may be produced.

Formaldehyde

Formaldehyde is used as a disinfectant and sterilant in both liquid and gas forms. It is used as an aqueous solution known as formalin. It is a bactericide, tuberculocide, fungicide, virucide and sporicide. It should, however, be regarded as a carcinogen and is a COSHH-regulated chemical. Employee exposure must be strictly controlled. Its use as a disinfectant is therefore severely limited except in the sealed controlled environment of a low-temperature steam and formaldehyde sterilizer, or as a preservative for tissue specimens.

Glutaraldehyde

Glutaraldehyde is a saturated dialdehyde that has gained wide acceptance as a high-level disinfectant. Aqueous solutions of glutaraldehyde are acidic, and in this state are not sporicidal. The solution needs to be 'activated' (made alkaline) by an agent to a pH of 7.5–8.5 to make it sporicidal. Once activated the solution has a shelf life of 14 days. Other glutaraldehyde formulations,

such as glutaraldehyde–phenate, potentiated acid glutaraldehyde and stabilized alkaline glutaraldehyde, have been produced to prolong the shelf life to 28–30 days. Its antimicrobial activity, however, is also dependent on a number of other factors, such as dilution and organic stress. The use of these solutions has become widespread because of their many advantages. These include excellent bactericidal properties and non-corrosive action on endoscopic, rubber and plastic equipment. Glutaraldehyde is usually used as a high-level disinfectant for medical equipment such as endoscopes, respiratory and anaesthetic equipment. It is non-corrosive to metal and does not damage lensed instruments. Excessive dilution of the solution frequently occurs, and staff need to ensure that it is not overused and that the degree of dilution is regularly checked. Also, healthcare staff can become sensitized to elevated levels of glutaraldehyde vapour, particularly when carrying out disinfection procedures in poorly ventilated areas, when using the solution in open immersion baths or when spills occur. This is a COSHH-controlled chemical and the occupational exposure limit (OEL) must not exceed 0.2 ppm (parts per million). At this level it is irritating to the eyes and nasal mucosa.

There are many other antiseptic and disinfectant products on the market. Their use, and the risks associated with that use, should be thoroughly investigated prior to their introduction in the operating theatre environment. The advice of the infection control team and the COSHH adviser should be sought if there is any concern.

When deciding on appropriate methods of cleaning and disinfection the following recommendations should be followed:

1. Prior to disinfection and/or sterilization of all patient care equipment a thorough cleaning process must take place to ensure removal of all organic material, such as blood, tissue etc., and other residues.

2. Indications for sterilization and high-level disinfection:

Critical items
• Critical medical devices or patient care equipment that enter normally sterile tissue or

the vascular system, or through which blood flows, must be sterile prior to use.

- Endoscopic accessories, biopsy forceps or other cutting instruments that break the mucosal barrier must be sterile before use. Other endoscopic equipment should be sterilized after each patient use; if this is not feasible then they require high-level disinfection.

- Laparoscopes, arthroscopes and other scopes which enter normally sterile tissue should be sterilized before each procedure where at all possible. If not possible, then they must receive high-level disinfection. Disinfection must be followed by thorough rinsing with sterile water.

- Equipment that touches mucous membranes, e.g. endoscopes, endotracheal tubes, respiratory therapy equipment and anaesthetic breathing circuits, should where possible be sterile or receive high-level disinfection after each use.

- When sterilization is indicated and steam, heat or ethylene oxide cannot be used, then glutaraldehyde or chlorine or chlorine dioxide may be used in a safe environment following the manufacturer's instructions.

Semicritical items
- Where possible these items should be sterile, as either recycled or disposable products. Where sterilization is not possible then high-level disinfectants may be used following thorough cleaning.

- There has been some debate over the years on the length of exposure time to disinfectants. This must be a controlled process and the current recommendations when using glutaraldehyde are:
   — 10 min immersion for the disinfection of the majority of potential microbiological contaminants, including hepatitis B and HIV
   — 30–60 min immersion for the disinfection of possible tubercle bacilli contamination
   — 3–10 hours' immersion if sterilization or the removal of bacterial spores is necessary.

- Where high-level disinfectant solutions are used it must be remembered that they will be subject to dilution over a period of time. It is recommended as part of the practice protocol that regular efficacy testing is carried out and that disinfectants are discarded after the recommended period of time if not overused, and, after a defined number of uses to prevent overuse or overdilution.

Non-critical items
- Any of the above methods may be used if disinfection is felt to be necessary.
- Where disinfection is not felt to be necessary then a thorough clean with warm water and a neutral detergent is sufficient.

It must also be remembered that with all methods of wet disinfection or cleaning a critical part of the process is to ensure that all equipment is dry immediately after cleaning and during storage.

PROCESSING HIV- OR HBV-CONTAMINATED EQUIPMENT

Standard sterilization and disinfection procedures, as recommended above, have been shown to be effective. No changes in procedures need to be made.

Non-critical items and environmental surfaces contaminated with visible blood and/or body fluids should be initially disinfected with a hypochlorite preparation. They can then be cleaned with normal cleaning agents. Staff should wear disposable gloves.

The selection and use of disinfectants is continually changing and products not mentioned above may become available in the future. It is recommended that before they are introduced the relevant scientific literature is read and the advice of the infection control team and the COSHH adviser sought.

This chapter has attempted to introduce the concept of risk management and to illustrate this with a number of critical issues which closely affect operating theatre staff, patients and visitors. It does not claim to be an all-encompassing review but to highlight those critical issues which are likely to have the greatest impact on effective risk management.

Latex sensitivity

With the emergence of HIV in the early 1980s, concern among healthcare staff regarding the potential hazards and modes of transmission of infection led to the rapid increase in the use of barriers for personal protection, with powdered latex gloves forming the primary method of protection.

Today an increasing number of healthcare staff and members of the public are affected by contact with irritants and chemical reactions caused by exposure to medical and non-medical products made of natural rubber latex. In the healthcare setting the risk of latex allergy is exacerbated by the use of powdered gloves which increase exposure to latex allergens, not only to the user but also to sensitized individuals in the vicinity. When powdered gloves are used during a surgical procedure the powder will be introduced into the patient's body or come into contact with mucosal surfaces causing subsequent allergic reactions. There is well documented evidence of postoperative complications related to glove powder.[44,45,46]

Sensitivity to glove powder or the latex may result in a wide variety of symptoms, such as pruritus, erythema, non-urticarial rash, urticaria (localised, e.g. hands, or generalised), angio-oedema, rhino-conjunctivitis, dyspnoea, asthma, bronchospasm, stridor, hypotension, intra-operative anaphylaxis and even death.[47]

It must also be remembered that gloves will not be the only source of latex exposure within the normal health care environment (Box 3.1).[48]

CURRENT SITUATION

Data from several American and European studies have revealed an increased incidence of both latex and glove powder allergies among healthcare staff and certain patient groups.[49,50,51] It has also been suggested that some of the latex products have not been subject to appropriate quality assurance procedures. In the UK there are no authoritative statistics at present. However, anec-

Box 3.1	Common equipment with a significant latex content[47]	
Adhesive tape	Stretcher mattresses
Ambu-bags	Neonatal incubators
Bulb syringes	PCA syringes
Colostomy pouches	Protective sheet
Condom type continence aids	Rubber gloves
Elasticated bandages	Stethoscope tubing and BP cuffs
Electrode pads	Stomach and GI tubes
Enema tubing	Tourniquets
Fluid warming blankets	Multi-vial bungs
Haemodialysis equipment	Wound drains

dotal evidence suggests that the prevalence and incidence of natural rubber latex and powder allergies have increased significantly.[52]

An allergy is an abnormal physiological response to any substance normally considered harmless. Natural rubber contains a variety of proteins which may act as allergens to the sensitized individual. In latex gloves there are also chemical accelerators used in the process of turning liquid latex into rubber. These chemicals are largely washed out in the manufacturing process but if the washing is inadequate some of the chemicals will remain. The corn starch powder used to make it easier to put gloves on may also be an allergen. In addition, the powder can leach some of the latex proteins from the gloves, creating an allergen-laden product which will not only sensitize on contact with the skin but which can be released into the atmosphere where it may be inhaled, possibly sensitizing others.

HYPERSENSITIVITY

Hypersensitivity is an 'immunological response of the body which results in tissue damage'.[53]

The body will have had previous contact with

the allergen and the individual's immune system will mount a defence when exposed again. When this response becomes excessive the individual is then hypersensitive.

Latex sensitivity is mainly classified as type 1 or type 4. In type 1, the immune system produces immunoglobulin E (IgE) antibodies on exposure to the allergen. This binds on to receptors on mast cells and basophils, and subsequent exposure to the same allergen may cause the release of the cell contents. Symptoms appear rapidly and type 1 is sometimes called 'immediate' hypersensitivity. This may cause the most severe symptoms following contact with the allergen.

In type 4 hypersensitivity there is no antibody formation; 'T' cell lymphocytes and macrophages are activated by the allergen, resulting in tissue damage. This may take some time to develop and type 4 is often referred to as cell-mediated or delayed hypersensitivity. Symptoms include reddening of the skin and itching, sometimes confused with irritant contact dermatitis. Type 4 is the more common reaction to latex sensitivity. Once sensitivity occurs it lasts for life.

Despite the above, to ensure staff protection when in direct contact with blood and body fluids, particularly during invasive procedures, latex gloves still appear to be technologically superior and provide better protection from potential pathogens than gloves made from synthetic materials.

In order to minimize the occurrence and effects of latex allergy, the Medical Devices Agency (MDA) issued guidance to emphasize the importance of making adequate provision for a safe working environment for all healthcare staff and appropriate arrangements for known sensitized patients.[54]

MANAGEMENT OF THE RISKS

To address the above issues it is recommended that each health care facility establishes a working group within their organization to address key issues and make recommendations to the management. It is recommended that the group consists of representatives from:

- Occupational Health department
- Infection Control Team
- Operating department staff
- General wards and departments
- Supplies.

The following issues will need to be addressed:

- regulatory requirements, including MDA, quality standards, biological safety, etc.
- informed selection and purchasing, particularly an awareness of risks and problems by purchasers and users
- possibly litigation risks – RCN test cases
- individuals with hypersensitivity should be considered. The organization needs to inform staff of the risks, both pre- and post-employment
- healthcare staff education on minimizing the risks, particularly ensuring effective hand care
- the patient care environment – must be safe for patients and staff
- identification of latex-sensitive patients and the development of care procedures to minimize the risks for these patients
- consider the purchase of powder-free gloves and agree a criteria for purchasing gloves with the lowest possible latex protein levels.

Each department which purchases and uses gloves will need to consider:

- purchasing issues – not ordering the cheapest on the market
- staff guidance on the appropriate type and use of gloves
- effective hand care and cleansing after wearing gloves, especially if they are damaged during use
- safe disposal of waste
- possible patient risks and care planning for sensitized patients including identification of sensitized patients preoperatively (Box 3.2)
- protecting contract/locum/agency staff.

PREOPERATIVE PLANNING

As the numbers of sensitized patients increase there will be a need not only to identify patients who may be at risk but also to prepare the oper-

---

Box 3.2 Patients in particular risk[47]

Spina bifida sufferers may be as high as 39–65%

Persons with genitourinary anomalies

Healthcare professionals (e.g. dentists, dental hygienists, surgeons, theatre nurses and nurses)

Patients who undergo multiple surgery, particularly in childhood

Patients with a history of allergies (e.g., eczema, asthma, etc.)

Latex industry workers

---

ating department staff to adequately care for these patients. It will be necessary to:

- formulate guidelines

- provide training for **all** department staff on the seriousness of latex allergy and the measures which need to be taken to minimize the risks
- ensure there is an adequate stock of latex free products to be used in place of those used routinely
- prepare and display a reference chart in each theatre on the management of latex hypersensitivity
- ensure adequate identification of latex sensitive patients both on their armband and in their clinical notes
- consider the provision of an emergency box either within the department or each anaesthetic room of latex-free items to be used in an emergency.

REFERENCES

1. Jackson MM, Lynch P 1985 Applying an epidemiological structure to risk management and quality assurance activities. Quality Review Bulletin: Joint Commission for Accreditation of Hospitals Organization 306–312
2. Balck B 1991 Quality and risk management: an integrated approach. NAQA Conference Papers: Issue 4, 17–19
3. Health and Safety at Work Act 1974. HMSO, London
4. Management of Health and Safety at Work Regulations 1992. HMSO, London
5. Workplace (Health, Safety and Welfare) Regulations 1992. HMSO, London
6. Provision and Use of Work Equipment Regulations 1992. HMSO, London
7. Personal Protective Equipment at Work Regulations 1992. HMSO, London
8. Display Screen Equipment Regulations 1992. HMSO, London
9. Manual Handling Regulations 1992. HMSO, London
10. Control of Substances Hazardous to Health Regulations 1988, 1994. HMSO, London
11. Dodds RDA et al 1988 Surgical glove perforations. British Journal of Surgery 75: 966
12. Orr NWM 1981 Is a mask necessary in the operating theatre? Annals of the Royal College of Surgeons of England 63: 390
13. Gerberding JL 1990 Risk of exposure of surgical personnel to patients' blood during surgery at San Francisco General Hospital. New England Journal of Medicine 322: 1788
14. Expert Advisory Group on AIDS 1994 AIDS/HIV-infected health care workers: guidance on the management of infected health care workers. UK Health Departments. HMSO, London
15. Recommendations of the Advisory Group on Hepatitis 1993 Protecting health care workers and patients from hepatitis B. UK Health Departments. HMSO, London
16. Humphreys H 1993 Infection control and the design of a new operating theatre suite. Journal of Hospital Infection 23: 61–70
17. Waste management – the duty of care – a code of practice 1991. HMSO, London
18. The Environmental Protection Act 1990. HMSO, London
19. Health and Safety Executive 1992 Safe disposal of clinical waste. HMSO, London
20. Health and Safety Executive 1995 Hospital Laundry: Arrangements for used and infected linen HSG (95) 18. HMSO, London
21. Lo Cicero J et al 1961 1987 Health hazards in the operating room: and update. Bulletin of the American College of Surgeons 72: 7–9
22. Garibaldi RA et al 1991 Predictors of intraoperative acquired surgical wound infections. Journal of Hospital Infection 18 (Supplement A): 289–298
23. Garner JS 1985 CDC guidelines for the prevention and control of nosocomial infections: guidelines for the prevention of surgical wound infections. American Journal of Infection Control 14: 71–79
24. Dripps RD et al The role of anaesthesia in surgical mortality. Journal of the American Medical Association 178: 61–266
25. Glass DC 1989 The control of substances hazardous to health: guidance for the initial assessment in hospitals. HMSO, London
26. Health and Safety Executive 1993 Guidance note EH 40/93: Occupational exposure limits. HMSO, London
27. Campbell M, Cripps NF 1991 Environmental control of glutaraldehyde. Health Estates Journal November: 2–6
28. Jackson MM 1986 Rituals without reason. Patterns in specialism: challenge to the curriculum. USA National League for Nursing, Washington

29. Bowel B 1992 Protecting the patient at risk. Nursing Times 88(3): 32–35
30. Electricity at Work Regulations 1989. HMSO, London
31. Ionising Radiations Practice Regulations 1985 & 1988. HMSO, London
32. Ionising Radiations Approved Code of Practice 1985. HMSO, London
33. Health Service Use of Ionising Radiations 1989 HN (89) 18
34. Administration of Radioactive Substances Act 1978. HMSO, London
35. Laser Protection Regulations. HMSO, London
36. Consumer Protection Act 1987. HMSO, London
37. Active Implantable Medical Devices Directive 1993. HMSO, London
38. Medical Devices Directive 1993. HMSO, London
39. Medical Devices Agency 1997 Reporting of adverse incidents relating to medical devices. MDA SN 9701.
40. Department of Health 1990 Management of Equipment. Health Equipment Information HEI(90)
41. Microbiology Advisory Committee 1991 Decontamination of equipment, linen or other surfaces contaminated with hepatitis B and/or HIV. Department of Health. HMSO, London
42. Department of Health 1989 Guide to good manufacturing practice for NHS sterile services. HMSO, London
43. Spaulding EH 1968 Chemical disinfection of medical and surgical materials. In Block S S (ed) Disinfection, sterilization and preservation. Lea & Febiger, Philadelphia, 517–531
44. Bauer X, Jager D 1990 Airborne antigens from latex gloves. Lancet 335: 912
45. Sussman G 1992 Latex allergy: Its importance in clinical practice. Allergy Proc 13: 67–69
46. Ellis H 1990 The hazards of surgical glove dusting powders. Surgery (Gynaecology and Obstetrics) 17: 152–527
47. Kelly KJ 1993 Latex sensitivity in operating theatre surgery. Medicine Group Journals Ltd, 2–4
48. Moore A 1994 Latex allergy; implications for patients, healthcare workers and NHS suppliers. Bandolier Special Bulletin for NHS Supplies, 1–12
49. Yassin MS, Lieri M, Fischer T et al 1994 Latex allergy in hospital employees. Annals of Allergy 72: 245–249
50. Turjanmaa K 1987 Incidence of immediate allergy to latex gloves in hospital personnel. Contact Dermatitis 17: 270–275
51. Food and Drug Administration 1991 Allergic reactions to latex containing medical devices. Medical Alert, March 29
52. The Nursing Times/Regent Hospital Products 1994 Occupational Health Nursing Survey
53. Thompson G, Ruane-Morris M, Lawton S 1994 Lines of defence. Nursing Times 90: 41, 48–51
54. Medical Devices Agency 1996 Latex sensitisation in the health care setting. (Use of latex gloves) MDA DB 9601, April

4

Anaesthetic practice

R. King

October 16th 1846, one of the great dates in the history of medicine. Before it the screams, the cries, the moans of the operating theatre. After it the peace and quiet of modern surgery. The surgeon picked up his knife, dissected out the cyst, nothing happened, not a murmur. Was he [the patient] alive or dead? Within a minute or two he stirred and sat up, the crowds went wild. Warren turned to them and said 'gentlemen this is no humbug'.

The birth of modern anaesthesia, as described by Professor Harold Ellis during the programme 'Courage to Fail – Nerves of Steel' (BBC 1987), was indeed a historical date in medicine. It sparked the genesis of what today is a highly specialized branch of medicine. Now, over 150 years after the events described above, an increasing number of specialist skills, knowledge and understanding are required from the practitioner to provide assistance in the delivery of an anaesthetic. This chapter aims to provide theatre practitioners with an understanding of their role in the care of the patient, the equipment and the pharmacology related to delivering an anaesthetic in the operating theatre.

Role of the anaesthetic practitioner

The title and role of the practitioner was defined in Chapter 1. In anaesthetic practice, recognition of who is considered qualified to provide competent assistance at the delivery of an anaesthetic has been addressed by the Association of Anaesthetists.[1] The document resulted from a working party and identifies three qualifications considered appropriate for undertaking the role of qualified anaesthetic assistance. These are:

- the English National Board awards for anaesthetic and surgical nursing
- the City and Guilds London Institute (CGLI) award for operating department assistants
- the National Vocational Qualification for Health Care – Operating Department Practice Level 3.

In order to maintain safe levels of patient care throughout any surgical or anaesthetic procedure, the practitioner must have a current and adequate level of knowledge, competence and understanding in the field of anaesthetics.

The role of the anaesthetic practitioner is classically seen to be in the operating department, although they should be able to apply their skills to other areas and situations, such as accident and emergency, intensive care units and X-ray departments.

The role of the anaesthetic practitioner is to:

- assess, plan, deliver and evaluate patient care, primarily within the operating department
- prepare for and participate in the areas where the anaesthetic is to be delivered, maintained, reversed, and where the patient is recovered.

It therefore involves the following:

- All aspects of direct patient care, from reception of the patient into the operating department to handover of the care of the patient to other healthcare professionals
- Preparation of the environment, including cleaning and adjustment
- Checking and fault finding of the equipment to be used, as well as any emergency equipment that may be required
- Preparation of agents to be given to the patient in accordance with the national and local policies and practice
- Reception of the patient, including any relevant checking of medical or nursing records to ensure correct identification of the patient for the specified procedure. This is outlined in Chapter 6
- Acting as a member of the theatre team to ensure the safety of the patient, visitors and other members of staff
- Providing assistance to the anaesthetist with the induction, airway management and maintenance of an anaesthetic
- Participating as a member of the theatre team in safely and correctly positioning the patient
- Providing assistance to the anaesthetist in the monitoring of the patient's vital signs
- Supplying, checking and assisting in the use of any additional equipment, medicines or fluids, as may be required
- Participating in the reversal or maintenance of anaesthesia, and subsequent transfer to the recovery area or intensive care unit; ensuring that the patient's needs are met until care has been handed over to another practitioner
- Carrying out decontamination and cleaning, disposal and restocking of equipment
- Liaison with persons in charge of the operating theatre, to ensure the smooth running of the operating list
- Updating knowledge of developments in the field of anaesthetics, extending knowledge and skills where appropriate and participating in the development of others.

These roles will be discussed in this chapter.

Patient care

There is a large amount of literature devoted to the care of the patient in the operating department, including discussions defining care and debate about who is best qualified to provide that care.

Practitioners must develop knowledge and practical skills in relation to many aspects of patient care, and be able to transfer and apply their knowledge and skills to new situations. This expertise must be gained from formal teaching in colleges, from clinical situations and from working alongside experienced members of the surgical and anaesthetic teams. This should allow the practitioner to develop a professional attitude and good communication skills, as well as the ability to provide physical and psychological patient care.

The essential aspects of patient care in the anaesthetic room are:

- communication
- reassurance and explanation
- comfort and dignity
- cultural and religious considerations
- consideration of patients' special needs
- care of the patient during induction, maintenance and reversal of anaesthesia.

Other relevant activities are reception of the patient in the operating department.

COMMUNICATION

Communicating with the patient is an essential skill the theatre practitioner must develop. Barriers often exist which inhibit effective communication between staff and patients, which the practitioner must consider and aim to remove.

- **Effects of premedication** One desired effect of a premedication is to induce a feeling of calm relaxation in the patient, usually making them drowsy. The practitioner must therefore assess the effects of the premedication and provide explanation and reassurance. A patient who is

relaxed and drowsy may need minimal explanations, but a patient who is awake or who has not had premedication may need much more information.

- **Background noise** The design and environment of modern operating departments, with no soft furnishings and many hard surfaces, means that background noise is enhanced. Although this is normal for staff, it can be alarming for the patient. The practitioner should therefore be aware of how the patient's perception of noise and the environment may be dramatically different from their own. A simple explanation that the noises are normal and no cause for concern should be given. The anaesthetic room should be a quiet and calm environment, to enhance the effects of the premedication and prevent startling the patient, as hearing is the last sense to be lost during induction of anaesthesia. Entry to the anaesthetic room should not be allowed when the patient is being induced, and notices should be displayed to this effect. The personnel present during induction should be kept to only those required and learners.

- **Theatre clothing** Clothing worn by theatre staff, particularly masks, hats and coloured suits, may further interfere with effective communication. The patient should have been given a simple explanation of theatre clothing preoperatively. The practitioner must ensure that masks are never worn in the anaesthetic room when the patient is awake, the one exception being when maintenance of sterility is required, such as for spinal anaesthesia. Practitioners must be aware of these barriers to communication, and take steps to compensate for their effects on the patient.

REASSURANCE AND EXPLANATION

The concept of holistic care involves considering the person as a whole, i.e. not just as a patient with physical conditions, but as a person with physical, physiological, social, spiritual and psychological needs. These are all relevant in the anaesthetic room, with patients often needing a great deal of reassurance and explanation, especially if they are feeling frightened or anxious. This should be appropriate to their needs, as discussed in relation to premedication, and other factors such as age and previous experience of surgery. A patient who has a check cystoscopy on a 6-monthly basis is likely to need less explanation than an anxious patient having their first operation. The practitioner must also consider the severity of the patient's illness: if the surgery is an emergency, the explanation must be adapted accordingly. The principle aim of reassurance is that the patient should understand that procedures undertaken in the anaesthetic room are normal, and not be alarmed by them in any way. The practitioner should also carefully consider the language they use: for example, the attachment of electrodes can be explained as 'to monitor your pulse', rather than 'to measure your heart'. Although it is the anaesthetist who will utilize equipment and induce anaesthesia, explanation by the practitioner is often valuable in informing the patient of events. It is rare that the insertion of even a narrow-gauge cannula, without the use of a local anaesthetic agent, will not hurt. Being honest and describing some of the sensations in terms of pushing, pulling and sharpness may allow the patient to anticipate what to expect.

COMFORT AND DIGNITY

The time the patient spends in the anaesthetic room is often a time of heightened awareness that they may remember clearly. It is helpful if they can be made as comfortable as possible. There may be limitations to this, owing to the nature of the trolley, operating table or bed, but every effort should be made to ensure the patient is comfortable while awake. This may involve adjusting their head or body position slightly, although they will need to be returned to the supine position for the induction of a general anaesthetic, or ensuring that they are warm

enough and not exposed in any way. The practitioner should be aware of the loss of dignity the patient may feel by being dressed in a hospital gown, without normal apparel such as clothes, make-up and jewellery. This may be felt particularly by patients who have removed dentures, wigs or other prostheses in readiness for surgery. The response to the patient and comfort they require are aspects of care left to the individual. Some patients may need support by contact, such as holding hands, or a hand on the shoulder. The practitioner should be able to meet the needs of the patient regardless of gender, religion, sexual orientation, colour, race or creed.

CULTURAL AND RELIGIOUS CONSIDERATIONS

The concept of respect for the patient's cultural, religious or ethnic background has certain practical considerations in the anaesthetic room. The removal or handling of items of religious or cultural significance may cause the patient great distress and even offence. Such items include:

- certain items of jewellery
- specific head wear, such as a turban
- wedding rings
- worry beads or rosary beads
- underwear.

In areas of the country where there are diverse cultural and religious influences, operating departments should have specific policies to identify correct procedures. Practitioners in such areas should aim to understand the relevant cultures and religions, in order to provide a high standard of holistic patient care.

CONSIDERATION OF PATIENTS' SPECIAL NEEDS

The theatre practitioner should consider any special needs the patient may have which may need intervention in the anaesthetic room. These will obviously vary greatly, but may include the following:

- learning disabilities
- mental illness

- physical disability
- partial or complete hearing loss
- partial or complete loss of vision
- partial or complete inability to speak
- inability to speak or understand English
- little understanding of the impending event, e.g. children of various ages.

The practitioner should assess the patient's needs preoperatively in order to provide practical aids such as positioning and comforting equipment and interpreters if needed. Effective communication with ward staff and a preoperative assessment is obviously essential with patients who have special needs, in order to plan and implement care thoroughly. The carer of a patient with special needs, for example those with learning disabilities, should accompany the patient until the induction of anaesthesia is complete. The setting of standards for children undergoing surgery has been addressed by Action for Sick Children. The areas addressed include:

- the decision to operate
- the rights of the child
- admission: elective and emergencies
- preparation for the operation
- ward procedures
- going to theatre
- the anaesthetic room
- the recovery room
- after the operation
- home again.

Four useful appendices include guidelines for parents accompanying their children to theatre and visiting in the recovery room.[2]

CARE OF THE PATIENT DURING INDUCTION, MAINTENANCE AND REVERSAL OF ANAESTHESIA

This includes:

- protection of the eyes
- correct positioning
- administration of drugs
- observation of the surgical team
- preparation of anaesthetic equipment
- staffing and managerial considerations.

Once the patient is anaesthetized the anaesthetic team maintain homoeostasis via the equipment and drug regimen. In addition, the patient's well-being must be observed.

Protection of the eyes, specifically the prevention of corneal abrasions, from equipment and/or drapes should be considered. The use of tape to maintain eyelid closure, or purpose-made eye protection pads, depends on the anaesthetist's preference and surgical requirements. The potential hazard of exceptionally sticky tape or allergic reactions must be considered.

In order to ensure safe administration of drugs and fluids, the monitoring and orderly placement of peripheral lines leading to the patient are a major consideration. There are often coloured plastic tags packed with manometer tubing for labelling, but more often tape is used to identify lines. It is important for the practitioner to be as familiar with the system as the anaesthetist, as disconnection and reconnection, emergency administration of large volumes of fluids and blood and the moving of the patient are aspects over which the practitioner may have some autonomy.

Observation of the surgical team is required as inadvertent leaning on the chest of the patient, shifting of the arm board in excess of 90° and standing on anaesthetic tubing are some of the potential complications to the maintenance of a safe general anaesthetic.

It appears from the author's experience that many patients have a fear of needles and find the array of specialist equipment in the anaesthetic area daunting. It is advisable to prepare the anaesthetic area prior to the patient's arrival. The setting up of i.v. fluids and giving sets, drawing up of drugs with hypodermic needles and cleaning and decontamination of equipment are some of the duties that may make the patient feel nervous and unimportant. Consideration for the patient and communication and explanation will help allay any anxiety they may feel.

Practitioners develop their own system of working to prepare the environment and equipment for a routine operating list. Depending on local staff and departmental policies, the initial task may be to check and ensure that the clinical area is clean: this may involve damp dusting. Even in departments where damp dusting is carried out by domestic assistants, the anaesthetic machines and other equipment may not be part of that routine. Familiarization with the proposed operating list, and to a certain extent with the particular anaesthetist, will often lead to the initial collecting and setting up of the required equipment. A definitive list of what to prepare is impossible to compile, as needs will vary between patients and anaesthetists; what should be routine, however, is a system of working and checking. Once the set-up for a routine list is complete, it is worth taking a few seconds to run through what is most likely to happen to the patient. One method is to look at each step, including all the intermediate stages, such as is strapping/securing tape available. In constructing a logical sequence of events, the risk of poor preparation is reduced. It follows that the initial collecting and setting up should have a logical sequence: the easiest general rule is to complete one task at a time. Practical experience and observing the routines of others is the advice often given to students, in order for them to develop their own style.

The availability of skilled assistance during reversal of the anaesthetic is essential, and the continuing trend of having theatre practitioners with experience in both surgery and anaesthesia will assist in the formulation of local policies to ensure the safety of patients.

RECEPTION OF THE PATIENT IN THE OPERATING DEPARTMENT

The role of checking and receiving the patient should be able to be undertaken by all operating department practitioners. This is often the culmination and focus of a patient's stay in hospital. Communication with and response to the individual patient by the practitioner is often the first step in the assessment of that patient, and will lead to further planning, delivery and evaluation of care.

Guidelines for ensuring that the patient has the correct operation are given in Chapter 6; this chapter focuses on the necessary anaesthetic considerations. Although these are important areas to check, the practitioner must bear in mind that the patient will have had the same questions asked many times during the previous few minutes or hours, which in addition to the effect of any premedication, may increase their anxiety and irritability.

Many departments use a checklist when receiving the patient, many aspects of which are related to ensuring the patient has the correct operation. Items that affect the safe delivery of an anaesthetic are:

- medical and nursing records
- blood test results
- investigation details and results
- prescription chart/medications
- physical checks.

Medical and nursing records

These should indicate the patient's previous medical history and any previous anaesthetic records. These are necessary to establish whether the patient has any medical conditions or any anaesthetic problems. They will be assessed by the anaesthetist preoperatively, but the practitioner should also be aware of them in order to plan effective care.

Blood test results

Any blood tests undertaken should be reported on before surgery and the results included in the medical records. The practitioner should look at these and alert the anaesthetist to recent results. The usual blood tests undertaken preoperatively include haemoglobin, urea and electrolytes, sickle cell and blood group and cross-matching.

Investigation details and results

Routine investigations may include an electrocardiogram and X-ray results, particularly for patients over 55 years old. These should accompany the patient to theatre and be reviewed by the anaesthetist, in order to check the patient's cardiac and respiratory condition.

Prescription chart/medications

It is necessary to check the patient's medications, the time of premedication and any drug allergies, which should be noted here as well as in the medical notes.

Physical checks

- Time of last food and drink intake: if less than 4–6 hours previously, confirm that the anaesthetist is aware of this.
- Make-up should be removed, as foundation cream and lipstick may disguise any changes in the patient's colour, for example cyanosis.
- Nail varnish should be removed, as coloured – and to a certain extent clear – nail varnish will distort or disguise changes in the patient's peripheral colour, as indicated by the nailbed.
- Any prosthesis, for example wigs, dentures, false eyes, glasses, contact lenses or artificial limbs, should be removed for safe keeping and generally retained on the ward. If the patient so desires it is often a practical policy to allow them to retain hearing aids, either throughout the anaesthetic or during induction; they can be removed for surgery and returned for recovery. Some anaesthetists request that secure-fitting dentures remain *in situ* as long as the anaesthetic team are aware of their existence.
- Jewellery should be removed and kept on the ward or given to relatives. Rings may become loose if the patient's temperature drops in theatre, and all metal jewellery carries electrical conduction risks (see Chapter 5). If a wedding ring is worn it must be securely taped.
- Dental crowns, caps and loose teeth should be identified and noted by the practitioner, as these may be damaged or dislodged during intubation.
- Any allergies should be noted and the surgical team informed. Common substances that may cause an allergy include iodine, Elastoplast and medications such as antibiotics.

The following guidelines identify important aspects of patient care during transfer and reception to the operating department:

- When the patient arrives at the transfer area, the appropriate theatre staff are informed.
- The reception area is prepared with appropriate patient transportation. All patient trolleys and beds must be clean and checked in accordance with local policy procedure.
- Confirm that the name of the patient and the procedure correspond with those on the operating list. Check essential patient details, as outlined in Chapter 6. It is often more appropriate to check the operative site once in the anaesthetic room, to preserve the patient's dignity.
- Check anaesthetic considerations as outlined previously:
  — medical and nursing records
  — blood results
  — investigation details and results
  — prescription chart
  — physical checks:
    – nil by mouth time
    – make-up and nail varnish
    – prostheses
    – dental crowns and caps
    – allergies.

Policies should identify how these checks should take place. It may be more appropriate to check them with the escorting nurse in order to avoid disturbing a sleeping or sedated patient.

- Stand next to the escort nurse. Do not communicate across the patient, or place notes and X-rays on the patient.
- Explain to the patient what is happening during any physical transfer.
- Protect the patient's elbows.
- Slides should be used to assist in the movement of patients according to the manufacturer's instructions, ensuring that there are sufficient staff to move the patient safely.
- It may not be necessary to move patients from their beds until after the induction of anaesthesia.

• The escort nurse (and parent or guardian for children) may remain throughout the transfer until the patient is settled on the trolley, or stay with the patient until induction.

• The patient must not be left unattended: protocols may be developed for chaperoning.

The principles for the reception of patients into the operating department remain the same, even where the procedures differ.

Principles and practice of anaesthesia

The principles and practice of anaesthesia discussed here relate primarily to general and regional anaesthesia as undertaken in hospital operating departments. It must be recognised, however, that these two defined types of anaesthesia may be used in conjunction with each other. The definitions of a general anaesthetic and a regional anaesthetic are given for the purposes of discussion. It is the responsibility of the practitioner to have a working knowledge and understanding of both aspects of anaesthesia.

GENERAL ANAESTHESIA

A general anaesthetic can be defined as the administration of an agent or agents to render the patient unconscious and insensitive to pain, and thereby non-reactive to the diagnostic or therapeutic procedure.[3] A general anaesthetic may be divided into two categories:

1. A general anaesthetic without an endotracheal tube. This involves the patient spontaneously breathing the gases and anaesthetic agents via the breathing system, a mask with or without an oral or nasal airway, or a laryngeal mask.

2. A general anaesthetic with an endotracheal tube. The placement of an endotracheal tube is one of the most effective methods of maintaining the airway. In order to intubate a muscle relaxant is usually required. In terms of airway management and respiration, this type of general anaesthetic can be considered to take one of three forms:

• spontaneous respiration (patient's natural respiration)
• assisted ventilation (by anaesthetist when required)
• controlled ventilation (by connection to a ventilator with IPPV (intermittent positive pressure ventilation)).

REGIONAL ANAESTHESIA

Regional anaesthesia is defined and discussed in three categories: conductive anaesthesia, infiltration anaesthesia and intravenous anaesthesia.

Conductive anaesthesia

Peripheral nerve blocks. The injection of a local anaesthetic agent such as lignocaine, percutaneously into the neurovascular bundle around the major peripheral nerves or plexuses of the upper or lower limbs. An example is the brachial plexus nerve block used for surgery or manipulations on the shoulder joint, arm, forearm and hand.

Central nerve blocks:

Epidural anaesthetic. The injecting of a local anaesthetic outside the dura, in the thoracic, lumbar or sacral levels of the spinal cord.

Spinal anaesthetic. The injection of a local anaesthetic into cerebrospinal fluid in the subarachnoid space around the spinal cord.

Central nerve blocks are used for intra- and post-operative analgesia, including analgesia for 'awake' surgical procedures such as lower section caesarean sections.

Infiltration anaesthesia

This can be either surface or epithelial, and is the injection of a local anaesthetic in or around the site of the proposed incision or incised tissue. This is often carried out by the surgeon for surgical procedures, and by the anaesthetist prior to large-bore or arterial cannulation in the conscious patient.

Intravenous anaesthesia

The most common procedure is the Bier's block, i.e. the intravenous injection of a local anaesthetic via an indwelling cannula, distal to a tourniquet that is applied to a limb. Used for surgery on, or manipulation of, most frequently the upper limb.

The practicalities of assistance with the administration of each of the above categories of anaesthesia are dealt with in this chapter. Anaesthesia has been described as a complex and highly developed science.[4] Any further information regarding the complex and detailed aspects of anaesthesia, pharmacology and associated equipment should be sought from the myriad specialist books available, as well as manufacturers' specification sheets. In order to assist in the delivery of a safe anaesthetic of any type, it is the responsibility of the practitioner to understand anatomy and physiology, the equipment and pharmacology related to the procedure, and to be aware of any adverse events that may occur during the procedure, generally classed as emergencies.

Anaesthetic equipment

The range and complexity of equipment associated with the delivery of an anaesthetic is vast. Anaesthetic equipment is considered in three categories:

- equipment for the delivery of a general anaesthetic
- equipment for the delivery of a regional anaesthetic
- equipment for monitoring the physiological state of the patient.

EQUIPMENT FOR THE DELIVERY OF A GENERAL ANAESTHETIC

As it is recognized that the most important person in the operating department is the patient, so it is often stated that the most important item of equipment for the delivery of any anaesthetic is the suction apparatus.

Suction

There are two types of suction equipment, portable and fixed. Manual and electrical units are common forms of portable suction apparatus; fixed units are driven by a centrally located compressor connected to a piped system. All mechanical forms of suction apparatus should be able to create a pressure below that of atmosphere that is variable through a range of pressures. A subatmospheric pressure of at least 600 mmHg (80 kPa) or higher is required for the efficient removal of vomitus.

The three main components of suction apparatus are:

- a vacuum source
- a reservoir
- tubing, which may also be a nozzle, catheter or some specialist attachment.

In order for suction equipment to function adequately the apparatus must be able to move sufficient volumes of air in order to create a vacuum. The following factors are important:

- the volume of displaced air
- the range of negative pressures the apparatus is able to attain
- the time taken to achieve adequate suction
- the length and diameter of the tubing must be such as not to compromise the efficiency of the previous criteria.

The vacuum source is usually a pump, which may consist of pistons, rotating fans, bellow or compressed gases using the Venturi principle.

The reservoir is commonly a collapsible plastic liner enclosed in a rigid container, with some system of filter and float to prevent substances reaching the pump.

The delivery tubing, usually single use and wide bore for anaesthetic purposes, is attached to a sterile rigid or flexible catheter. Anaesthetic suction catheters should have a smooth tip to prevent any mucosal damage. Rigid suction catheters are commonly used for the removal of pharyngeal and bronchial secretions, as well as blood from the nasal and oral cavities. Flexible suction catheters are used in the removal of fluids from the trachea and main bronchi – endobronchial suction catheters.

To minimize the risk of contamination prior to the handling of any component of the suction apparatus, the operator must wear protective gloves. Developments have led to a catheter design that is handled through a plastic sleeve, thereby reducing risk to both patient and theatre staff. As regards the disposal of body fluids recovered by suction apparatus, the tubing and suction attachment are just as great a potential source of contamination as the reservoir itself, and the appropriate considerations and precautions should be adopted.

The procedure for checking suction is as follows:

Electric suction
- Connect clean tubing and sterile suction end.
- Check tubing and container fittings secure.
- Check that filter is clean, dry and fitting securely.
- Switch on suction at wall and machine.
- Clamp tubing and observe dial for vacuum pressures between 400 and 600 mmHg.
- Switch off suction at wall, leave machine turned on, or vice versa depending on policy.

If desired vacuum pressure is not reached, check:

- Suction is turned up fully.
- All connections and covers are secure.
- Container is switched to correct bottle if a twin bottle unit is used.

If faults exist:

- List faults.

- Remove machine.
- Report with list of faults.

Pipeline suction
- Connect clean tubing and sterile suction end.
- Check tubing and container fittings secure.
- Check that filter is clean, dry and fitting securely.
- Plug in pipeline and switch on suction.
- Clamp tubing and turn suction control, observing dial for pressures:
  - LOW: 50–100 mmHg
  - MED: 250–400 mmHg
  - HIGH: 400–600 mmHg.

The anaesthetic machine

The anaesthetic machine is probably the largest and most varied item of anaesthetic equipment. In order for the practitioner to come to terms with the wide range of types and styles of anaesthetic machines, it is worth remembering what an anaesthetic machine is and what it should do.

The anaesthetic machine is basically a trolley that facilitates the transportation and delivery of specific gases and vapours to the patient as part of the anaesthetic regimen. In the years since Boyle designed some of the first anaesthetic machines the gas/vapour delivery system has become very sophisticated, as have the safety features. The premise of the anaesthetic machine being a trolley has allowed the shelf sections to be used as storage for the increasing range of monitoring equipment. Modern anaesthetic machines are often designed with integrated monitoring equipment (Fig. 4.1).

Despite the sometimes dramatic changes in the additional functions and design of anaesthetic machines the fault-finding and safety checks follow the same principle, and rely on the practitioner understanding what they are checking for, and proceeding through a logical sequence of events. An example of a checking procedure is a single hose test.

Single hose test or qualitative test for anaesthetic gases
- Detach all pipelines from pendent sockets or from wall sockets.

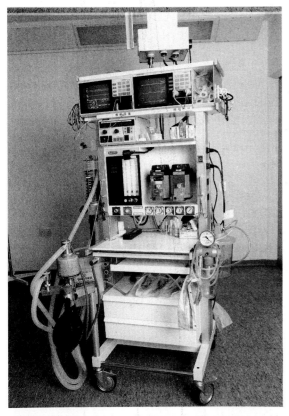

Figure 4.1 A Datex Flexima anaesthetic machine with integrated monitor. (Reproduced from Aitkenhead & White 1996, with permission.)

- Close all cylinder valves.
- Open all rotameter valves.
- Open OXYGEN cylinder valve:
  Only oxygen rotameter should be activated with a continuous flow.
- Close OXYGEN cylinder valve.
- Audible Oxygen alarm should sound.
- Open NITROUS OXIDE cylinder valve:
  Only nitrous oxide rotameter should be activated with continuous flow.
- Close NITROUS OXIDE valve.
- Repeat steps using CARBON DIOXIDE cylinder if fitted.

Note: If any abnormality is observed during the above stages, reject the machine.

- Connect OXYGEN pipeline hose:

Only the oxygen rotameter should be activated with continuous gas flow.
- Disconnect OXYGEN pipeline hose.
- Audible Oxygen alarm should sound.
- Connect NITROUS OXIDE pipeline hose:
  Only nitrous oxide rotameter should be activated with continuous gas flow.

Note: If any abnormality is observed during the above stages, reject the machine.

- Leaving NITROUS OXIDE pipeline connected, **turn off all rotameters.**
- Reconnect OXYGEN pipeline.
- Using OXYGEN gas flow, carry out all circuit checks.

To assist all anaesthetic personnel, the Association of Anaesthetists of Great Britain and Ireland have published a checklist,[5] which is a comprehensive check to be undertaken at the beginning of each operating theatre session, utilizing an oxygen analyser, checking medical gas supplies, vaporizers, breathing systems, ventilator and suction apparatus. The publication states that the check procedures are the responsibility of the anaesthetist. The role of the practitioner in undertaking the above qualitative hose test is therefore a preliminary fault-finding exercise and extra safety measure for not only the anaesthetic machine, but also for all other anaesthetic equipment.

Gas delivery

Gases are supplied to the anaesthetic machine either via cylinders attached to the frame of the machine or via pipelines which draw upon a central hospital supply. In the UK hospitals that have a pipeline supply usually deliver oxygen and nitrous oxide at 4 bar (400 kPa/60 psi). The pipeline supply is connected directly to the inlet of the flowmeters. The pressure of the gases within the cylinders, however, is higher and requires the use of pressure regulators, which are located between the cylinder outlet and the inlet to the flowmeters. Gas cylinders and anaesthetic equipment are fitted with a 'pin index' system which prevents incorrect connection to the regulators.

Pressure regulators perform the following functions:

- Reduce the high pressure of gas within the cylinder to a safe working pressure; this in turn prevents damage to the equipment and working components of the anaesthetic machine.
- Maintain a constant output pressure to the anaesthetic machine, regardless of the fall in pressure within the cylinder as the gas is used.

Thus the gases supplied to the anaesthetic machine, via different methods, reach the flowmeter at a constant pressure.

Flowmeters are a method of increasing/decreasing the flow rate of gases to the patient via needle valves that allow accurate adjustment. Needle valves open to allow the passage of gas to the flow meter tubing. These flowmeters – most commonly rotameters – are calibrated to read the flow of gas in litres per minute (l/min). In each glass rotameter tube is a bobbin; readings are usually taken from the top of the bobbin against the calibrations on the glass tube. The angled grooves cut into the top collar cause the gas passing the bobbin to rotate, thus indicating that it is in a free-flowing current of gas, and not stuck to the side of the glass tubing by particles, static electricity or magnetic influences. As the gas flow (flow rate) is increased by opening the needle valve the bobbin is raised higher. This allows higher flow rates to pass the annulus, as the glass tubing has a larger diameter at the top than at the bottom.

As the properties that influence the displacement of the bobbin change from gas to gas, the bobbins and glass rotameter tubing are specifically calibrated for the gas they are to carry (Fig. 4.2).[6]

'Quantiflex'™ systems may be used to maintain a constant ratio between oxygen and other gases used. They do not allow hypoxic mixtures to be delivered, regardless of the change in flow rates set (Fig. 4.3).

At this stage the gases are often referred to as carriers (although nitrous oxide is effectively the carrier gas), as the next stage of their journey generally includes picking up any volatile agents required. In order to do this the gas flow must

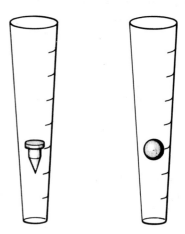

Figure 4.2 A diagrammatic representation of the bobbin (left) and ball (right) flowmeters. (Reproduced from Aitkenhead & White 1996, with permission.)

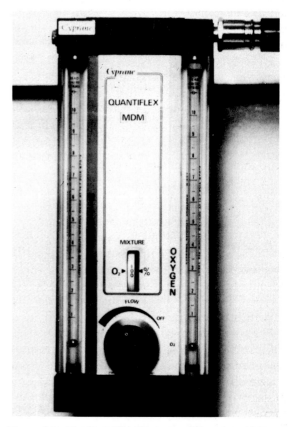

Figure 4.3 The Quantiflex flowmeter. (Reproduced from Aitkenhead & White 1996, with permission.)

pass over or through the agent, and thus become partly or fully saturated with it.

Vaporizers have developed into sophisticated devices that meet the needs of specific volatile anaesthetic agents. Early methods of delivery for inhalational anaesthetic agents involved open drop and semi-open drop methods.

In present-day anaesthetics the gases passing over the liquid agent take up the vapours and pass on to the patient. Each inhalational agent has a specific vaporizer calibrated for only that agent, as each agent has its own physical and anaesthetic characteristics. There are many 'bottle' types of vaporizer, although their regular use in the UK is probably rare. Generally these are used for ether, methoxyflurane and trichloroethylene, but the use of these agents has now virtually ceased. One of the most popular types was the Boyles vaporizer; others include Goldman, Rowbotham and McKesson. Some more innovative examples recorded include metal cans with holes and a 4 oz (125 g) empty instant coffee jar, as described by Ward.[6]

Present-day vaporizers are temperature compensated, which allows accurate percentages of anaesthetic agent to be added to the carrier gas. This is achieved by designs that take into consideration the factors that affect the vaporization rates of anaesthetic agents. These can be summarized as:

- boiling point and vaporization rate
- temperature of the liquid
- temperature of carrier gases
- flow rate of gases
- surface area contact of gases and liquid
- shape and volume of space above the liquid.

To reduce the temperature effects of the above factors, features such casing material and design, and the bimetallic strip are incorporated into vaporizer technology.

The vaporizer is a relatively heavy item of equipment owing to the large mass of metal in the housing. This bulk of metal goes some way to ensure that the ambient temperature does not dramatically affect the vaporizing chamber and consequently the vaporization rate. The bimetallic strip is essentially a temperature compensating device, consisting of two strips of different

metals bonded together; it relies on the principle that different metals expand at different rates and by different amounts when heated. When the temperature within the vaporization chamber falls or rises, thus affecting the vaporization rate, the bimetallic strip triggers a valve, increasing or reducing the total amount of gas flow through the chamber. This allows the gas flow to be regulated to compensate for excessive changes in temperature and thereby ensures accurate concentrations. Vaporizers that have some form of *te*mperature *c*ompensation are often referred to as Tec vaporizers (Fig. 4.4).

Vaporizers fall into two categories, depending on how the fresh gas flow is generated: 'drawover' and 'plenum'.

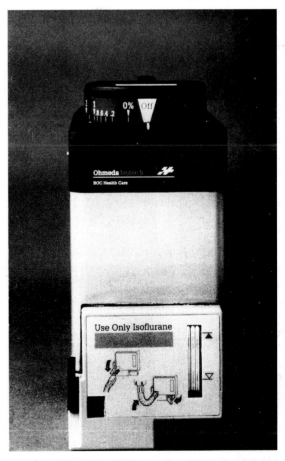

Figure 4.4 The Mark 5 TEC vaporizer. (Reproduced from Aitkenhead & White 1996, with permission.)

'**Drawover' vaporizer** If a negative pressure is created downstream from the vaporizer, either mechanically or by the patient's respiration, gas is drawn through the vaporizer chamber (Fig. 4.5).

'**Plenum'** If the unidirectional gas flow is generated upstream from the vaporizer, creating a positive pressure, it forces the gas to flow through the vaporizing chamber. The series of vaporizers from this category generally available are referred to, in chronological order, as Mark 3, Mark 4 and Mark 5. The most recent development is the Tec 6 (Fig 4.6) which is designed solely for the addition of desflurane to inhalational anaesthetic gases. It must be connected to a Selectatec series manifold and an appropriate electrical mains supply. The filler is designed with a fitting specific for the agent. A liquid crystal display indicates low levels of volatile agent in the sump. The control dial allows concentrations to be set between 1% and 18%. The vaporizer is required to warm up and

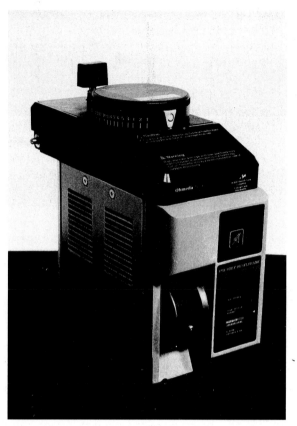

Figure 4.6 The TEC 6 vaporizer. (Reproduced from Aitkenhead & White 1996, with permission.)

the volatile agent will not be available until the correct temperature is reached.

The potential hazards of filling vaporizers with the wrong agent are reduced by each anaesthetic vapour having a specific colour-coded and filling lock system, known as the key filling system (Fig. 4.7).

The **pressure relief valve** may be located downstream of the vaporizer on anaesthetic machines with regulated pressures of 45 or 60 psi (~ 300 or 400 kPa). This valve opens at 5 psi (~ 34 kPa) to prevent damage to the equipment upstream (see above) if a high pressure is created by obstruction.[6]

A **non-return valve** may be incorporated into some machines to prevent any back pressure caused by ventilators such as the Howells' or Manley. Back pressure created in the vaporizer leads to a potentially high vapour concentration.[6]

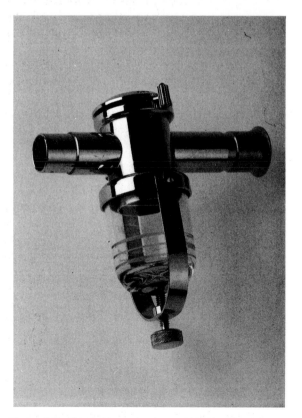

Figure 4.5 The Goldman drawover vaporizer. (Reproduced from Aitkenhead & White 1996, with permission.)

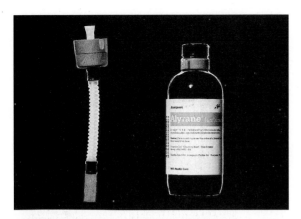

Figure 4.7 Key filling system. (Reproduced from Aitkenhead & White 1996, with permission.)

Oxygen bypass All anaesthetic machines should have an oxygen bypass (flush) control. This allows the delivery of high flow rates (35 l/min) of oxygen in an emergency. It receives its supply directly from the oxygen pressure regulator, bypassing the vaporizers and nitrous oxide supply to deliver pure oxygen. The flushing switch should be protected against inadvertent use, which can cause cycling problems with ventilators such as the Manley.

One disadvantage of the oxygen bypass flush is that the flow rate of oxygen is not indicated by the rotameters, but the delivery of 35 litre/min should make enough noise to notify a member of the team that it has been turned on, either deliberately or accidentally.

Further uses of the oxygen flush are:

- to rapidly inflate a reservoir bag while trying to ventilate a patient
- to flush out circuits
- for preoxygenating the reservoir bag and circuit prior to preoxygenating the patient.

Patient outlet Once the gas flow has passed from the flowmeters along the back bar, where the vaporizers are usually located, it arrives at the patient outlet. The patient outlet may be in the form of a 'Cardiff swivel', which allows horizontal rotation of the outlet, giving positioning flexibility to any connection. The patient outlet is the final stage of the fresh gas flow through the anaesthetic machine, and the point where a breathing system is attached.

Breathing systems The names of the components that make up equipment for the delivery of gases from the anaesthetic machine to the patient are often confusing. Ward[6] clarifies them as follows:

The term *Breathing system* should be used in the abstract, and describes the method by which gases are delivered to the patient.

Breathing attachments are the actual group of interconnected components used to complete a *breathing system*.

The *breathing circuit*, he suggests, should refer only to a system in which gases pass through various channels and some or all of them return to the point from which they came.

Breathing attachments

Reservoir bags ('rebreathing' bags)

The bag is constructed from black rubber and is available in a range of sizes, but generally 0.5 litre and 2 litre bags are used. Two-litre reservoir bags are available with a single looped end or an extended looped end, which may be cut off to create a double-ended bag. The loop at the closed end of the bag, in addition to allowing it to be stored, can be folded over and attached to the pin on the bag mount to reduce the volume of the bag.

Expiratory valves

Expiratory valves, also called adjustable pressure-limiting valves by the British and International Standards, are to facilitate the escape of patient-expired gases from the circuit. The pressure at which the valve opens should be low enough to allow expired gases to exit, but at the same time not allow the reservoir bag to empty owing to lack of resistance. The most common is the 'Heidbrink valve', which has a screw top that allows control of the opening pressure of the spring-loaded disc inside.

Breathing tubes

Breathing tubes are generally corrugated, allowing flexibility without kinking, and must be of sufficient diameter to offer low resistance to the gas flow. Traditionally this tubing, often called elephant tubing, has been made of rubber or neoprene, although various plastics are frequently used. Plastic tubing has the advantage of being lighter, transparent or semitransparent, cheaper and single use. Tubing is available in various lengths, or in a large roll. The ends of the tubing allow the attachment of tapered connectors. These are standard fittings, 22 mm/15 mm, male to female to which other components are fitted.

Face masks

Face masks are designed to fit over the nose and mouth or, in the case of nasal masks, just the nose, and therefore come in a range of sizes. Masks have either specific contours, air-filled cuffs or flanged cuffs, to form the seal. They should create a leak-free junction with the patient with the minimum of pressure.

Catheter mounts

The catheter mount forms the junction between the breathing circuit and the patient's tube. It usually consists of a short piece of narrow-gauge smooth or corrugated tubing, with a right-angled 15 mm connector for the patient's tube at one end and a female 22 mm tapered fitting at the other.

Endotracheal tube connectors/right-angled connectors

The right-angled endotracheal tube connector may have a suction port incorporated: examples of this are found in the Cobbs and Magill connectors. It is situated between the endotracheal tube and the catheter mount (as described above). With the increased use of plastic connections, being lightweight and easily connected and disconnected from the endotracheal tube, right-angled connections without suction ports are more common (Figs 4.8 & 4.9).

Breathing systems

Mapleson classified breathing systems in 1954; this has led to six variations, commonly referred

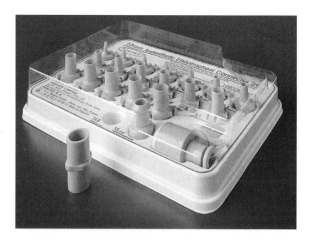

Figure 4.8 Anaesthetic tracheal connector set.

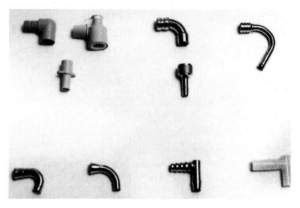

Figure 4.9 A variety of tracheal tube connectors. Clockwise from top left: Portex and Portex swivel with 15 mm tracheal tube connector, Nosworthy, Worcester, Cobbs, Rowbotham, Magill oral, Magill nasal. (Reproduced from Aitkenhead & White 1996, with permission.)

to as Mapleson A, B, C, D, E and F (Fig. 4.10). This classification appears to be widely accepted.[7,8]

The following are brief descriptions of the common terms used when discussing breathing systems.

• **Drawover** The drawover system has been described above, under Vaporizers. Examples of this type of system are the EMO ether vaporizer, the AE Fluothane vaporizer and the Oxford Miniature vaporizer.

• **Open and semi-open** These systems are described above, under Vaporizers.

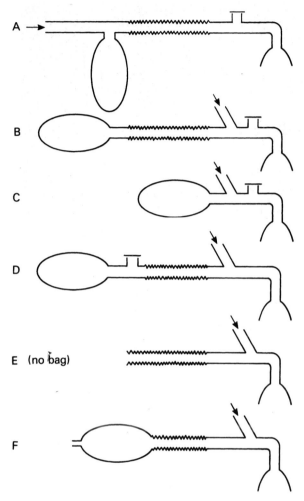

Figure 4.10 Mapleson classification of breathing systems. (Reproduced from Aitkenhead & White 1996, with permission.)

• **Closed** The design of these systems deliberately allows partial or total rebreathing, so there should be the facility for carbon dioxide absorption. The flow rate of oxygen is low, but still essential to allow for metabolic use and the inevitable leakage.

• **Semiclosed** This category includes systems such as the Magill, where rebreathing, particularly of alveolar gas, is not intended.

• **Assisted** An example is the use of a Venturi injector to advance the flow of gases through the system to the patient.

• **Dead space** The term dead space can be applied to both anatomy and apparatus. The anatomical dead space is said to be that volume of the respiratory system occupied by gases which does not take part in the alveolar gaseous exchange (external respiration). Endotracheal intubation reduces the anatomical dead space, which in the average adult is approximately 150 ml. Apparatus dead space is the volume of anaesthetic equipment that contains exhaled gases at the end of expiration; these are designated to be inhaled during the next inspiration. In most systems gases contained in the apparatus dead space have not been involved in external respiration.

• **Scavenging** Scavenging is the safe removal of waste gases and vapours from the breathing system. There are various systems available, both active and passive.

Maintaining the airway

Maintenance of the airway in the semi- or unconscious patient is a basic skill taught in cardiopulmonary resuscitation programmes as well as operating department training and education programmes.

The maintenance of the airway in a clinical environment, with the array of artificial airways, requires a wide range of skills from both the anaesthetist and the practitioner. A patent airway may not always be achieved without additional equipment, which may include the following.

Manual movement of the anatomy

The simple action of pushing upwards and backwards, elevating the mandible, on the supine patient may free the obstructed airway. Often, however, lifting the angles of the mandible forward, flexion of the neck and extension of the head are the most effective methods of maintaining the airway in the unconscious or anaesthetized patient. This latter action, often referred to as 'sniffing the morning air', lifts the tongue forward from the posterior pharyngeal wall.

The oropharyngeal airway

The most popular of these airways is the Guedel: these are positioned in the upper airway and are used primarily to either maintain an airway, often in conjunction with a mask, or to relieve airway obstruction. Additional benefits include preventing the patient biting the endotracheal tube and facilitating suction of the oral cavity and oropharynx.

The nasopharyngeal airway (Fig. 4.11)

This type of airway is inserted via the external nares. Constructed from supple latex, the flanged end prevents complete insertion into the nose. It allows a patent nasal airway in circumstances where the oral airways may be contraindicated, i.e. with loose or capped teeth.

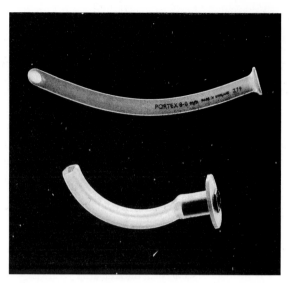

Figure 4.11 Nasopharyngeal airway (above) and Geudal oropharyngeal airway (below). (Reproduced from Aitkenhead & White 1996, with permission.)

The laryngeal mask/airway (Fig. 4.12)

Also known as the Brain airway (after its designer, Dr A. Brain), this device has made a major impact on airway management in the last few years. The oval head is inserted into the pharynx and lies posterior to the laryngeal opening, with a cuff inflated to form a seal. It is available in a range of sizes, from 1 for neonates and infants under 6.5 kg to 5 for large adults. A reinforced version is available which is designed to prevent kinking of the tube section. Suggested uses of the laryngeal mask are as follows:[3]

- routine inhalation anaesthesia
- inhalational anaesthesia, where the maintenance of a mask in place is difficult
- airway maintenance, in known and unexpected difficult intubations
- emergency management of a failed intubation
- cardiopulmonary resuscitation.

The endotracheal tube

This is probably the most common method of securing the airway in patients who require neuromuscular blockade. The range of sizes, shapes and construction materials for endotracheal and tracheostomy tubes is vast, and the choice lies

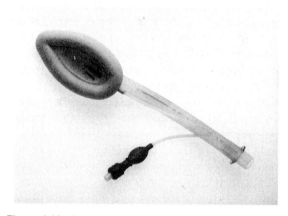

Figure 4.12 Laryngeal mask. (Reproduced from Aitkenhead & White 1996, with permission.)

with the anaesthetist. The criteria that may influence the decision to use an endotracheal tube are as follows:

- when maintenance of the airway is difficult or it is likely to become obstructed (e.g. owing to the positioning of the patient) or unable to be achieved by any other means
- when the operative procedure requires the abolition of muscle tone, and therefore artificial ventilation is required

- when the operation requires placing the patient in a position that obscures the anaesthetist's view or limits access
- to prevent the passage of any foreign substances, gastric contents, blood, etc., into the trachea and subsequently further into the respiratory passage
- as part of a resuscitation procedure, as in cardiac arrest
- where the operative site is to be shared, or is in close proximity between the surgeon and the anaesthetist
- in circumstances where artificial ventilation is required, either during or after the operation, and when the patient may require specialist treatment postoperatively, i.e. transfer to the intensive care unit
- if the thoracic cavity is to be opened.

If any of the above criteria are met, endotracheal intubation should be performed.

The introduction of an endotracheal tube is facilitated by the use of a laryngoscope or, in difficult circumstances, a fibreoptic intubating bronchoscope. Traditional, standard endotracheal tubes were made from red rubber or latex, but plastic tubes are increasingly being used. The use of plastic endotracheal tubes removes the need to collect, decontaminate, check, pack and sterilize, which is required for red rubber and latex tubes.

Disposable plastic (polyvinyl chloride) endotracheal tubes (Fig. 4.13) are presterilized and packaged with a connector, and may need to be cut to size before presentation to the anaesthetist. The distance from the distal tip of the tube is marked out in centimetres on the tube's length. The choice of endotracheal tube is the anaesthetist's decision, and will include consideration of cuffed or non-cuffed, size and length.

The division between oral and nasal tubes is lessening in significance with the advent of disposable plastic tubes, but traditional cuffed red rubber oral tubes often have the pilot tubing (connecting the cuff to the inflating port) running on the external surface of the endotracheal tube, whereas the cuffed red rubber nasal tube has this pilot tubing running within the wall of the endotracheal tube, thus reducing the likelihood of

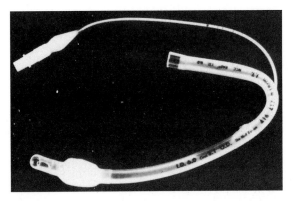

Figure 4.13   A pre-formed tracheal tube. (Reproduced from Aitkenhead & White 1996, with permission.)

trauma to the mucosal membranes of the nasal cavity. Most plastic tubes have the pilot tubing within the wall and may be used orally or nasally.

The most common standard shape of endotracheal tube is the continuous curve of the Magill cuffed endotracheal tube. The Oxford tube, with its distinctive 'L' shape, conforms to the oral pharynx profile and the reinforced tube, containing a spiral of metal or nylon within the wall, prevents any kinking.

The purpose of the inflated cuff at the distal end of the endotracheal tube is to maintain a seal between the cuff and the mucosal membrane of the trachea, thus allowing positive pressure ventilation as well as preventing the inhalation of pharyngeal or gastric secretions (Fig. 4.14 A & B).

The plastic disposable endotracheal tubes have a one-way valve at the inflating port of the pilot tubing which eliminates the need to clamp off the cuff tubing, as used to be required with red rubber tubes. However, when deflating the cuff the inflating device, usually a 20 ml syringe, needs to be reinserted in order to aspirate the air. Some practitioners attempt to deflate the cuff by pulling off the pilot tubing, but this may actually prevent deflation by effectively sealing the tubing. All modern tubes include a small 'pilot' balloon at the inflating port to indicate that the cuff has been inflated. The volume of air that is required to inflate the cuff correctly is that which is just enough to maintain the seal within the trachea.

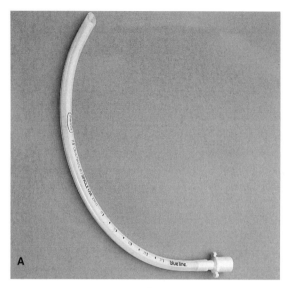

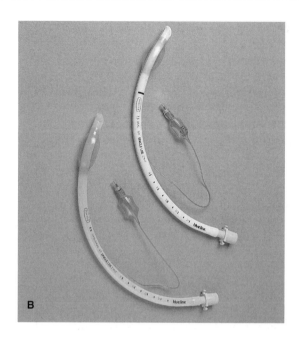

Figure 4.14 A: Plain or uncuffed endotracheal tube. B: Standard cuff endotracheal tube.

One method of identifying that this seal has been achieved is to listen for the back flow of air caused by the anaesthetist ventilating while slowly inflating the cuff. As this sound ceases so inflation of the cuff should cease. This crucial aspect of safe intubation is practical and students should utilize the opportunity to discuss and identify such methods with experienced staff at the earliest opportunity. The device that was specifically designed for inflation of an endotracheal cuff is the Mitchell's inflator. Most plastic tubes have a Luer fitting on the inflating port. If syringes are to be used for inflating endotracheal tube cuffs they must be clearly marked as such to ensure that they are not used for any other purpose.

There is no specific length to which endotracheal tubes should be cut for adults, although

Ward[6] gives an indication of normal requirements. A general rule of thumb is 21 cm for females and 23 cm for males.

Table 4.1 outlines the importance of gauging the correct length of endotracheal tubes.

The size of an endotracheal tube is designated by its internal diameter. There is a popular formula for identifying the correct diameter of endotracheal tubes for children over 1 year old:

$$\frac{\text{age in years}}{4} + 4.5 \text{ mm}$$

Guidance on the correct size of tube for adults is given in Table 7.1 from the textbook by Ward;[6] as

Table 4.1 Hazards of incorrect endotracheal tube length

Too long	Too short
Risk of intubation of a bronchus (usually the right)	Risk of cuff lying above or at the level of the larynx
Excessive tube length protruding from the mouth/nose may cause kinking	Pulling of the connector and catheter mount causing kinking and movement of the tube
Difficulty of tying/taping in of the tube	Difficulty of tying/taping in of the tube
Potential for patient to bite on or through the tube prior to extubation	

a general rule a size 8 is used for females and a size 9 for males.

As mentioned above, the insertion of an endo-tracheal tube usually requires the use of a laryngoscope (Fig. 4.15). These usually consist of a detachable handle containing the power source for illuminating the bulb. Fibreoptic laryngoscopes have the bulb in the handle, which transmits the light through a fibreoptic bundle in the blade. The older style 'standard' laryngoscopes have the bulb in the blade. The blade is usually set at right-angles to the handle and is detachable.

There are two common types of blade (Figs 4.16 & 4.17):

• The curved blade, the Macintosh, has a Z-shaped cross-section. Its design facilitates the placement of the rounded tip anterior to the epiglottis.
• The straight blade, examples of which are the

Robertshaw, Soper and Seward, is designed to be placed posterior to the epiglottis.

These blades are available in a range of sizes. The Macintosh blade is often available with an angle of 135°, known as the 'polio' blade, which is useful when insertion into the mouth is hindered, e.g. by a barrel chest or enlarged breasts. It is particularly useful in obstetrics.[3]

There are a number of other aids to intubation, the most common of which are flexible bougies, stylets and forceps.

Bougies are most often made of gum elastic and tend to be long, often twice the length of an

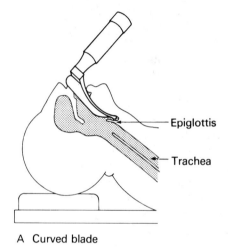

A Curved blade

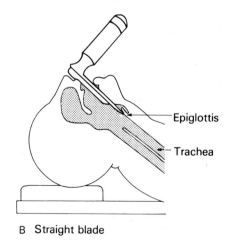

B Straight blade

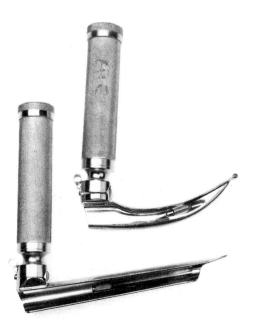

Figure 4.15 Laryngoscopes with Magill blade (above) and Macintosh blade (below). (Reproduced from Aitkenhead & White 1996, with permission.)

Figure 4.16 Use of the laryngoscope. (Reproduced from Aitkenhead & White 1996, with permission.)

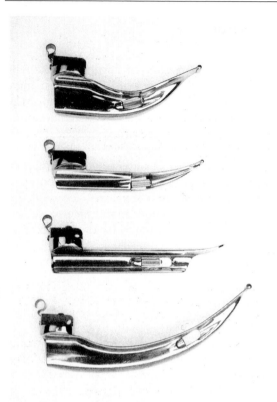

Figure 4.17 A selection of laryngoscope blades. From top: Macintosh infant, Robertshaw, Magill infant, large adult Macintosh. (Reproduced from Aitkenhead & White 1996, with permission.)

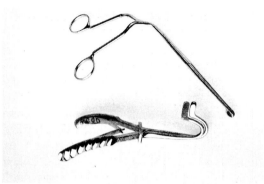

Figure 4.18 Magill forceps (above) and Ferguson mouth gag (below). (Reproduced from Aitkenhead & White 1996, with permission.)

uncut endotracheal tube. There are various methods of use, one being the introduction of the bougie, either blind or with the aid of the laryngoscope, and then passing the endotracheal tube over the bougie. The bougie should be lightly lubricated to facilitate removal once the tube is in place.

Stylets tend to be far more rigid and shorter than bougies. Their primary purpose is to hold the tube to a preset curve. They should always be lubricated prior to insertion into the tube, to ensure they can be withdrawn easily once the tube is in place.

Forceps are used to hold and guide the tube with the aid of the laryngoscope. The most common design is the Magill forceps, which are angled to facilitate easy insertion and manipulation of the tube (Fig. 4.18).

Once the airway is secure respiratory function is either spontaneous, assisted or controlled.

Ventilation and ventilators

Ventilation of the patient may be carried out, provided that the airway is maintained. The reservoir bag or Ambu-bag may be squeezed by hand, producing ventilation. Variations may be the rate of squeezing and how much of the bag is squeezed, relating to the rate of respiration and tidal volume. The expiration of gases depends on the elastic recoil of the lungs, as in normal physiology. Ventilators essentially perform the same functions as just described, but have the capability for fine adjustment and accurate measurement of the rate volumes of gas; in addition, they do not suffer from fatigue, as does the anaesthetist's hand.

Table 4.2 highlights the differences between spontaneous and artificial ventilation.

The driving source for ventilators is either an electric motor or gas pressure. The gas pressure may be provided by compressed air (e.g. Penlon Nuffield ventilator) or by the flow of gases from the anaesthetic machine (Manley ventilator). In the former the gas supply plays no part in ventilating – it is purely a power source. Most current ventilators work on the principle of intermittent positive pressure ventilation (IPPV). This, as its name implies, requires gas to be driven into the lungs under pressure, i.e. mechanical inspiration. Expiration is passive as in normal physiology. The phases of ventilation are divided into four cycles: inspiration, inspiration to expiration, expiration, and expiration to inspiration. The inspiration phase is a fundamental aspect of ventilation, and ventilators can be classified accord-

Table 4.2 Differences between spontaneous and artificial ventilation

Spontaneous	Artificial
Air is drawn into the lungs by reducing intrathoracic pressure (diaphragmatic and intercostal movement)	Air is passed into lungs by positive pressure
Under control of respiratory centre	Under manual/machine control
Pressure within thorax below that of atmosphere; this assists venous return to the heart	Pressure within thorax rises and thereby impedes venous return of blood to the heart, reduces blood pressure and increases central venous pressure
Air drawn in, warmed and humidified by nasal passages, which also remove particles to reduce risk of infection	Bypasses nasal structures and requires equipment to warm and humidify; increased infection risk

ing to how inspiration is produced. Classification of ventilators as either pressure generators, which deliver a predetermined pressure, or flow generators that deliver a predetermined flow of gas, was suggested by Mapleson in 1969.[3]

Flow generators The ventilators in this category have the common feature that they are powerful to compensate for low-compliance lungs and high airway resistance. Once source of power is a high-pressure gas flow, which may be delivered directly to the patient and intermittently interrupted. Alternatively, the high-pressure gas is used to compress a bellows containing the fresh gas; an example is the Ohmeda Modulus/7810 machine. The second source of power is an electric motor that will provide a constant gas flow.

Pressure generators In these ventilators gases are delivered to the lungs via the patient's airway until a preset pressure (for example 1.5 kPa) is reached. The volume of gas delivered is derived from the pressure set and the patient's lung compliance. The inspiratory pressure is created by a weight on top of the bellows. The volume of gas in the bellows will cease to be driven into the lung when the pressure in the alveoli equals that created by the weight. Example of this type of ventilator include the Manley and East Radcliffe.

The current variety and sophistication of ventilators means that many of them can be used as both pressure and flow generators, as well as having a range of controls to change the cycling phases. The Siemens Servo 900 series and the Engström Emma are two examples.[3]

Care of the patient requiring ventilation

The practitioner must consider the following aspects of care for the ventilated patient throughout anaesthesia:

• Ensuring that adequate ventilation is being maintained by the ventilator is achieved by monitoring:
— check blood pressure and pulse
— monitor ventilator readings and functioning
— monitor expired CO_2 and pulse oximeter reading.
• Ensuring adequate removal of secretions from the trachea and bronchi may be achieved by:
— listening for abnormal respiratory sounds and the anaesthetist listening to the chest
— observation of decreased tidal volume and any increase in inflation pressure.
• Prevention of damage to the oral cavity and trachea can be prevented by:
— monitoring the position of endotracheal tubes and artificial airways (nasal/oral)
— monitoring the cuff of the tube by observation of the pilot cuff.
• Prevention of lung infection may be achieved by the use of:
— bacterial filters on ventilators.
• Humidification of inspired gases, if required, may be achieved by the use of:
— heat and moisture exchange equipment, such as the 'Swedish nose'.

Failure to maintain adequate ventilation

The practitioner must be aware of possible causes of ventilator problems in order to identify them quickly and act accordingly should they arise.

Causes within the ventilator
- Mechanical failure
- Leaks
- Inadequate setting of parameters.

Causes within connections between ventilator and patient
- Loose connections
- Dislodged/misplaced tube
- Kinking
- Water in tubing
- Leaks around the cuff
- Overinflated cuff.

Causes arising in the patient
- Sputum
- Spasm
- Reduction in lung compliance, e.g. pulmonary oedema
- Fighting the ventilator – spontaneous breathing.

Intravenous infusion equipment

Intravenous fluid is administered:
- for the replacement of fluid, electrolytes, proteins and cells or platelets
- to feed patients unable to take food by mouth, i.e. coma/alimentary tract problems
- as a route for drug administration
- as a method of altering body chemistry (e.g. diuretics, electrolytes).

The reasons for using an intravenous route are:

- Drugs reach the site of action more quickly than by any other route, and the action is more accurate. (Some agents are not absorbed in the alimentary tract.)
- In shock, the drugs may not be absorbed in the GI tract or from the muscles.
- Large volumes of fluid can be administered quickly.

The equipment required includes the intravenous fluid and a giving set consisting of piercing needle, filter, drip chamber, tubing, regulator and injection port. Access to a vein is through a plastic cannula, which is fixed in place by strapping or Opsite, etc. A skin disinfectant (antiseptic) and a drip pole or hanging facility are also required.

Hazards of intravenous infusion

The hazards of intravenous (i.v.) infusion are identified below, with the action required to avoid them:

- infection: adherence to aseptic technique is vital
- air embolism: all connections must be secure; no air in the giving settubing; air must be excluded when changing containers
- overinfusion: may cause left ventricular failure (circulatory overload). Close observation of infusion rate is necessary
- osmotic imbalance: hypertonic or hypotonic solutions may cause cellular dehydration or 'waterlogging' of tissues. Correct fluids to be given as per anaesthetist's instructions.

The warming of fluids – most often blood and blood products – can be achieved in two ways:

- **'Dry' method** This usually requires an extension tube to be attached to the giving set (with a filter in the drip chamber) and a purpose-made 'flat' flow channel pack. This pack is primed and fitted on to a warming plate, with a door closing to enclose the pack between two plates that are warmed to a preset temperature. These devices are electrically driven; the usual precautions and safety measures for electrical apparatus, in addition to the manufacturer's instructions, should be followed. There are cutout switches built into the blood warmer to ensure that blood is not overheated.
- **'Wet' method** This usually consists of a chamber filled with water, with a heating element in the chamber floor as in a kettle. It is electrically powered and the appropriate considerations apply, as well as the potential hazard of water being present. The chamber is attached to a drip stand or placed on a secure

surface. The giving set (including a filter in the drip chamber for the use of blood) requires a connecting coil of tubing to be immersed in the water chamber. It is important not to allow the connections at each end of the coil to become immersed as this carries an infection risk, even if sterile water is used. Often a further extension tube is attached to the distal end of the coil. As with the dry method the electrical apparatus should have a cutout switch built in to prevent overheating of the water.

Both the above methods may be inefficient if the extension tubing distal to the warming pack/coil is too long: the warmed fluid will become cooler before it reaches the patient.

Disposal of i.v. infusion equipment

Great care must be taken with equipment used in i.v. procedures. All needles, including the piercing end of giving sets, must be regarded as contaminated and disposed of in sharps containers, by the person who has used them. Used blood bags are also potential sources of infection and should be handled and disposed of carefully according to statutory guidelines.

EQUIPMENT FOR THE DELIVERY OF REGIONAL ANAESTHESIA

The principle of regional anaesthesia is the administration of drugs to secure analgesia and/or motor blockade to allow surgical or anaesthetic procedures to be carried out. This method has the advantage that the patient is conscious or only mildly sedated and, not having been subjected to the effects of a major general anaesthetic, is able to maintain their own airway, assist in positioning and in most cases verbally report their condition. These patients are usually able to return to the ward and early ambulation is achieved.

The potential hazards of regional anaesthesia include infection risk, neural damage, spinal headaches, dural tears, inadequate blocks, and fear and anxiety in the patient.

As with general anaesthesia the practitioner will need a basic knowledge and understanding of anatomy and physiology to be able to select the appropriate equipment and assist in the procedure.

As described earlier, for the purposes of this chapter regional anaesthesia is divided into conductive, infiltration and intravenous. The preoperative assessment by the anaesthetist is essential to reassure and to explain the rationale and the procedure for a regional anaesthetic technique to the patient, in addition to the physical assessment. The patient is often conscious during regional anaesthesia, and so the role of the practitioner in reducing anxiety, explaining procedures and requesting movement from the patient, particularly during epidural and spinal procedures, continues throughout the operation. It is often left to the practitioner to stay with and reassure the patient, passing on their responses to the surgical team.

Equipment to enable immediate resuscitation should be prepared in any area where a local or regional procedure may take place. This should include:

- a system for delivering oxygen under pressure via a face mask or endotracheal tube
- a laryngoscope with at least two sizes of blades
- intubation aids, stylets and bougies
- a facility for tilting the trolley/table head down
- suction apparatus
- intravenous cannulae, giving sets and fluids
- thiopentone or diazepam for convulsions
- drugs for hypotension (ephedrine).

In addition, intravenous access by placement of a suitably sized cannula prior to the procedure is advisable.[8]

The preparation of the patient for any form of regional anaesthesia should begin with the explanation and assessment, followed by obtaining their consent. The patient must be positioned appropriately for the anaesthetist to administer either an epidural or a spinal anaesthetic. The exact positioning depends on the patient's ability to flex the spine, the anaesthetist's preference and the planned site of the epidural/spinal needle. The common positions are lateral and sitting: the lateral position will depend on whether hyperbaric solutions are to be utilized. Lateral positioning will require trolley/table stability, room for the anaesthetist and sterile surface maintenance. Operating department trolleys should have secure sides that can be used to prevent the patient falling forward; further assistance may be required to maintain the patient's position. The patient is manoeuvred so that the dorsal aspect lies parallel to the edge of the table, with the knees brought up to the chest and the head and neck tucked into the chest to allow maximum flexion of the spine. The sitting position will depend on the environment and equipment available. Often the patient sits on the table/trolley, legs hanging over the side with a stool for the feet, and flexing the spine by bending the head and neck forward (Fig. 4.19). Other regional anaesthetic techniques include peripheral nerve blocks, which can be at various sites on the body. For a majority of peripheral nerve blocks the patient will be required to lie supine, occasionally with a limb extended. The prime safety aspects of these positions are patient stability and equipment security. The role of the team in reassuring, reducing anxiety and keeping the patient informed is a major factor in the success and speed of the procedure.

An aseptic technique is essential to ensure that the procedure carries no risk of introducing infection to the patient. The area should be prepared beforehand and the appropriate equipment be ready for use.

Spinal anaesthesia

Spinal anaesthesia, sometimes referred to as subarachnoid block or spinal analgesia, is achieved by the administration of a local anaesthetic drug within the subarachnoid space, usually at the lumbar interspace. The interspaces most often used to gain access to the subarachnoid space and hence the spinal nerves are L3–4, L4–5 and L5–S1. The mixed spinal nerve conveys a variety of functions – motor, pain, temperature, autonomic activity, touch, pressure and proprioception – all of which are affected to a greater or lesser extent. Indications for the use of spinal anaesthesia include surgery of the lower extremities, lower abdomen and perineum, and vaginal and caesarean delivery.

In preparing to assist with a spinal technique the practitioner should consider the following equipment:

- full resuscitation facilities, including a vasopressor such as ephedrine
- intravenous fluid (1 l), giving set, large-bore cannula (16 or 14 gauge), securing tape. The blockade of sympathetic nerve fibres causes vasodilatation at and below the level of the block; in cases of hypotension initial treatment is via the infusion line

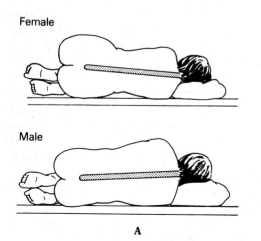
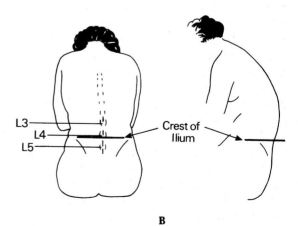

Figure 4.19 Spinal curvature in: A, lateral; B, sitting positions. (Reproduced from Aitkenhead & White 1996, with permission.)

- appropriate equipment to secure the patient during the procedure
- surface or trolley cleaned and prepared to receive a sterile field
- skin preparation solution, sponges/swabs and forceps for application
- paper towels
- drape and towel clips, or disposable fenestrated drape with adhesive strips
- syringes (sizes to be discussed with the anaesthetist)
- filling needle or quill and filter for drawing up drugs
- local anaesthetic agents (as specified by the anaesthetist)
- hypodermic needle
- spinal needle (size as specified by the anaesthetist).

All the above, including ampoules of local anaesthetic drugs, are available in sterile packs. This means that only the items required need be opened, which is cost-effective as well as allowing for the differing techniques of anaesthetists. The above is not a definitive list: it is the responsibility of the anaesthetic practitioner to fully understand the procedure, discuss the anaesthetist's needs and prepare accordingly. Having cannulated and secured intravenous access, with the attachment of an intravenous fluid the patient may be positioned as described above. The anaesthetist will often identify landmarks to ascertain the correct level and insertion point, and may mark the site before preparing to scrub up. The procedure must be carried out aseptically. The anaesthetist should scrub, gown and glove as for any surgical procedure, and utilize aseptic techniques. The practitioner is effectively carrying out the circulating duties. The skin is prepared with an aqueous antiseptic solution and draped. Landmarks are used to identify the correct interspace. The skin and subcutaneous layers are anaesthetized, usually with lignocaine. The spinal needle is inserted until the resistance offered by the ligamentum flavum and the dura mater is encountered. The sudden loss of resistance following piercing of the dura mater implies that the tip of the spinal needle is lying in the subarachnoid space. Confirmation of correct placement is sup-

ported by a slow leak of cerebrospinal fluid (CSF) from the hub of the needle. The selected local anaesthetic drug is then administered. Following withdrawal of the spinal needle the puncture site should be cleaned or sprayed with an antiseptic solution. A waterproof dressing will give some protection to the wound. The effects of a successful subarachnoid block will occur within 3–5 minutes, although the maximal effect may take up to 30 minutes.[3] Various methods are used to ascertain the effectiveness and level of the blockade, including pricking the skin with a needle and spraying with ethyl chloride. There is a range of size spinal needles available, from 19 to 31 G; sizes 22–29 G are most commonly used. A 32 G catheter has been introduced to allow further administration of drugs. Although the technique appears successful, the equipment is difficult to handle and has recently been implicated in nerve damage after repeated injections of local agents. Continuous spinal infusions are no longer used so much.[3]

Epidural anaesthesia

Epidural anaesthesia, also referred to as extradural, is accomplished by injecting a local anaesthetic drug into the epidural space. The siting of the epidural depends upon the level of blockade required: the choice of site is usually quoted as a prefix; i.e. lumbar, thoracic, caudal or cervical epidural. The action of the local anaesthetic is not necessarily in the epidural space: drug action may take place at the paravertebral and subarachnoid levels of nerve roots or on the spinal cord. The nerves affected are as described for spinal anaesthesia. Advantages of the epidural technique over the spinal include a lower risk of postspinal headache, and the placement of an epidural catheter allows control of the commencement and duration of analgesia. The ability to safely block a wider range of levels and administer further doses allows pre- and postoperative analgesia to be given. The onset of action of local anaesthetic agents is slower and less intense than with the spinal technique.

In preparing to assist with an epidural anaesthetic the practitioner should consider the fol-lowing equipment:

- Full resuscitation facilities, including a vasopressor such as ephedrine
- Intravenous fluid (1 l), giving set, large-bore cannula (16 or 14 gauge), securing tape. The blockade of sympathetic nerve fibres causes vasodilatation at and below the level of the block; in cases of hypotension initial treatment is via the infusion line
- Appropriate equipment to secure the patient during the procedure
- Surface or trolley cleaned and prepared to become a sterile field
- Skin preparation solution, sponges/swabs and forceps for application
- Paper towels
- Drape and towel clips, or disposable fenestrated drape with adhesive strips
- Syringes. The anaesthetist may require separation of the syringes used for local infiltration and those used for the epidural. There are various methods for this, particularly as the same size syringes are used for more than one purpose. In order to correctly identify which syringe is for what, the anaesthetist may:
  — discard the infiltration syringe and hypodermic needle once used and before the epidural local is drawn up
  — request glass and plastic syringes
  — request only one of each size of syringe
- Filling needle or quill and filter for drawing up drugs
- Local anaesthetic agents (as specified by the anaesthetist)
- Hypodermic needle
- Tuohy needle, epidural catheter and filter.

In addition to the above items supplied sepa-rately, epidural packs are available commercially (Fig. 4.20). The sterile packs containing epidural equipment and the cost considerations described for spinal anaesthesia apply. Again, the above is not a definitive list: it is the responsibility of the practitioner to fully understand the procedure, discuss the anaesthetist's needs and prepare accordingly. Having cannulated and secured intravenous access, with the attachment of an

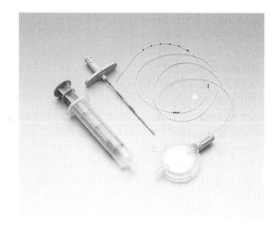

Figure 4.20 Epidural pack.

intravenous fluid the patient may be positioned as described above. The anaesthetist will often identify landmarks to ascertain the correct level and insertion point, and may mark the site before preparing to scrub up. As described above for spinal anaesthesia, the procedure must be carried out aseptically. The anaesthetist should scrub, gown and glove. The skin is prepared with an aqueous antiseptic solution and draped. Landmarks are used to identify the correct level. The superficial and deep tissues are infiltrated with a local anaesthetic via the hypodermic nee-dle and syringe. The Tuohy needle is inserted until the resistance offered by the ligamentum flavum is encountered. There are various meth-ods for identifying the correct level of insertion of the Tuohy needle, recognizing that there is often a negative pressure in the extradural space. A technique called the 'hanging drop' requires a drop of saline in the hub of the needle; this is drawn into the needle when the extradural space is encountered (provided there is negative pres-sure).[3] The use of low-resistance (glass) syringes with saline or air in the barrel is probably more common. As the needle is advanced slight pres-sure is applied to the plunger; as the tip of the needle enters the extradural space the resistance is lost. With the use of air, aspiration will give an indication whether a dural tear has occurred by the presence of CSF. Catheter insertion is through the Tuohy needle, which is marked at 1 cm inter-vals and has a blunt tip with a curved bevel to identify direction. Tuohy needles are available between 16 and 19 G; the epidural catheter is usually 16 G, although 18 G are available. The catheter is usually primed and then inserted, the needle removed and the catheter left in the patient, checked by the marked graduations. Usually 2–5 cm of catheter is left in the patient. Application of a 0.2 μm filter to the administration end of the catheter is carried out by the anaesthetist before removing sterile gloves. The catheter is secured, the area sprayed with antiseptic or plastic and a swab and waterproof plaster applied. The remaining length of catheter is secured to the patient's back. The selected local anaesthetic drug is then administered. Bupivacaine takes approximately 15–20 minutes to become effective, and lasts for 1.5–2.5 hours. Bupivacaine 0.25–0.75% and lignocaine 1–2% are the agents most commonly used. Similar methods to those described for spinal anaesthesia are used to assess the effectiveness and level of the blockade. Injection of a local anaesthetic agent into the sacral canal, which is a continuation of the epidural space, is often referred to as a caudal. Caudal should be administered using an aseptic technique. The needle is usually 19–21 G, and either bupivacaine 0.25–0.5% or lignocaine 1–2% is used.

Combined epidural/spinal

This is a technique that combines the rapid onset and effectiveness of a spinal anaesthetic with the advantages of epidural catheterization. The technique involves the insertion of an epidural needle, as described above. Once this is in place, a long fine spinal needle is passed through the epidural needle which acts as guide. The spinal needle is just longer than the epidural needle, so as to allow it to pierce the arachnoid mater into the subarachnoid space. A spinal anaesthetic is then delivered and the spinal needle withdrawn. An epidural catheter is then introduced in the usual way. The aseptic considerations outlined above for both spinal and epidural anaesthesia also apply to this technique.[9]

The use of opioid analgesics via spinal or epidural routes is gaining popularity, allowing pain relief without the loss of motor function.[9] This technique is often referred to as a 'mobile epidural'. Research is ongoing towards patient-controlled analgesia via opioid epidurals.

Peripheral nerve blocks

Peripheral nerve blocks are also referred to as somatic nerve blocks, and are commonly used for surgical procedures or manipulation as well as for postoperative pain relief. The title of the block usually defines the site or area of injection; a short bevelled needle is used to reduce the risk of nerve contact. Some of the more common nerve blocks include brachial plexus, ulnar nerve, digital nerve, axillary, median nerve and femoral.

Infiltration anaesthesia

Infiltration anaesthesia can be epithelial (subcutaneous) or intradermal, and involves the introduction of a local anaesthetic agent around a lesion or proposed incision. This technique is often used for minor surgery, suturing, or the introduction of a feeding line. The use of diluted solutions of local anaesthetic is common, particularly for extensive surgery, to anaesthetize deeper tissues. Consideration must be given to the maximum safe dosage and the time required for the agent to work. Subcutaneous infiltration of a local anaesthetic agent is often advisable before large-bore intravenous cannulae and arterial cannulae are introduced into conscious patients.

Intravenous anaesthesia

This technique is often referred to as intravenous regional anaesthesia (IVRA) and in general the most common procedure is the Bier's block. Full resuscitation equipment must be available, owing to the potentially fatal effects of a large volume of local anaesthetic agent, administered intravenously, gaining rapid access to the systemic circulation. The toxic effects may range from convulsions to death caused by respiratory and/or cardiac depression. Deaths from IVRA techniques have been attributed to errors in administering the correct drug, incorrect dosage, inappropriate technique, and incompetence and/or inadequate resuscitation methods.[8] The aim of an intravenous regional anaesthetic is to allow relatively short surgical procedures to be performed in a bloodless field with maximal analgesia on a conscious patient. Surgical procedures performed under this technique include manipulation and reduction of Colles' fracture and carpal tunnel decompression. Premedication is generally not required.[8] The equipment required to perform a Bier's block includes:[8]

- full resuscitation equipment
- intravenous cannulae (20 or 22 gauge) × 2
- padding for the tourniquet
- exsanguination equipment (Esmarch's bandage, Rhys-Davis exsanguinator)
- single or double pneumatic tourniquet
- local anaesthetic agent
- monitoring equipment.

The practitioner must be familiar with the procedure in order to prepare and assist the anaesthetist and deliver care to the patient. The following is a general outline of the procedure for administering a Bier's block to the upper limb.

Resuscitation equipment is prepared and the equipment to be used for the block checked, particularly the tourniquet for leaks. Monitoring equipment is applied to the patient: the purpose of the equipment and any sensation that the patient may experience should be clearly explained. Regular monitoring of the blood pressure and recording of the ECG with the attachment of a pulse oximeter are probably minimal requirements. A cannula is inserted into the dorsal aspect of both the right and the left hand of the patient. The cannula in the contralateral limb is for the administration of emergency drugs if required. The use of needles is contraindicated as when the limb is exsanguinated the needle may pass through the vein. An orthopaedic bandage is applied to the proximal end of the limb, where the tourniquet is to be applied. A single- or double-cuff

tourniquet is applied. The limb is exsanguinated by either:

- raising and occluding the brachial artery in cases where the use of equipment may cause trauma and pain to the patient
- the use of a Rhys Davis exsanguinator; or
- the use of Esmarch's bandage.

A single- or double-cuff tourniquet is applied and inflated. The inflated pressure of the tourniquet must be higher than the patient's systolic blood pressure: texts suggest either 100 mmHg above systolic or twice the systolic. As with other surgical uses of tourniquets, the pressure and time of inflation must be recorded. The local anaesthetic agent is then slowly injected over a period of about 2 minutes. Prilocaine 3 mg/kg (0.6 ml/kg of a 0.5% solution) is usually the drug of choice, although lignocaine can be used. Bupivacaine is contraindicated owing to its toxicity. The patient may sense paraesthesia initially in the proximal end of the limb. The motor and sensory nerve fibres are usually blocked in 5–10 minutes. Throughout the procedure the pressure of the tourniquet should be monitored, in addition to the routine monitoring of the patient. The tourniquets should be left in place and inflated for at least 20 minutes regardless of the surgical time. In the case of a prolonged surgical procedure the cannula should be left *in situ*. After an hour the tourniquet cuff may be deflated for a period of 5 minutes, and then the limb re-exsanguinated and a second injection of half the original dose of local anaesthetic agent given. This method ensures that the tourniquet time is not exceeded. The first signs of toxic effects from the local anaesthetic may be paraesthesia of the tongue and lips. If convulsions occur, treatment with thiopentone or diazepam via the cannula in the contralateral limb and administration of 100% oxygen may be required. A similar method may be used on the lower limbs, although the result may be less effective and larger volumes are required. Caution should be exercised in patients with severe arteriosclerosis, hypotension, or who are obese, and the technique is contraindicated in cases of sickle cell anaemia.[3,8]

EQUIPMENT FOR MONITORING THE PHYSIOLOGICAL STATE OF THE PATIENT

The term monitoring has become synonymous with all aspects of patient care in delivering an anaesthetic – indeed, the word derives from the Latin *monere*, 'to warn',[6] which should be the primary function of monitoring equipment, allowing action to be taken in time to maintain the patient's wellbeing.

Direct observation

Despite continual developments in the sophistication of modern monitoring equipment, it is unlikely that we will be able to replace the most reliable and immediate source of monitoring, trained personnel and their senses. The anaesthetist and the practitioner are able to use sight, touch, smell and sound to continually assess the patient's condition, as well as monitoring the anaesthetic equipment. One important aspect of this is that the anaesthetic team should have physical and visual access to some part of the patient. Most often this is the head and neck or arm and hand, or at worst, part of the foot, but some part of the patient's surface area must be able to be accessible to the anaesthetic team to enable the use of touch and vision as part of the assessment. The mechanical – usually electrical – equipment should be seen as adjuncts to direct observation. However, together humans and machines should be able to create a high degree of safe patient monitoring throughout any clinical procedure.

Electrocardiograph

Electrocardiograph (ECG) machines monitor the electrical activity of the cardiac muscle. The reading can give different 'views' of cardiac activity, depending on the lead configuration. More importantly, what makes the ECG worthwhile is the interpretation and analysis of the reading. What the practitioner will interpret from the trace will depend on their knowledge, interest and experience. As with a majority of physiological monitoring it is important to recognize the baselines of the physiological parameters for the individual patient, and be able to act accordingly. The rate and rhythm of the ECG are basic parameters of which the practitioner should have a clear knowledge.

Routine interoperative ECG monitoring generally utilizes one of the potential 12 recordings: CM5 appears to be the most popular, as it reveals ST segment changes within the QRST complex. CM5 stands for chest/central, manubrium and V5/5th left intercostal space; in practice this involves one active lead attached to the electrode at the top of the sternum or joint of sternum and right clavicle; the second active lead is attached to the electrode placed on the left side of the chest, just under the left nipple. The inactive lead is usually attached to the electrode placed on the left shoulder. Depending on the exact location these are variations of lead II or V5 of the 12-lead ECG recording. During routine cardiac monitoring under anaesthesia the aforementioned configurations are most useful for detecting myocardial ischaemia (as this usually affects the left ventricle), dysrhythmias, and inadequate anaesthesia, as this most commonly presents as tachycardia.

It should be remembered, however, that an ECG trace showing normal sinus rhythm does not necessarily mean adequate cardiac output, or even peripheral blood flow, therefore other parameters should be taken into consideration in assessing the cardiovascular state of the patient.

Blood pressure

Blood pressure is the result of the force of the blood against the vessel walls. The influences on blood pressure are:

- pressure exerted on the system by the contraction of the left ventricle of the heart
- peripheral vascular resistance
- circulating volume
- stroke volume of cardiac output.

In the surgical patient other factors may have a direct effect on the blood pressure, such as:

- positioning
- drug regimen (epidural)

- anxiety
- medical condition
- loss of muscle tone.

The unconscious ventilated patient may be susceptible to at least four of the above five.

Monitoring and measurement of blood pressure

Clinical blood pressure is measured in millimetres of mercury (mmHg), and may be monitored directly (invasive) or indirectly (non-invasive)

Invasive The equipment required for invasive blood pressure monitoring consists of a cannula, a connecting catheter and a transducer. The cannula is usually a Teflon parallel-sided cannula size 20–22 G and is placed into an artery, most often the radial artery unless the patient's condition contraindicates this.

The connecting catheter (manometer tubing) between the cannula and the transducer should be short, i.e. less than 200 cm, to reduce potential dampening of the signal, and have a compatible connection (Luer lock) at both ends. The catheter is primed with heparinized saline (e.g. 1000 units heparin in 500 ml of sodium chloride 0.9%).

The transducer usually consists of a chamber of heparinized saline continuous with the catheter tubing. One wall of the chamber is a membrane/diaphragm that is connected to an electrical circuit. Pressure fluctuations in the patient are reflected in the heparinized saline, causing movement of the diaphragm, which in turn causes electrical changes in the circuit, changing resistance. These changes are displayed as reading of pressure, as a digital display and/or as a continuous waveform.

As with any invasive procedure the preparation for introducing a cannula into an artery should conform to an aseptic technique. Emphasis should be placed on dressing and labelling of the arterial line. The dressing should be such as to prevent infection of the site from external sources and secure the indwelling cannulae. Labelling of the arterial line should be clear to all involved in the care of the patient. Blue and red plastic indicators for the manometer line and the three-way taps are often included in the manufacturer's packaging.

The practitioner often plays a crucial role in arterial cannulation, resulting in a smooth, aseptic, blood-free procedure. As with any procedure that may involve blood and/or body fluids, the use of gloves is necessary and should be part of local policy. However, palpation of the artery and the use of adhesive tape is awkward when gloved.

The practitioner occluding the cannulated artery until the cannula is connected to manometer tubing, the anaesthetist safeguarding the cannulation site and supporting the area/limb, followed by the practitioner ensuring that the area is free from blood and securing the cannula with the selected tape/dressing, is an example of anaesthetist and practitioner working together to reduce the risks of blood and body fluid contamination.

Non-invasive There are two common methods used for non-invasive blood pressure monitoring: the oscillotonometer and the automatic blood pressure monitor.

The oscillotonometer consists of two cuffs in a cover, the upper (proximal) cuff is the occluding cuff and the lower (distal) is the sensing cuff. The upper cuff corresponds to a normal cuff as found in a sphygmomanometer; the lower one corresponds to the palpating finger or stethoscope. The cuff is inflated to above systolic, a valve on the reading dial is slowly opened and a lever depressed, allowing air from the occluding cuff to leak out, and the sensing cuff records the systolic pressure by causing the needle to fluctuate on the dial.[9] The oscillotonometer is portable and reliable at average blood pressure values.

Probably the most often-used non-invasive blood pressure monitoring devices in anaesthesia are the automatic adaptations of the oscillotonometer, i.e. the Dinamap and Datascope. These allow visual readouts of systolic, diastolic and mean blood pressure, allowing the reading to be taken at preset intervals (Fig. 4.21).

Central venous pressure

Central venous pressure (CVP) measurement indicates the status of circulating volume during anaesthesia, and is equated with the right ven-

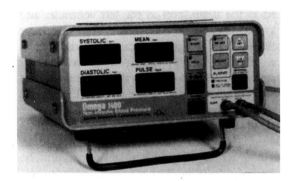

Figure 4.21 An automated oscillometer. (Reproduced from Aitkenhead & White 1996, with permission.)

tricular end-diastolic pressure. The measurement of the CVP is facilitated by the placement of a catheter, such that its distal end is lying in the lower end of the superior vena cava or in the right atrium. The measurement of CVP is affected by other factors and independent readings are of little value. The response of the CVP to a fluid regimen, taking into account other monitored values, allows assessment of circulating volume status. The value of CVP measurement is in allowing assessment of, and planning a regimen for, fluid and blood replacement.

Routes and sites for central venous cannulation

• **Right cephalic**. Introducing a long cannula (a drum catheter for example) is often difficult, partly because of the valves at the junction with the axillary vein. Abduction of the arm by the practitioner may ease the passage of the cannula.

• **The internal jugular vein** is one of the most popular routes and is reported to have the highest chance of correct catheter placement, at approximately 90%.[8] In addition to being uncomfortable in the conscious patient, however, potential hazards of internal jugular cannulation include pneumothorax, carotid artery puncture, brachial plexus/phrenic nerve damage and air embolus. A 5.5 inch, 16 or 14 G cannula is generally used for intravenous cannulation of the internal jugular.

• Other sites include the external jugular vein and the subclavian vein.

To measure the CVP a catheter is inserted via an arm or neck vein and advanced to reach the superior vena cava. Attached to this catheter are a saline drip and giving set, a 'T' piece (three-way tap and manometer tubing specifically designed for this purpose), a measuring rod and a length of manometer tubing. Before a reading can be taken from the manometer the patient is placed in a horizontal position (where possible) (Fig. 4.22). Using the spirit level on the rod attached to the vertical manometer tubing the zero of the scale is set to the level of the midaxillary line, this being taken to represent the level of the right atrium. The saline drip should be turned off when the readings are made and slight movements of the saline level with respiration may be seen. Readings are usually recorded as cmH_2O. As an alternative to the simple saline manometer, a pressure transducer (as for invasive arterial monitoring) may be used: this will give a continuous reading and allows identification of the CVP waveform.

NERVE STIMULATORS

The availability of a peripheral nerve stimulator (Fig. 4.23), whenever a general anaesthetic involving neuromuscular blocking agents is used, is recommended by the Association of Anaesthetists.[10] The nerve stimulator, in monitoring the degree of neuromuscular blockage, should ensure that the patient receives adequate ventilatory support and is not allowed to become partially paralysed. Nerve stimulators cause depolarization of nerve fibres by applying an electrical current to a peripheral nerve. A current of 50 mA for a duration of between 0.2 and 1.0 ms may be required at a voltage of 50–300 V. This current is unlikely to cause adverse effects on cardiac muscle.[8] The response of electrical stimulation can be directly observed, palpated or recorded. The electrical stimulus can be delivered as single shocks, as a succession of high-frequency pulses, or as trains at lower frequencies.

There are a number of patterns of stimulation:

• single pulses
• tetanic stimulation
• posttetanic stimulation using single pulses
• train of four
• posttetanic count, usually for intense blockade
• double burst stimulus, used to assess recovery from non-depolarizing blockade.

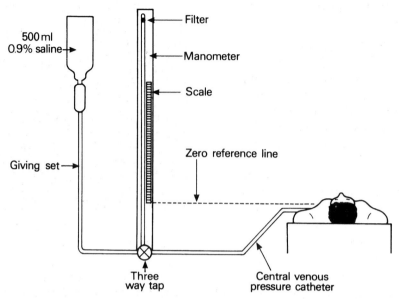

Figure 4.22 Measurement of central venous pressure using a manometer. The manometer tubing is filled from the infusion bag and the tap turned to connect the manometer to the central venous catheter. The fluid level in the manometer falls until the height of the fluid column above the zero reference point is equal to the central venous pressure. (Reproduced from Aitkenhead & White 1996, with permission.)

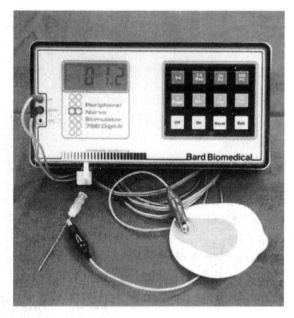

Figure 4.23 Nerve stimulator. (Reproduced from Aitkenhead & White 1996, with permission.)

The responses to stimulus observed are:

• Responding to single pulses reflects normal neuromuscular function, therefore no blockade exists.

• Twitches of equal strength but reduced in numbers, stimulated by single pulses or train of four, and sustained but reduced contractual movement, are indicators of a depolarizing blockade.

• The progressive fading of twitches in response to single pulses, leading to no response, indicates a non-depolarizing blockade. The more complete the neuromuscular blockade, the fewer the twitches. This can be roughly equated to the percentage of blockade by using the train of four stimulus:

— No twitches = 100% blockade
— 1st but no 2nd, 3rd or 4th twitch = 90% blockade
— 1st, 2nd but no 3rd or 4th twitches = 80% blockade

— 1st, 2nd and 3rd but no or reduced 4th twitch = 75% blockade.

In addition to mechanical assessment of neuromuscular blockade, patient movement can be used as an indictor. A sustained head lift for 5 seconds can indicate a blockade of less than 30%; the patient's ability to grip with the hand, protrude the tongue or open the mouth are additional indicators of neuromuscular blockade.[3]

The practitioner needs to be aware of the purpose of nerve stimulators and the patterns of stimulation used and, practically, the types of stimulator and the placement of electrodes. Although surface and needle electrodes are available, for routine monitoring, surface electrodes – usually ECG electrodes – are used. Three common sites for placement are:

- The ulnar nerve: two electrodes are placed along the ulnar aspect of the forearm: a stimulus applied should cause adduction of the thumb.
- The facial nerve: stimulation by two electrodes placed anterior to the ear is possible, although facial muscles have reduced sensitivity to neuromuscular blocking agents which may lead to underestimation of the degree of blockade.[3]
- Lateral to the neck of the fibula, relating to the common peroneal nerve: stimulation gives rise to foot dorsiflexion.

Pulse oximetry

The introduction of pulse oximeters into routine clinical practice has created an economical, compact, non-invasive and efficient method of monitoring both pulse rate and oxygen saturation in the patient. The convenience of pulse oximetry has increased the range of patient monitoring routinely carried out during the induction of anaesthesia. Particular advantages during induction are where preoxygenation is required, during emergency anaesthesia and during difficult intubations.

The pulse oximeter connection to the patient is via a small lead, attaching a probe usually to a digit or earlobe (Fig. 4.24). The principle behind oximetry is that oxygenated haemoglobin and

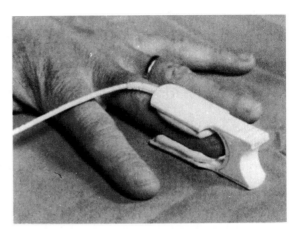

Figure 4.24 Pulse oximeter finger probe. (Reproduced from Aitkenhead & White 1996, with permission.)

deoxygenated haemoglobin have different absorbable spectra at different light wavelengths. Comparison of absorbencies at different wavelengths leads to an estimation of relative concentrations of oxygenated and deoxygenated haemoglobin. Microchip technology allows a rapid interpretation, resulting in pulse oximeters recording oxygen saturation of arterial blood. Within the probe diodes emit light, usually in the red/infrared wavelength: the transmitted light is detected on the other side of the probe by a photodetector. The signal from the probe is converted into a reflection of pulsatile arterial blood flow and amplified. The signal is often shown as a continuous trace and a numerical reading (Fig. 4.25).

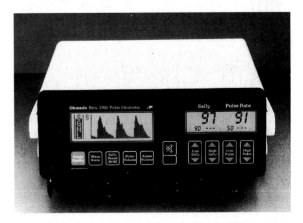

Figure 4.25 Pulse oximeter display module. (Reproduced from Aitkenhead & White 1996, with permission.)

The readings from pulse oximeters can be inaccurate if other forms of haemoglobin are present. Inaccurate readings may result when arterial oxygen saturation is less than 50%, if nail varnish or colouring is present, and if venous congestion occurs.

Pulse oximeters are generally straightforward to use, do not need time to calibrate or warm up, are non-invasive, and work regardless of skin pigmentation. Oximetry provides an overall assessment of the oxygen regimen being delivered to the patient's internal and external respiration mechanisms. In addition to being advantageous during all stages of anaesthesia, the use of pulse oximeters is particularly beneficial in recovery areas, in one-lung anaesthesia, in intensive care units, in areas where anaesthetized patients have to be monitored in poor lighting conditions, and in paediatric anaesthesia. There have, however, been reports of burns, particularly with the prolonged use of finger probes on children.[3]

Gas analysers

Carbon dioxide

The measurement of carbon dioxide levels in the final portion of exhaled gases roughly equates to the alveolar partial pressure of carbon dioxide. The continuous measurement and pictorial display of carbon dioxide concentration is known as capnography, giving rise to the common term capnographs for carbon dioxide analysers. Most capnographs work on the principle that carbon dioxide absorbs infrared radiation, as do any gases that consist of molecules with two or more different atoms. An infrared analyser can be used to measure the concentrations of other gases, such as nitrous oxide and the volatile anaesthetic agents. The presence of nitrous oxide in anaesthetic gases can lead to inaccurate readings of carbon dioxide concentration, and so analysers compensate automatically or require the operator to manually log in the percentage of nitrous oxide being used.

Capnographs have two methods for sampling the end-tidal gases to measure carbon dioxide concentration: mainstream and sidestream

systems. The mainstream requires a special connector to be inserted into the patient's breathing apparatus that includes a shaped pathway lined with sapphire glass. The analyser is located over the connector and the infrared beam is passed directly through the expired gases. The signal is then relayed to the electrical processor for display. Although connector and analyser are bulky compared to the sidestream system, the advantage is that there is no transit time for gas samples. The sidestream system requires a gas sample to be drawn from an inline connector, through narrow-bore tubing, often with a moisture trap, before entering the analyser. The transit time for the sample to reach the analyser, should, with the correct tubing, only add 1 second or less to the response time of the analyser, with no significant modification of the signal.[11] The display of a continuous trace of end-tidal carbon dioxide concentration is more valuable for interpretation by anaesthetists than values alone.

Capnography is useful in the assessment of adequate ventilation and allows the monitoring of any modification to normocapnia when desired. The measurement of end-tidal carbon dioxide concentration is useful in the diagnosis of oesophageal intubation, embolism (air, pulmonary or fat), rebreathing, disconnection and malignant hyperpyrexia. Some capnographs also measure nitrous oxide, oxygen and respiratory rate.

Oxygen

In monitoring the oxygen concentration of inspired gases the anaesthetist can ensure that the required percentage of oxygen is being delivered to the patient. This usually requires the use of a galvanic oxygen analyser (Fig. 4.26) placed in the inspiratory limb of the breathing system. These analysers are relatively cheap, are battery powered, not affected by humidity, and are calibrated using air.

Respirometer

Expired gas volumes may be measured by a respirometer. The Wright anemometer is one of

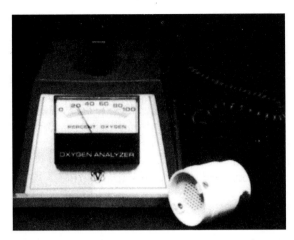

Figure 4.26 Galvanic oxygen analyser. (Reproduced from Aitkenhead & White 1996, with permission.)

the most popular, measuring volume as expired gases pass over the vanes within the respirometer (Fig. 4.27). The rotation rate of the vanes is proportional to gas flow, as indicated by a needle and dial. At high tidal volumes the Wright respirometer may overread, and underread at low volumes. Inaccuracy and malfunction may occur if the vanes become damp, as when in continuous use with expired – and hence humidified – gases. Electrical types of respirometer are available but are rarely used in routine clinical practice, owing to the expense and the exacting calibration.[3,8]

Temperature monitoring and regulation

The potential problem of intraoperative hypothermia exists for many patients undergoing long surgical procedures. Age and ambient temperature are probably the most influential factors. Other relevant factors have been indicated, such as the duration of surgery and anaesthetic drugs. The delivery of a general anaesthetic depresses the thermoregulatory centre and represses the patient's capacity to maintain body temperature. The use of muscle relaxants ablates striated muscle tone, one of the major sources of heat production in the body. Other potential reasons for hypothermia include:

- the use of anaesthetic agents
- the use of neuromuscular blocking agents
- the use of morphine
- surgical exposure
- ambient theatre temperature

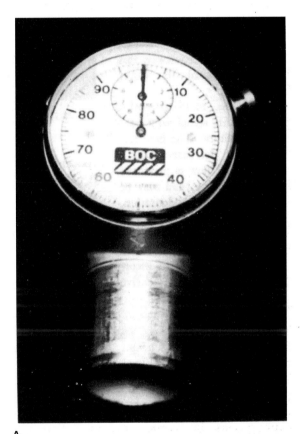

A

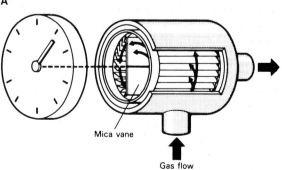

Mica vane

Gas flow

B

Figure 4.27 A: Wright respirometer. B: Diagrammatic representation of the mechanism. (Reproduced from Aitkenhead & White 1996, with permission.)

- decreased central nervous system activity due to premedication
- type and length of surgery
- age (old and young patients are particularly susceptible)
- inactivity (long intraoperative times)
- unconsciousness
- spinal and epidural anaesthesia, causing vasodilatation and loss of muscle tone.

There are a number of steps that can be taken to assist in maintaining the patient's body temperature, such as control of the environmental temperature, the use of blankets, the use of a space blanket and the use of a warming mattress on the operating table.

There are two main considerations in temperature monitoring: the patient's core temperature and their peripheral temperature. Core temperature is the central body temperature, and is influenced far less than peripheral temperature by the external environment. It is classically defined as the temperature of the blood leaving the heart.[12] Core temperature may be monitored but needs invasive methods: common sites are the lower oesophagus, nasopharynx and rectum. Measurement and monitoring is usually via single use or reusable temperature probes, which are mostly used in cardiac surgery, other major cases and intensive care units.

Peripheral temperature monitoring will reflect the influence of the external environment temperatures on the body 'shell', and is liable to much greater variation. These variations will be most extreme at the peripheral sites, such as the hands and feet, and reflect the fact that normal body temperature varies according to the site at which it is measured.[12] Thermometers, infrared and electronic monitoring devices are available, but the initial assessment of patient temperature for most routine cases is by vision and touch by members of the theatre team.

Levels of monitoring

The minimum levels of monitoring may vary according to the type of surgery to be undertaken and the individual patient's condition. The preoperative assessment of the patient by the anaesthetist, along with the expected changes due to surgical or anaesthetic procedures, will indicate the type of monitoring required. Table 4.3 categorizes the types of operative procedure and suggests monitoring as either essential or desirable. The standards published by the Association of Anaesthetists of Great Britain and Ireland[10] are becoming generally accepted, superseding those of Sykes.[13]

Table 4.3 Essential and desirable patient monitoring.

Operation category	Monitoring	
	Essential	*Desirable*
Minor		
Less than 30 minutes Inhalational face mask GA	Pulse: palpation stethoscope, finger plethysmograph, ECG Indirect arterial pressure	Pulse oximeter
Medium		
Less than 3 hours Relatively healthy patient blockade,	As for minor Expired volume if IPPV employed	End tidal carbon dioxide, Neuromuscular
Endotrachael anaesthesia Blood loss <10% of blood volume		Temperature
Major		
	ECG	Neuromuscular blockade
Longer than 3 hours	Pulse oximeter	
Blood loss >10% of blood volume	Direct arterial pressure	
Operations on: chest central nervous system cardiovascular system	Central Venous Pressure Blood loss measurement Urine output Temperature: patient, blood warmer, mattress, inspired gas Blood gas analysis Serum potassium concentration Coagulation status	

From Sykes[13]

Pharmacology

The anaesthetic drug cupboard contains a vast array of drugs, reflecting the variety of types of anaesthetics, the fact that more than one drug is available for any one purpose, and that research is continuing to search for the ideal drug.[14]

Names of drug groupings, such as premedication, triad of anaesthesia, reversal agents, hypotensive agents, locals and emergency drugs, are commonly used for the categories of drugs that contribute to an anaesthetic. The following section is not intended solely to specify drugs and their actions, but to briefly outline the rationale for their use.

The practitioner does not need to know anaesthetic pharmacology to the same depth as that of the experienced anaesthetist, but may need to know the individual preferences of many anaesthetists; this requires a working knowledge of a wide variety of drugs. The research stages of new pharmacology often involve anaesthetic practitioners assisting the anaesthetist with trials and research. With this in mind some drugs are included that have just been or are about to be launched at the time of writing. Drug names will be in the format of the British Pharmacopoeia nomenclature.

PREMEDICATION

Ideally this part of the anaesthetic should be prescribed by the anaesthetist who will be delivering the general anaesthetic. The anaesthetic preoperative assessment will highlight any predisposing factors that may influence the premedication and subsequent anaesthetic management. The anaesthetic regimen for an individual patient may be discussed with the practitioner, particularly when the patient requires unusual or non-routine management. As discussed earlier in this chapter, an important aspect of receiving and checking a patient into the department is the identification of any prescribed premedication, specifically the drug dosage and the time it was given. The practitioner should be familiar

enough with the routine drugs of premedication, the rationale for their use and their desired effects and possible side effects, to be able to evaluate the status of the patient and plan their care. The following considers the rationale of premedication and some common drugs used as premedicants.

- **Allay anxiety** It is increasingly recognized that the preoperative visits from both medical and non-medical staff play a significant role in relieving the anxiety of the patient.[8] If the visit from the anaesthetist has not done so an antiolytic may be prescribed: often a benzodiazepine is most effective.[8]
- **Reduction of secretions** Anaesthetic agents such as ether and ketamine are known to stimulate bronchial and pharyngeal secretions; although these agents are used far less now, the use of anticholinergic drugs counteracts this effect. Anticholinergics are still prescribed, as secretions are also stimulated by the presence of an airway or endotracheal tube in the oral/nasal cavities and by gaseous inductions in small children. A drying agent may be prescribed for predictable events, such as oral and nasal operations, or unpredictable events such as laryngeal stridor and coughing, caused by vocal cord irritation by secretions. The commonly used anticholinergics are atropine, hyoscine and glycopyrronium.
- **Sedation** Sedation does not always imply relief of anxiety. Sedative drugs are often only given on the request of adult patients. The use of a sedative as part of a premedication may reduce the amount of induction agent required and allow a smoother induction,[3] but these drugs often have a fairly long action and may still be effective after the anaesthetic has been discontinued. The opiate analgesics, benzodiazepines and phenothiazines, all produce some sedation. Midazolam given orally 20 minutes before the operation ensures a relaxed, drowsy patient. Although it is only available in injection form in the United

Kingdom (oral use is outside the product licence) it is often used in oral solution outside the United Kingdom, particularly in children.

• **Reduce postoperative nausea and vomiting** The reduction of postoperative vomiting and nausea may be achieved by an antiemetic premedication. However, opiate drugs given during the procedure are often the cause of postoperative vomiting and nausea. Therefore, antiemetics given intravenously during the anaesthetic would have more effect.[8] Droperidol and the phenothiazines, along with metoclopramide, have a different site of action from the antihistamine and anticholinergic drugs, but all can be used as antiemetics. Ondansetron (Zofran) 8 mg orally given with premedication drugs, or 4 mg i.v. perioperatively, is effective in reducing postoperative nausea and vomiting, especially in gynaecological procedures.

• **Produce amnesia** The use and effectiveness of a premedication to produce amnesia is an area of debate, particularly regarding children. There is a question as to whether retrograde amnesia is achievable, whereas amnesia after administration of the benzodiazepine drugs, such as midazolam and particularly lorazepam, is occasionally desirable.[8]

• **Reduce amount, and increase pH, of gastric contents** In patients with a higher risk of vomiting and regurgitation, consideration may be given to reducing the pH of gastric contents and/or promoting gastric emptying. Sodium citrate 0.3 M may be used to neutralize the acidity of the stomach contents, and metoclopramide will promote gastric emptying, in addition to its antiemetic properties.[8]

• **Diminish vagal reflexes** In order to diminish vagal reflexes, specifically bradycardia, during surgery, anticholinergic drugs such as atropine may be prescribed. Vagal bradycardia may be caused by traction of the eye muscles, which may lead to arrhythmias. The use of opiate and some non-depolarizing muscle relaxants, such as atracurium and vecuronium, together with some surgical stimulus, has been associated with bradycardia, as has the induction of anaesthesia with halothane, particularly in children. A second bolus of suxamethonium,

which may also lead to asystole, has also been implicated. Atropine should always be given prior to a second dose of suxamethonium.[8]

• **Reduce sympathoadrenal responses** Endotracheal intubation is sometimes accompanied by a sympathoadrenal stimulus causing tachycardia and hypertension. These reactions are not welcome in the healthy patient and are potentially hazardous or fatal in the compromised patient. Beta-blocking drugs may be considered to preclude the above reactions, but caution should be exercised with asthmatic patients.

Drugs commonly used for premedication are:

• papaveretum and hyoscine (scopolamine)
• lorazepam: very long-acting
• diazepam (occasionally with metoclopramide): long-acting
• temazepam: shorter-acting than lorazepam
• midazolam: very short-acting
• morphine and atropine
• promethazine and atropine.

INTRAVENOUS INDUCTION AGENTS

The term induction has been defined by Yentis et al[3] as 'transition from the awake to the anaesthetised state, although the end point is difficult to define'. Intravenous induction agents are widely used for routine anaesthetics in adults, and almost all take effect in one arm–brain circulation period.[8] Intravenous induction allows the rapid onset of anaesthesia, masking the excitable stage of anaesthesia. Aitkenhead and Smith[8] list 17 ideal properties of an intravenous anaesthetic agent, only to conclude that none of the agents presently available meets all these requirements. Research continues to identify an ideal drug for a specific purpose, but owing to the numerous facets of anaesthesia, there is no such thing as the ideal drug that will do everything.[14]

Since its first use in 1934, sodium thiopentone has been the most widely used intravenous induction agent; however, the regular use and ever-increasing popularity of propofol over the last 7 years has proved it a major rival. Sodium thiopentone has been popular because of its well researched, relatively stable properties. In addition to Aitkenhead et al's list, Jameson[15] identifies similar characteristics. However, of relevance to the practitioner is the further feature identified by Yentis et al[3] of propofol being water soluble, and not requiring reconstitution before use. The short-acting barbiturates thiopentone and methohexitone both require reconstitution, which is often a task requested of the anaesthetic practitioner. Both thiopentone and methohexitone, once reconstituted, should be stored in a refrigerator and used within 24 hours. The main advantage of propofol over both the barbiturates and other intravenous induction agents is its rapid recovery time, with little hangover effect, which is useful in the ever-increasing number of day-case surgical procedures. The disadvantages of propofol are pain on injection and reported marked drops in blood pressure.[14] The latest intravenous induction agent currently undergoing extensive clinical trials is pregnenolone. Its advantages seem to be no pain on injection, a rapid and smooth induction, a short duration of action and cardiovascular stability. If pregnenolone meets expectations it is likely to become very popular; like propofol, it is formulated in soya bean emulsion and therefore presents as a white milky liquid.[14]

The intravenous induction agents are:

- **Barbiturates**
  —Thiopentone: ultrashort acting (5–10 minutes), is generally a smooth induction, with dose-related depression of myocardium and respiratory centre;
  —Methohexitone: shorter acting than thiopentone, useful when brief anaesthesia is required, cardiovascular depression less pronounced than with thiopentone.

Both these barbiturates have a rapid induction time, no first stage and a brief second stage of anaesthesia. Dangerous in hypovolaemia, especially if given rapidly. Adult dosages: thiopentone 3–6 mg/kg i.v.; methohexitone 1–1.5 mg/kg i.v.

- **Etomidate** Non-barbiturate intravenous induction agent with little cardiovascular depression. Pain on injection with potential excitatory effects. Adult dosage: 0.3 mg/kg i.v.; gives narcosis lasting 6–10 minutes.

- **Ketamine** An intravenous agent said to produce dissociative anaesthesia; with good analgesic properties, it preserves pharyngeal and laryngeal reflexes. It has a stimulating effect on the heart, increasing the rate and raising the blood pressure by up to 25%. It may cause vivid dreams or hallucinations, which can be frightening, most commonly in patients 20–60 years old. Contraindicated in patients with a history of cardiovascular accidents, hypertension or psychiatric instability. Ketamine is presented in solutions of three different strengths, 10 mg/ml, 50 mg/ml and 100 mg/ml. Dosage is 1–2 mg/kg i.v. for induction, administered slowly.

- **Propofol** First clinical use was in 1986. Propofol allows a smooth induction with rapid recovery and no hangover. Reports of pain on injection are common: some anaesthetists may give a prior injection of lignocaine, or add lignocaine to the propofol. A rapid recovery and reorientation make it the agent of choice for day-case surgery and short operations. It has also been identified as suitable for total intravenous anaesthesia and intravenous sedation.[3] Propofol has some antiemetic effect and hypotension is common. Not licensed for children under 3 years, nor for sedation of children of any age. Adult induction dosage 1.5–2.5 mg/kg i.v.

MUSCLE RELAXANTS

Muscle relaxants were first used to produce neuromuscular blockade in the early 1940s, when D-tubocurarine was introduced. They can be categorized as either depolarizing or non-depolarizing. By specific impairment of the neuromuscular junction all muscle relaxants enable light levels of anaesthesia to be induced with adequate relaxation of the skeletal muscles. Patients who have received a muscle relaxant require assisted or controlled ventilation until the drug has been inactivated or antagonized. Table 4.4 outlines some of the properties of muscle relaxants.

Table 4.4 Properties of muscle relaxants

Drug	Initial dose (mg/kg)	Onset time (min)	Duration of action (min)
Alcuronium	0.15–0.3	3–5	20–40
Atracurium	0.3–0.5	1.5–2	20–30
Doxacurium	0.025–0.08	4–5	100–200
Gallamine	1–2	1–2	20–30
Mivacurium	0.07–0.15	1.5–2	10–15
Pancuronium	0.05–0.1	2–3	40–60
Pipecuronium	0.07–0.08	2.5–3	90–120
Rocuronium	0.06–0.08	1–2	30–50
Tubocurarine	0.25–0.5	3–5	30–50
Vecuronium	0.05–0.1	1.5–2	20–30
Suxamethonium	1–1.5	0.5–1.5	2–5

Non-depolarizing muscle relaxants

The earlier non-depolarizing muscle relaxants, tubocurarine, gallamine, alcuronium and pancuronium, are giving way to vecuronium and atracurium. These agents, however, all have a different duration of action and varied side effects, and so the choice is based on the patient's condition and the duration of relaxation required. The onset of action is an average of 2–3 minutes, and duration varies between agents from 20 to 60 minutes.[3] The reversal of non-depolarizing muscle relaxants is required by the administration of an anticholinesterase. Mivacurium and rocuronium are the most recent of the non-depolarizing agents, and clinical trials are being carried out on doxacurium and pipecuronium.

- **Alcuronium** Temporary hypotension may follow injection. Anaphylactic reactions have been reported. Excretion via renal system.
- **Atracurium** Histamine release may occur. The drug is without vagolytic or sympatholytic properties. Advantage over other non-depolarizing muscle relaxants in patients with renal or hepatic impairment, as it is degraded by Hofmann elimination (the rate of degradation relying on body pH and temperature), thus excretion is not dependent on the function of the renal or hepatic systems. Duration of action may be prolonged in hypothermia.

- **Doxacurium** Advocated for long surgical procedures where cardiovascular stability is necessary. Similar to pancuronium but with cardiovascular stability, depending on dosage neuromuscular blockade may last up to 3 hours. It is excreted via renal and hepatic routes unchanged.
- **Gallamine** Causes marked tachycardia. Crosses the placental barrier more readily than other muscle relaxants. Renal elimination.
- **Mivacurium** Histamine release may occur with large doses. Minimal cardiovascular changes. Proposed as an alternative to suxamethonium, particularly in children, as onset and recovery are faster than in adults although not faster than suxamethonium. Eliminated rapidly, mainly via the renal system.
- **Pancuronium** No significant histamine release or significant changes in blood pressure. May cause increases in heart rate. Renal and hepatic elimination.
- **Pipecuronium** More potent than pancuronium and displays similar actions, although with fewer cardiovascular effects. No histamine release, with less than 50% excreted via kidneys.
- **Rocuronium** Fast onset of action. Good intubating conditions: 30–90 seconds following administration. Minimal cardiovascular effects and no significant amounts of histamine released. Excreted via hepatic system.[14]

- **Tubocurarine** Histamine release is common and may cause an erythematous rash. May cause ganglion blockade associated with vasodilatation hypotension. Excretion renal and hepatic.
- **Vecuronium** Minimal histamine release, sympathetic blockade and vagolytic effects, therefore minimal effect on blood pressure and pulse rate. Renal and hepatic elimination.

Depolarizing muscle relaxants

The only depolarizing agent in current clinical use is suxamethonium, which gives rapid and profound muscle relaxation, allowing for rapid intubation; it has a brief duration of action (3–5 minutes in the average patient). One characteristic of suxamethonium absent from non-depolarizing agents is the initial period of muscle fasciculation following administration. The disadvantages are the potential side effects, such as arrhythmias, bradycardia after a second dose, hyperkalaemia, postoperative muscle pain, and with prolonged administration the blockade resembles that of a non-depolarizing agent (dual block).

Reversal of muscle relaxants

All of the non-depolarizing muscle relaxants are reversed by the action of anticholinesterase agents. Clinically the major acetylcholinesterase inhibitor is neostigmine, which is active within 1 minute of administration. Neostigmine is routinely administered intravenously with anticholinergic agents such as atropine or glycopyrronium. These counteract the muscarinic actions of neostigmine, particularly bradycardia and increased bronchial and pharyngeal secretions. Neostigmine is also used to treat myasthenia gravis.

Neostigmine causes muscarinic stimulation, which presents as bradycardia, increased gut motility, salivation, sweating and potential bronchospasm. These side effects may cause postoperative problems and delay full recovery of the patient. Dosage for the reversal of non-depolarizing blockade is 0.04–0.08 mg/kg i.v. with 0.02–0.04 mg/kg atropine or 10–20 µg/kg glycopyrronium.

Depolarizing muscle relaxants do not require the administration of a reversal agent. They are metabolized in and around the neuromuscular junction with the aid of the enzyme plasma cholinesterase. Plasma cholinesterase is normally found in sufficient concentrations to metabolize suxamethonium. Patients sensitive to the actions of suxamethonium, with lower levels of plasma cholinesterase, may present with respiratory paralysis for 2 hours or more: treatment is to prolong the anaesthesia with artificial ventilation until recovery occurs. This complication of suxamethonium is often referred to as scoline apnoea.

INHALATIONAL ANAESTHESIA

Ether and chloroform were the original, and often the only, anaesthetic agents used. Pharmacological and pharmacokinetic developments, along with aspects such as the flammable nature of ether, have led to the limited use of these early agents in most western countries. This section will consider anaesthetic inhalational agents, both volatile and gaseous.

Oxygen

Oxygen is the most important inhalational agent delivered to the patient: the methods of oxygen delivery are discussed elsewhere in this chapter. Oxygen is a tasteless, colourless and odourless agent, presenting as a gas at pressures of 1 atmosphere and temperatures exceeding –183°C. Hospitals that use more than 150 000 litres of oxygen per week are often supplied by a liquid oxygen tank. The liquid oxygen is surrounded by a double-layered casing, with either a vacuum similar to a thermos flask or insulating particles between the layers. Liquid oxygen is stored at a temperature of –150 to –175°C. Portable supplies are available in cylinders.

Oxygen has various characteristics the practitioner should be aware of:

- Oxygen supports fuel combustion.
- The use of grease or oil as lubricants is highly dangerous, as they form an explosive mixture with oxygen under pressure.

- Increases in the oxygen content of arterial blood lead to direct vasoconstriction.
- The delivery of high percentages of oxygen to patients with chronic bronchitis may lead to carbon dioxide narcosis, owing to the patient's adjusted physiology to high carbon dioxide retention. This may affect central and peripheral chemoreceptors and lead to ventilatory failure.

Nitrous oxide

Nitrous oxide is a faintly sweet-smelling colourless agent, available in cylinders. Pipeline nitrous oxide is supplied via a manifold of cylinders. This agent is non-irritant and is not flammable, but will support combustion of fuels where there is no oxygen, as in high temperatures (above 450°C), when nitrous oxide breaks down into oxygen and nitrogen. It is recognized as a good analgesic, hence its use in Entonox, but has poor anaesthetic properties. It has a minimal effect on the heart rate and blood pressure, and no effect on renal or hepatic function. Nitrous oxide expands in body cavities containing air, passing from the blood into cavities much quicker than nitrogen can diffuse out, as it is 40 times more soluble. Used as a carrier gas for volatile agents and oxygen in concentrations of 50–66%.[3] Uptake and recovery times are rapid and it is excreted unchanged via the lungs.

Carbon dioxide

Carbon dioxide is a colourless agent with a pungent aroma. It is produced commercially and is available in cylinders. Until recently it was used mainly to increase the rate and depth of respiration during anaesthesia and to assist blind nasal intubation by causing hyperventilation. Recent literature seems to suggest that the use of carbon dioxide is potentially hazardous owing to the effects of hypercapnia. It has been suggested that to avoid such hazards, cylinders of carbon dioxide are removed from anaesthetic machines. Some of the effects of hypercapnia are increases in tidal volume, respiratory rate, heart rate and arterial blood pressure. The practitioner should be aware of any local policies regarding the anaesthetic use of carbon dioxide cylinders. Delivery of 5% or less will cause an increase in rate and depth of respiration in the healthy; over 10% causes drowsiness; and at 30% the patient becomes comatose. High concentrations initiate the onset of vasodilataton, raised blood pressure, flushed appearance and rapid pulse, followed by cardiac irregularities and falling blood pressure, potentially leading to death. Carbon dioxide is used in laparoscopic surgery to inflate the abdominal cavity (see Chapter 5).

Entonox

Entonox is a combination of 50% oxygen and 50% nitrous oxide, supplied in cylinders. The primary use of Entonox is in maternity departments for obstetric analgesia, although it is carried on board paramedic/ambulance transport for trauma-related analgesia. It is usually self-administered by patients via a demand valve: if the patient loses consciousness the mask is dropped and ambient air is inhaled. There are minimal cardiovascular, neurological or respiratory side effects. Entonox in cylinders that have been allowed to become cool (0 to 7°C) will separate out. The nitrous oxide will liquefy, so that if the cylinder is used oxygen will be delivered first, followed by nitrous oxide in dangerous concentrations that may cause death. Cylinders must therefore be kept horizontally at a constant temperature above 5°C. Cylinders that have been exposed to cold conditions must be rewarmed according to recommendations and guidelines from the manufacturer.

Helium

Helium is an inert gas which is less dense than nitrogen. The flow of a mixture of oxygen and helium is greater than that of oxygen and nitrogen, thus the supply of alveolar oxygen in upper airway obstruction will be more efficient with a helium/oxygen mixture. Supplied in cylinders as helium and as a 21% oxygen and helium mixture.

Halothane

Halothane (fluothane) was first used clinically in 1956, and gained in popularity owing to its advantages over ether and cyclopropane of greater potency, non-irritancy and non-flammability. Unfortunately, 2 years after its introduction the first report of halothane hepatitis was published. Since 1958 the link between halothane and hepatitis has caused debate and controversy. Halothane is currently available, although its use has declined; it is still considered to be the agent of choice for upper airway obstruction.[3] A controversial recommendation from the Committee on Safety of Medicines in 1986 advised that halothane should not be used following a history of previous exposure and adverse reactions; previous exposure within 3 months, unless the indications are felt to be clinically overriding; a history of unexplained jaundice/pyrexia after previous exposure to halothane.

Halothane is a colourless liquid, said to have a pleasant smell. Inhalational induction with halothane is rapid and generally smooth, as is recovery. It is a poor analgesic and has significant effects on the heart rate and blood pressure. Arrhythmias may occur and the myocardium is sensitized to catecholamines, particularly injected adrenaline. Relaxation of skeletal muscle is common and the action of non-depolarizing muscle relaxants may be enhanced. Gravid uterine muscle is relaxed (dose related), and so halothane should be avoided in pregnancy. Halothane is non-irritant and the cough and swallow reflexes are lost early in inhalational induction, together with inhibition of secretions and bronchodilation; the benefits for difficult airway and upper airway obstruction are thus seen. Shivering may be observed during recovery. Induction with halothane often requires a gradual increase in the concentration of 0.5–5%; maintenance of anaesthesia is sustained with 0.5–2%. The colour coding for safe identification and filling procedure for halothane is red.

Enflurane

Enflurane (ethrane) was introduced 10 years after halothane and is a colourless volatile liquid

with an aroma not dissimilar to ether. Induction and recovery is rapid, although less potent and with less effect on the heart and circulation than with halothane. It potentiates the effects of non-depolarizing muscle relaxants to a greater degree than halothane or isoflurane, with dose-dependent uterine relaxation. There are reports of swings in depth of anaesthesia, particularly in children, and incidences of hiccoughs. Enflurane is best avoided in patients with a history of epilepsy, as convulsions may be triggered. Respiratory depression is greater than with halothane or isoflurane and tachypnoea is common, with reduced tidal volume and bronchodilation. Concentrations of 1–3% are generally used for maintenance of anaesthesia, with higher doses for inhalational induction. The colour coding for the safe identification and filling procedure for enflurane is orange.

Isoflurane

Isoflurane (forane) has the most stable cardiovascular properties of these three most popular volatile anaesthetic agents, but some hypotension is caused by peripheral vasodilatation. Synthesized in 1965 but not introduced until 1980, isoflurane has gained popularity despite being nine times as expensive as halothane.[3] Compared to the above two volatile agents isoflurane is irritant, and therefore coughing is more likely to occur. Small amounts (less than 0.2%) of isoflurane are metabolized within the body, therefore it has the lowest risk of hepatic impairment. Isoflurane is a colourless liquid with a strong aroma similar to ether. Uterine relaxation is dose dependent, with possible enhancement of non-depolarizing neuromuscular blockade. With induction concentrations ranging between 0.5 and 5%, maintenance of anaesthesia requires 1–2.5%. The colour coding for the safe identification and filling procedure for isoflurane is purple.

Desflurane

Desflurane (suprane) has a less powerful aroma than isoflurane and a very fast induction and recovery time. Inhalational induction may utilize concentrations of between 4 and 11%, giving surgical anaesthesia in 2–4 minutes. Maintenance of narcosis for surgery is between 4 and 6% when nitrous oxide is used. Desflurane is not recommended as an inhalational agent in paediatric anaesthesia owing to the potential of breath holding, apnoea, laryngospasm, coughing and increased production of pharyngeal and bronchial secretions. Neuromuscular blockade agents are potentiated. The main disadvantage appears to be expense and the specialized vaporizers required.

Servoflurane

Servoflurane is not yet licensed in the United Kingdom. There are reports of difficulty with its use in closed circuits, it being slightly inactivated by soda lime, although adverse results have yet to be reported. Servoflurane has similar clinical properties to isoflurane, with the advantage of being non-irritant and having a pleasant smell.[3,14]

ANALGESIA

Analgesia is one of the components of the triad of anaesthesia, thereby making it a basic constituent of general anaesthesia. Analgesia in its own right, however, plays a role in most western people's lives: the relief of pain is part of most cultural and sociological attitudes. The availability of mild pain-relieving agents from high-street pharmacists is taken for granted. This attitude to pain, and anticipated freedom from it, extends to patients' expectations of hospital treatment. The perception of pain, from 'Will the needle hurt', to major postoperative pain relief, demands a high degree of consideration from both prescribing and non-prescribing healthcare staff. The physiology of pain is closely connected with the psychological, hence the importance of individual patient care described earlier. Each of us has a personal perception of pain, based on environmental, sociological and physiological influences, in addition to our own pain threshold. Study of these aspects of pain has led to an increase in the number of pain clinics and the

development of equipment such as patient-controlled analgesia machines. The analgesic agents available to the anaesthetist are considerable in number, some of which will be described here. One method of describing an analgesic agent in relation to anaesthesia is proposed by Yentis et al[3]: 'Analgesic drugs are distinguished from anaesthetic agents by their ability to reduce pain sensation without inducing sleep'. The authors further discuss the difficulty of making the separation in clinical practice, i.e. opiates in sufficiently high doses will cause loss of consciousness. This semantic/practical dilemma highlights the potential side effects and interactions of analgesic agents.

Opiates are, by definition, drugs derived from opium. Pain relief and euphoria have been obtained from opium and morphine for centuries. Synthetic opiates have been available in increasing numbers from the 1930s, and current terminology for anaesthetic analgesia appears to be opioids or opioid analgesic drugs.

- **Morphine** is used as the baseline against which other opioids are compared, and so its properties are well described. Morphine is a very good analgesic, and although it has some side effects that are not desirable, it remains one of the most popular. Morphine has an effect on both the peripheral and the central nervous system, with stimulating and depressing effects on the central nervous system. Pain relief from morphine is wide ranging, but it is particularly effective against nagging dull pain rather than sharp occasional pain. Psychological and emotional effects from pain are depressed, the pain threshold is raised, leading to euphoria and drowsiness. The respiratory centre is depressed, affecting the rate rather than the tidal volume, with the very young and the old being most sensitive. Stimulation of the vagus nerve may cause bradycardia, and miosis is caused by stimulation of the oculomotor nerve. Other unwanted side effects include excessive histamine release, irritation, peripheral vasodilatation, constipation and delayed gastric emptying. The standard adult i.v. dose is 0.1–0.15 mg/kg.
- **Diamorphine** is an opioid analgesic which has less severe side effects than morphine, but

which is far more liable to cause addiction. Diamorphine acts for about half as long as morphine, but is about twice as strong.

• **Papaveretum** has effects akin to those of morphine and is used in analogous situations. Since 1991 preparations of papaveretum containing noscapine were contraindicated for women of childbearing age. However, preparations of papaveretum (Omnopon) were reformulated in 1993, excluding the agent noscapine. Side effects are similar to those of morphine, but papaveretum is about half the strength of morphine.

• **Pethidine** is a synthetic opioid analgesic about 0.1% of the strength of morphine, with similar effects but causing less respiratory depression and less likely to cause nausea and vomiting.

• **Fentanyl** is a synthetic opioid analgesic derived from pethidine and has very little effect on the cardiovascular system. Its uses are mostly intraoperative and it causes significant respiratory depression, being up to 100 times as strong as morphine.

• **Alfentanil** is significantly less potent than fentanyl, with a faster onset time and shorter duration of action. Similar effects and side effects to fentanyl.

• **Sufentanil** has similar effects to fentanyl and is over five times as potent as the latter. Although not available in the United Kingdom, it is used in the USA. The drug of choice in hypodermic darts for sedating elephants and rhinos.

• **Phenoperidine** is a synthetic opioid analgesic related to pethidine. Effective analgesic with respiratory depression and potential vasodilatation and hypotensive effects.

• **Buprenorphine** is 25 times more potent than morphine, compared to which it has a slower onset time but a much longer duration of action. Causes respiratory depression that cannot easily be counteracted by naloxone.

• **Meptazinol** has partial antagonistic properties for the respiratory depression caused by morphine. The analgesic effects are mostly reversed by naloxone, with less respiratory depression and sedation than morphine, compared to which it is 10 times less potent.

• **Nalbuphine** is an opioid analgesic used for premedication, interoperative analgesia and pain relief.

• **Remifentanil** is a synthetic opioid analgesic agent still undergoing trials and evaluation. It is claimed to be short-acting with a very fast elimination time. Not licensed for use in the United Kingdom.

In addition to the opioid analgesic agents, many non-steroidal anti-inflammatory drugs (NSAID) are available to provide analgesia. This group of drugs also provides anti-inflammatory and antipyretic actions, and their use ranges from the treatment of mild pain to postoperative analgesia. The possible side effects include rashes, defective coagulation and gastrointestinal disturbance. The effectiveness of these drugs on individuals is variable.

• **Naloxone** is an opioid antagonist used to counteract the unwanted side effects of opioid analgesic agents, but in doing so it reduces or abolishes the analgesia provided by the analgesic agent.

ANTIEMETICS

Nausea and vomiting, caused by some opioid analgesic agents and/or anaesthetic/surgical trauma, is a potential postoperative problem. Drugs such as metoclopramide and prochlorperazine have for some time been popular antiemetic agents. Ondansetron, a new antiemetic introduced in 1990, along with Granisetron, appears to be particularly effective in cases of severe vomiting.[14]

LOCAL ANAESTHESIA

Chemical agents employed for local anaesthesia generally have the same mode of action. Low concentrations have a delaying effect; high concentrations completely block the movements of ions across nerve cell membranes. This effect is not specific to nerve cells: other cells which are capable of excitation can also be affected. This leads to the rationale for the use of lignocaine in the control of cardiac arrhythmias. Smaller nerve fibres are easier to block than larger ones; autonomic, sensory and motor nerve fibres are usually blocked in a sequence. The sequence identifies initial sensory loss of temperature and pain followed by loss of motor function. As the action of these agents is primarily on nerve axons, the nearer the injected agent to the nerve the more effective it is. Higher concentrations and dosages equate to faster onset time and duration of action.

Local analgesia may be accomplished in three main ways: intravenously, by infiltration (surface or epithelial) and by conduction (regional blockade).

Intravenous regional anaesthesia (IVRA) was first described in 1908 by the German surgeon Karl Bier. IVRA is a technique whereby a limb, isolated from the circulation by use of a tourniquet, is injected with a local anaesthetic agent via a vein. One of the most popular techniques of intravenous regional anaesthesia is referred to as a Bier's block. The procedure usually involves the siting of an intravenous cannula into each hand. The limb is then exsanguinated, a double-cuff tourniquet is applied and the proximal cuff inflated, often to twice the systolic blood pressure. The local anaesthetic agent is then injected slowly; after 5–10 minutes the distal cuff may be inflated and the proximal deflated: this helps to reduce any discomfort the patient may experience.

Precautions regarding the use of tourniquets must be applied. The administration of a Bier's block has many potential hazards, and preparation of the patient and equipment is the obvious factor that will reduce the associated risks. All the equipment must be tested for leaks, all routine monitoring apparatus should be available, as should resuscitation equipment and drugs. Where possible the patient should be starved, and may also be sedated during the procedure. The technique should not be used in patients with sickle cell anaemia or trait, and careful consideration must be given to obese patients or those with severe hypertension and arteriosclerosis. The IVRA technique may be used on the lower limbs, although larger volumes may be required with possibly less effect. Lignocaine may be used as the local anaesthetic agent, although prilocaine (0.6 ml/kg of a 0.5% solution) is more popular and safer.[3]

Topical application was first described in 1884 by Koller, when he demonstrated the analgesic properties of cocaine in ophthalmology, at the suggestion of Freud.[7] Until recently the technique was only reliable when mucous or membranous tissue was selected, and it was widely used to facilitate intubation or in minor surgery of the eye or nose. The method of administration may be via pastes, ointments, soaked swabs or sprays, and the agents often used are cocaine, amethocaine and lignocaine. The topical application Emla cream (Eutectic Mixture of Local Anaesthetics), consists of lignocaine and prilocaine in a lanolin base and relies upon a reaction between the two agents which allows it to permeate through the skin. The application is covered by an occlusive dressing and provides analgesia 1–1.5 hours after application. Emla cream is particularly useful in paediatric anaesthesia prior to intravenous cannulation. Infiltration anaesthesia was first introduced by Schleich in 1892.[7] Prior to the introduction of Emla this technique was the only reliable method of anaesthetizing the skin and underlying tissues. Infiltration anaesthesia is useful for minor surgery and suturing, and may be used by the surgeon for deeper tissue manipulation.

The above techniques, although useful, have limitations in the size of the area that can be anaesthetized safely. Conduction anaesthesia overcomes this by blocking the sensory, and occasionally motor, nerves supplying an entire area. This may be achieved in one of several ways. The nerve may be blocked at a major branch by direct infiltration of the local anaesthetic agent, for example brachial plexus block, stellate ganglion block and facial nerve block. Alternatively, the nerves may be blocked where they enter the central nervous system, for example spinal and epidural techniques.

The agents used for the above types of local anaesthesia are as follows:

- **Cocaine** The first analgesic used in clinical practice. Unlike the other agents it has a marked vasoconstrictive action. Owing to the toxicity of cocaine its use is mainly surface, particularly in nasal surgery, occasionally in nasal intubation to prevent bleeding, and in ophthalmic surgery. The maximum safe dosage is 3 mg/kg, with a duration of action of up to 1 hour.

- **Procaine (Novocaine, Planocaine)** Seldom used because it is rapidly metabolized (short acting) by pseudocholinesterase. It is, however, only one-quarter as toxic as cocaine but has no topical effect. It has a marked vaso-dilatory action and is sometimes used during surgery on small vessels to combat arteriospasm. Maximum adult dose 500 mg and duration of action 30–45 minutes.

- **Lignocaine (Xylocaine, Lidocaine, Duncaine, Xylotox)** Probably the most frequently used local anaesthetic agent, owing to its favourable safety aspects compared to previous agents.[3] It has a rapid onset of action via all routes, is a very stable solution and is the standard against which all other local anaesthetic agents are compared. A range of strength solutions are available: injection and infiltration usually require a 0.25–0.5% solution, 1–2% for nerve blocks and epidurals, 4% (usually coloured pink) for topical anaesthesia of respiratory mucous membranes, and 10% spray for topical anaesthesia. The maximum recommended dose is 3 mg/kg plain and 7 mg/kg with adrenaline. A 1% solution has a duration of action of 1 hour, increasing to 1.5–2 hours with adrenaline. The primary use of lignocaine is probably infiltration, often combined with adrenaline, although it is a useful antiarrhythmic drug in ventricular tachycardia. Lignocaine is a constituent of Emla cream.

- **Prilocaine (Citanest)** Prilocaine is less toxic than lignocaine, and because of this it is recommended for use in intravenous regional anaesthesia as a 0.5% solution. The maximum safe dose is 5 mg/kg and 8 mg/kg with adrenaline. The duration of action is half again that of lignocaine, but the onset time is slower. It is a constituent of Emla cream.

- **Bupivacaine (Marcaine)** Although bupivacaine has a slower onset than lignocaine its duration of action is much longer – up to 4 hours in an extradural block and 12 hours in

some nerve blocks.[3] It is widely used in spinal and epidural anaesthesia, particularly for obstetrics, as it crosses the placental barrier more slowly and in smaller amounts than other agents. Solutions for conduction anaesthesia are generally 0.25–0.5%. Although a 0.75% solution gives a longer duration of action when given epidurally, this concentration is contraindicated in obstetrics because of its toxic effects.[3] Bupivacaine is contraindicated in IVRA as there is some indication that it may have a more toxic effect on the myocardium than other local anaesthetic agents.[8]

- **Amethocaine** Amethocaine is mostly used for surface analgesia, as it is rapidly absorbed from mucous membranes. It is contraindicated in inflamed, traumatized and highly vascular surfaces, and is used for spinals in the USA.

- **Addition of vasoconstrictors** Of the vasoconstrictors added to local anaesthetics, adrenaline is the most potent and popular. Adrenaline in a dilute solution (i.e. 1:200 000) is an effective vasoconstrictor when injected into the tissues. This is a valuable property when the drug is used with local anaesthetic agents, with the exception of cocaine. Adrenaline slows the absorption of the agent, thereby increasing its duration of action. In addition to this, because the agent is absorbed into the general circulation more slowly, the toxic effects are reduced and the safe dose is increased. The use of vasoconstrictors is absolutely contraindicated for use near end-arteries, digital ring and penile blocks, and in IVRA owing to the high risk of ischaemia.

- **Addition of hyaluronidase (Hyalase)** This is used as a 'spreading' agent. It is an enzyme which aids the dispersal and absorption of drugs through the interstitial spaces. Its use speeds the onset of analgesia and allows a greater area of analgesia to be produced for a smaller volume of solution. It may be of value in plastic surgery procedures where the injected local anaesthetic solution might otherwise distort the anatomy. There is a decline in popularity of this agent as its benefits are debatable.[3]

- **Addition of dextrose** Adding dextrose to a solution of local anaesthetic increases its specific gravity relative to that of the cerebrospinal fluid.

This technique is useful in order to utilize gravity and patient positioning to achieve or emphasize a spinal blockade in a specific region.

Hazards and complications

One of the first things to consider is infection. Infection following epidural or spinal anaesthesia may be catastrophic. It is therefore essential that strict asepsis be observed in all local techniques. Epidural and spinal procedures should be approached in the same manner as a surgical operation, with the anaesthetist gowned and gloved and the practitioner assisting in maintaining a sterile field and observing aseptic techniques.

The action of local anaesthetic agents depends on the pH of extracellular fluid. The pH of infected tissue is lower than normal, and therefore the effects of a local anaesthetic agent are reduced. Dental abscesses, for example, have to be treated before extraction can take place with the use of local anaesthetic drugs.

The toxic effects of infection can be alarming, and include either depression or stimulation of the central nervous system, with unconsciousness and/or convulsions. There may be vasomotor collapse and vomiting. Cardiac depression and even arrest may result. It is therefore essential that patients for local anaesthesia are adequately prepared, including being fasted. Barbiturates, muscle relaxants, vasopressors and equipment for artificial ventilation should always be readily available. Convulsions may be treated with reduced amounts of thiopentone (50 mg) or diazepam (2.5 mg).

VASOPRESSORS

These drugs cause vasoconstriction; some also affect the heart, the ultimate aim being to increase arterial blood pressure during anaesthesia. Vasopressors, particularly adrenaline, may also be used to extend the duration of action of local anaesthetics. Vasoconstriction is generally achieved by the sympathomimetic actions of these agents. The most commonly used include adrenaline, dopamine, dobutamine, ephedrine and methoxamine.

VASODILATORS

These agents are generally used to reduce blood pressure, which may be achieved by action on the vascular muscle of the veins, the arteries or both, to reduce the systemic vascular resistance. Drugs in this category include glyceryl trinitrate, sodium nitroprusside, isosorbide, hydralazine, salbutamol, labetalol and clonidine hydrochloride.

ANTIBIOTICS

These are drugs used to prevent or treat bacterial infections by killing bacteria or inhibiting bacterial replication. This group of drugs has a wide spectrum of bactericidal activity. Prophylactic antibiotics are an important aspect of patient care for many operative procedures. The timing of preoperative doses of antibiotics is critical: administration should be less than 1 hour before surgical procedure for maximum effect.

Examples of some common antibiotics and the specialty often related to them are given in Table 4.5.

Table 4.5 Common antibiotics and their use in surgery

Cefuroxime 1.5 g + metronidazole 500 mg	Colorectal surgery
Augmentin 1.2 g	Gynaecological procedures
Amoxycillin 3 g	Patients with underlying endocarditis

INTRAVENOUS SOLUTIONS

The preparation and administration of intravenous fluids, including blood products, is a common routine for anaesthetic practitioners. The administration of any fluid requires the same knowledge, responsibility and consideration as other drugs. The checking and preparation of fluids should therefore involve the same rigorous procedures as required for drugs drawn up in a syringe. The information present on the blood or fluid pack needs to be considered. Intravenous fluids are often divided into two categories, colloids and crystalloids. For intravenous purposes a colloid is described as a fluid that will initially remain within the cardiovascular circulation, which is most useful for replacing blood loss and less effective for electrolyte imbalance, and more expensive than crystalloids. Colloids include blood products, Hetastarch, gelatin derivatives and dextrans.[3]

A crystalloid may be described as an intravenous fluid that will cross a semipermeable membrane, thus allowing movement of electrolytes to correct any imbalance. Examples of crystalloids are saline 0.9% (normal saline), dextrose and Hartmann's solution.

There follows a brief description of some of the fluids used, categorized into intravenous solutions and blood products.

Intravenous solutions

- **Dextrose 5%** A means of giving water without causing haemolysis; dextrose is added to make the fluid isotonic. Also provides a small amount of energy source.
- **Sodium chloride 0.9% (normal saline)** Isotonic but slightly acidic to body fluid as its pH is 7 (body fluid 7.4). Rapid infusion may raise blood pressure for a short period, but excessive administration raises the salt content of the body, leading to fluid retention and oedema.
- **Dextrose saline 4.3%** Dextrose with 0.18% saline. Provides calories (energy), salt and fluid.
- **Ringer's and lactated Ringer's solutions (Hartmann's)** Contains sodium, potassium, calcium, chloride and lactate. Similar in composition to extracellular fluid and are known

as a 'balanced salt solution'. Widely used and useful for general fluid replacement.
- **Mannitol 10%** An alcohol excreted by the kidneys. Used as an osmotic diuretic. Dehydrates tissue and stimulates urine production.
- **Sodium bicarbonate 8.4%** Used to reverse acidosis, which usually follows cardiac or respiratory arrest. Usually only administered after results of blood gas analysis have been reviewed.
- **Dextrans (40, 70 & 110)** These are polymer carbohydrate solutions prepared by fermentation of sucrose, with an average molecular weight of 40 000, 70 000 or 110 000. They are known as 'volume expanders' due to their high molecular weight. Used to maintain circulating volume after haemorrhage, remaining in the circulation for up to 24 hours. They also have anticoagulant properties and are sometimes used as a prophylactic treatment for DVTs.
- **Haemaccel and Gelofusin** Gelatin-based plasma substitutes, used to maintain circulating volume in massive haemorrhage when blood is not available.
- **Hespan 6%** colloidal solution for plasma volume expansion, which has properties approximate to those of human albumin. The expansion of plasma volume may improve haemodynamic stutus for 24 hours or longer.

Blood and blood products

- **Whole blood** is rarely issued nowadays as so many by-products are taken from it. Usually issued as packed cells. Used mainly for replacement following haemorrhage but also has specialist applications (e.g., in obstetrics). Best substance available for replacement following haemorrhage, but should be treated with the utmost respect as it is expensive and a mismatched transfusion may be catastrophic.
- **Plasma and albumin** are two freeze dried products which have to be reconstituted with sterile water for injection. It is made from blood that has passed its expiry date and has a specific use in restoring proteins (e.g., in cases of burns).
- **Human albumin 4.5%** (formerly known as Plasma protein fractions (PPF)) Liquid

preparation which has largely replaced freeze dried plasma.

- **Fresh frozen plasma (FFP)** separated and frozen from whole blood. It retains its clotting factors and is therefore useful in patients who have had a massive transfusion of stored blood during surgery.
- **Cryoprecipitate** prepared from FFP and containing the clotting agent Factor VIII used to treat haemophilia.
- **Hyperimmune globulins** are antibody preparations derived from donated blood and are used to protect against several specific diseases such as Chicken Pox and German Measles. Gamma globulin protects against Hepatitis A for up to 6 weeks.

CONCLUSION

Following a routine surgical list, with its share of traumatic and difficult anaesthetic procedures, a senior consultant anaesthetist once remarked that 'a boring anaesthetic is generally a safe anaesthetic'.

Working in the anaesthetic areas we can appreciate that an 'uneventful' anaesthetic is a well prepared and safe anaesthetic, without detracting from the skills and preparation demonstrated when the unexpected happens.

The anaesthetic practitioner in preparing themselves with knowledge and skills, and the environment with care and consideration, will be able to assist in delivering a high standard of patient care to all those who require an anaesthetic.

REFERENCES

1. Association of Anaesthetists 1988 Assistance for the anaesthetist. The Association of Anaesthetists of Great Britain and Ireland, London.
2. Hogg C 1994 Setting the standards for children undergoing surgery. Action for Sick Children, London.
3. Yentis S M, Hirsch N P, Smith G B 1993 Anaesthesia A-Z–an encyclopaedia of principles and practice. Butterworth Heinemann, Oxford
4. Brigden R J 1989 Operating theatre technique. Churchill Livingstone, Edinburgh.
5. Association of Anaesthestists 1990 Checklist for anaesthetic machines. The Association of Anaesthetists of Great Britain and Ireland, London
6. Ward C S 1989 Anaesthetic equipment: physical principles and maintenance. Ballière Tindall, London.
7. Atkinson R S, Rushman G B, Alfred L J 1987 A synopsis of anaesthesia. Wright, Bristol
8. Aitkenhead A R, Smith G 1996 Textbook of anaesthesia. Churchill Livingstone, Edinburgh
9. Carrie L, Simpson P 1990 Understanding anaesthesia. Butterworth Heinemann, Oxford.
10. Association of Anaesthetists 1989 Recommendations for standards of monitoring during anaesthesia and recovery. The Assocation of Anaesthestists of Great Britain and Ireland, London
11. Parbrook G D, Davis P D, Parbrook E O 1992 Basic physics and measurement in anaesthesia. Butterworth Heinemann, Oxford
12. Closs J 1992 Monitoring the body temperature of surgical patients. Surgical Nurse 5(1): 12–16
13. Sykes M K 1987 Essential monitoring. British Journal of Anaesthesia 59: 901
14. Holt B L 1994 New drugs in anaesthesia. The Hospital Pharmacist 1: 36–38
15. Jameson P 1994 Principles of general anaesthesia. Surgery 12(3): 58–60

FURTHER READING

Dobson M B 1988 Anaesthesia at the district hospital. World Health Organization, Geneva.
Goudsouzian N G, Karamanian A 1987 Physiology for the anaesthesiologist. Appleton-Century-Crofts, New York
Green J H 1985 Basic clinical physiology. Oxford University Press, Oxford
James Mather S, Edbrooke D L 1982 Basic concepts for operating room and critical care personnel. John Wright, Bristol
Ostlere G, Bryce-Smith R 1980 Anaesthetics for medical students. Churchill Livingstone, Edinburgh.
Ponte J, Green D W 1986 Anaesthetics, intensive care and pain relief. Hodder and Stoughton, London
Sykes M K, Vickers M D, Hull C J 1981 Principles of clinical measurement. Blackwell Scientific, Oxford

5

Surgical preparation

M. Taylor   C. Campbell

The function of the operating theatre is to provide a suitable environment for the surgical team to perform surgery.

The theatre practitioner is a vital member of the surgical team and provides necessary support to both the anaesthetist and the surgeon as they aim to achieve their primary function: high-quality patient care. Previous chapters have discussed the organization and management of the operating department, legal issues facing theatre practitioners, risk management and anaesthetics. This chapter focuses on the role of the theatre practitioner in relation to surgery and thus is geographically based in the operating theatre itself.

The chapter begins with guidelines on the preparation of the theatre for an operating list (or case), and includes an overview of basic theatre equipment and how it should be checked. The 'tools of the trade' of the theatre practitioner are then considered, i.e. items commonly used in all operating theatres for surgery. This includes surgical instruments, sutures and staples, surgical drapes, gowns and gloves, and is followed by a consideration of the large amount of supplies required in an operating theatre. This includes swabs, fluids, wound dressings and drains, and an overview of the various implants used in surgery.

Finally, specialized equipment will be discussed. It is important for theatre practitioners to gain an understanding of such equipment, as technology is developing rapidly and its use is becoming increasingly common.

The description of items used aims to provide

the theatre practitioner with a certain knowledge and understanding, including a definition, their functions and uses; requirements; types; handling and cleaning; supply and storage. The focus is therefore the provision of skilled assistance to the surgeon and the scrub team.

Preparation of the theatre

Preparation of the theatre and all equipment within it is essential in order to ensure a safe environment for both patients and staff. General principles to consider are as follows.

1. *The theatre should be clean and dust free.* This is vital to ensure that contamination of surgical wounds does not occur and give rise to the possibility of infection.

Prior to the start of each operating session the theatre furniture, lights, surfaces and floor should be cleaned with detergent. The risk of acquiring infection from floors in the operating theatre is low and cleaning alone is usually adequate.[1] Detergents will usually suffice as infection rates are not influenced by the use of disinfectants.[2] The floor should be cleaned thoroughly after each operating session. Blood or body fluid spillages should be removed immediately using disinfectants; normal cleaning should follow (see Chapter 3).

Floors may be cleaned routinely by mopping with detergent and water. The detergent should be freshly prepared in a clean, dry bucket and accurately diluted for use. Buckets should be emptied and stored dry after use. Mop heads should be clean and dry prior to use and laundered afterwards.[1] Each operating theatre should have its own bucket and mop clearly labelled.

Standards of domestic care should be set by the hotel services manager and agreed with the theatre manager. These should include policies for cleaning between operations and at the end of operating sessions. Domestic staff should be trained to undertake the cleaning of all clinical and ancillary areas.

Portering staff should be employed to assist with the transfer of patients and the collection or delivery of supplies, and may undertake domestic duties.

These tasks may be undertaken by support workers trained to NVQ Level 1.

A visual inspection for cleanliness should be undertaken by the theatre practitioner. Cleaning must be carried out in accordance with national infection control guidelines and local policies, thus ensuring that high standards are met.

Daily damp cleaning with detergent of the horizontal surfaces of the operating room, for example ledges and shelves, is necessary. Research has shown that 90–99% of microbial contaminants from the air and other sources are deposited on such surfaces.[3]

High wall washing should be built into the planned preventive maintenance programme for each department to ensure a good general standard of cleanliness. This should be carried out at 3–6-monthly intervals in the operating theatre.[1] Proper cleaning of theatre surfaces will contribute to the control of airborne microorganisms that are carried on dust and lint.

2. *The operating list should be clearly displayed so that the theatre practitioner can prepare all necessary equipment and supplies.* From this list he or she should be able to ascertain the planned operation, the site (i.e. left or right), and the patient's name, sex, age and hospital number. This information must be clear and unambiguous, for example no abbreviations should be used and sites of operation should be written in full as right or left, not R or L. Fingers should be described as thumb, index, middle, ring and little, and toes should be described as hallux (big), second, third, fourth and fifth (or little).[4] This information allows the theatre practitioner to arrange the theatre equipment and furniture appropriately as well as alerting them to the need for items required for patient care. For example,

the age of the patient may determine the need for temperature regulation or pressure area care.

3. *All theatre furniture and equipment and instrument trays must be present in theatre.* The basic furniture and equipment required for an operating list includes the following:

- operating table
- operating lights
- suction apparatus
- electrosurgical equipment
- instrument trolleys
- bowl stands
- Mayo table
- a means of swab counting and disposal
- anaesthetic and patient monitoring equipment (see Chapter 4)
- stools for both standing and sitting.

Practitioners should also be aware of any specialized equipment that may be required for the type of surgery being performed, for example:

- tourniquets
- power tools
- air cylinders
- endoscopic equipment, including monitors
- light source
- insufflator
- microscope
- laser.

Instrument trays and supplementary instruments for each operation on the list should also be present in the operating theatre.

4. *Consumable items must be available.* Items commonly used during surgery include:

- sutures
- scalpel blades
- draping packs
- swabs
- dressings
- wound drains
- suction tubing
- lotions and fluids
- clinical/non-clinical waste bags
- non-sterile gloves.

Any other items required, such as implants, should be made available before the operating list begins.

A minimum stock of consumables should be held in each theatre, relevant to the type of surgery performed and the individual operations on a list. Theatre practitioners should be aware of the stock requirements of an individual theatre and maintain this level. The theatre should be fully stocked at the beginning of the list to avoid unnecessary delays and danger to the patient owing to the unavailability of an item such as suction tubing, for example.

5. *The scrub area should be well stocked.* A consistent supply of surgical gowns, gloves, nail-brushes, scrub solutions, face masks and non-clinical waste bags is needed for any operating list. Further protective equipment may also be required if high blood loss or aerosol of blood or fluids is expected (see Chapter 3).

6. *The necessary documentation must be available.* This includes:

- patient care documentation forms
- swab charts (if used)
- specimen/laboratory forms
- computer patient data records
- operation costing forms
- surgeons' preference cards/kardex.

Care documentation forms will include the preoperative care plan as well as the intraoperative record of care given.

Computer patient data records have now replaced the operation record register in some departments.

Operation costing forms are in daily use in the private sector and this practice is now moving into NHS hospitals, especially those with Trust status. This allows a more precise method of costing individual operations as well as allowing managers to charge specialist theatres for surgical sundries used, leading to a more cost-effective use of items.

Cards indicating surgeons' preferences are used in most operating departments. This allows the theatre practitioner to prepare for each surgical procedure with individual surgeons' preferences taken into account. This includes the type of skin preparation used, positioning of patient and equipment, specialized equipment, specific supplementary instruments, sutures and dressings and will reduce the risk of an extended anaesthetic caused by an item not being available.

PREPARATION OF EQUIPMENT

The theatre practitioner should be familiar with the basic operating theatre equipment, its maintenance and safety checks. Although equipment varies depending on the manufacturer, general guidelines can be offered. The amount of equipment stored in an operating theatre should be kept to a minimum, as it may be a source and route of spread of infection.[5]

Operating theatre table

The operating table is used for all surgical procedures and is capable of adjustment to give a variety of positions. A variety of operating tables are available, either manually or electronically operated. They may be adapted with the addition of accessories for specific types of surgery. Basic features are:

* brakes/mobility mechanism
* raising and lowering mechanism
* lateral tilting mechanism
* Trendelenburg/reverse Trendelenburg mechanism
* adjustable head and foot sections
* antistatic sectional mattress
* rotation of table top
* the table base should minimize obstruction to the theatre staff
* break-back mechanism
* chair/sitting mechanism.

An example is the Eschmann J series (Fig. 5.1). Other specialist tables are available for orthopaedic surgery, neurosurgery, and urological/gynaecological procedures, for example the Eschmann RX system (Fig. 5.2).

Preparation of the operating table must include the following:

* the antistatic mattress must be intact
* the table positions must be attainable
* all featured mechanisms must be working
* the table must be clean and dust free.

When using an electronically controlled operating table the theatre practitioner must take care to follow the manufacturer's guidelines in respect to the cleaning and charging of the unit.

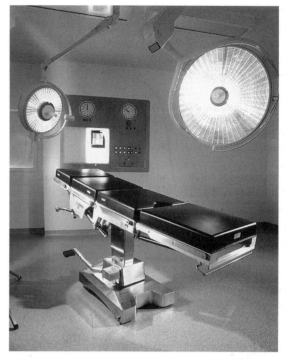

Figure 5.1 Eschmann J operating table.

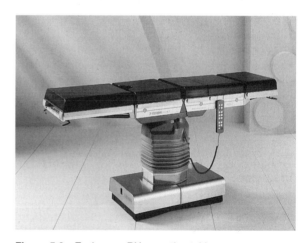

Figure 5.2 Eschmann RX operating table.

The depth of the antistatic mattress is an important consideration in preventing the formation of pressure areas. Operating table mattresses can be purchased in a variety of depths from 5 to 8 cm. Practitioners should be aware that British Standard

2891 (1992)[6] states that the depth of an operating table mattress should not be less than 7.5 cm.

There are many accessories available to assist with the safe positioning of the patient and ensuring surgical access. These include:

- arm boards/tables
- lithotomy poles
- arm gutters
- lateral positioning supports
- safety straps.

This is by no means an exhaustive list and theatre practitioners should familiarize themselves with other specialized accessories in use in orthopaedic and neurosurgical theatres.

After each use the table, mattress and accessories should be cleaned with detergent and warm water. Care should be taken when cleaning electronically controlled tables to avoid water entering the electronic mechanisms. If disinfection is required the use of aldehyde-based disinfectants and a hypochlorite solution (1000–5000 ppm) is recommended. Hypochlorite solution should not not come into contact with any metal components, which should be cleaned with alcohol, such as industrial methylated spirit 70%. The table should then be left to air dry.

The integrity of mattress pads should be checked regularly and at the end of an operating list they should be assembled on their edges on the table top to assist in drying out and to prolong mattress life. All table attachments should be stored on the accessory stand to avoid loss or damage. Any anaesthetic agents that spill on to the mattress should be wiped off immediately.

Theatre lighting

Good operating area illumination is essential in order to enhance surgical access. Operating theatre lights are designed to be shadowless and some can be focused. Basic features are:

- suspended from the ceiling
- single or multiple lights
- manoeuvrability – multiplicity of positions
- separate control panel away from operative site

- easily cleaned
- minimum maintenance
- sterile handle attachments for surgical team use
- shadow reduction owing to beams of light coming from a variety of angles.

Preparation of theatre lights must include:

- daily checking of function by qualified personnel and documentation of this
- if a multiple type of light is in use, all bulbs should be in working order
- light should be clean and dust free
- mobility should be checked
- stability should be checked, so that the light does not drift once positioned.

Suction apparatus

Suction apparatus is a source of negative pressure which allows the removal of particles from the surgical field. A variety of types of apparatus are available (Fig. 5.3):

- portable
- fixed
- disposable
- reusable.

Components required are:

- a suction unit, either wall mounted or portable
- suction tubing (sterile)
- a sterile sucker
- a suction bottle/liner.

Prior to the commencement of an operating list the following should be checked:

- cleanliness of the unit
- cleanliness of filter
- variable suction pressure attainable
- supplies of bottles/liners available
- availability of sterile tubing and suckers.

Electrosurgical diathermy units

Preparation of the diathermy units should include:

- regular maintenance and documentation
- equipment manuals should be available for staff information

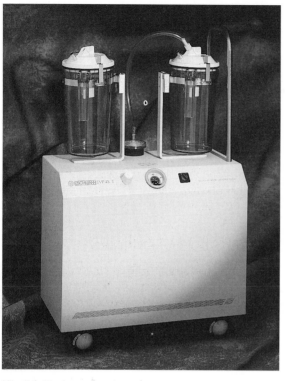
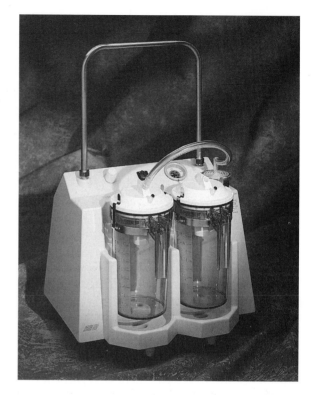

Fig. 5.3 Suction units.

- units should be clean and dust free
- availability of diathermy pads
- alarm system checked prior to patient's arrival
- wall socket checked for damage prior to use
- plug and lead checked for damage
- unit is plugged in
- foot pedals correctly attached and free from damage
- all connections securely attached
- power setting checked with the surgeon.

Other theatre furniture, including instrument trolleys, bowl stands, Mayo tables and stools, should be clean and dust free prior to the start of the operating list. Attention should be given to wheel mechanisms on trolleys and bowl stands to ensure free and smooth movement. Trolleys, Mayo stands and bowl stands should be made of stainless steel, aluminium or a steel covered in nylon. All trolleys should be abrasion and scratch free. The furniture should be correctly positioned for particular surgical procedures.

More detail on this and specialized equipment can be found later in this chapter.

REFERENCES

1. Ayliffe GAJ, Lowbury EJL, Geddes AM, Williams JD (eds) 1993 Control of Hospital Infection. A Practical Handbook, 3rd edn. Chapman & Hall, London
2. Danforth D, Nicolle LE, Hume K et al 1987 Nosocomial infections on nursing units with floors cleaned with a disinfectant compared with detergent. Journal of Hospital Infection 10: 229
3. Mallison GF 1975 Housekeeping in the operating suites. AORN Journal 21 February: 213–220
4. Medical Defence Union 1988 Theatre safeguards. Medical Defence Union, Medical Protection Society, Medical and Dental Defence Union of Scotland, National Association of Theatre Nurses, Royal College of Nursing, London.

5. Ayliffe GAJ, Collins BJ, Taylor LJ 1991 Hospital-acquired Infection. Principles and Prevention, 2nd edn. Butterworth Heinemann, Oxford

6. British Standards Institute 1992 British Standard 2891 Specification for operating table mattresses and mattress sections. British Standards Institute, Milton Keynes.

Instrumentation

Instruments vary in structure and design to fulfil a specific task, depending on the type of usage and the preferences of the individual surgeon. There is no standard nomenclature for surgical instruments and this can vary between hospitals, regions and manufacturers.

Most surgical instruments are made from a high grade of stainless steel, which appears to be the optimum material. Stainless steel is classified by the amount of iron, carbon and chromium it contains and the type chosen depends on the flexibility and malleability required for that particular instrument. It is the theatre practitioner's responsibility to know the particular function of each instrument and its proper use and care.

Instruments can be divided into six categories:

- sharps
- haemostatic forceps
- clamps
- grasping/holding
- retractors
- accessories.

SHARPS

Sharps include scalpels and scissors. Scalpels are used to incise and dissect: they are basically a handle to which disposable blades are attached. Examples are Bard–Parker handles, which are available in various lengths and sizes, with a range of disposable blades which are prepacked and sterile.

Scissors are also available in a variety of sizes for differing purposes and are used for dissection and for cutting of surgical materials. Scissor tips may be sharp or blunt and the blades straight or curved. Scissors used for

plastic or ophthalmic surgery may have a spring-action handle to ensure minimal hand movement and hold the blades in an open position (Fig. 5.4).

HAEMOSTATIC FORCEPS

These are generally called artery forceps and are used to achieve haemostasis. Most artery forceps have curved tips to allow visual access at the tip and all jaws are serrated. The serrations are of varying length and depth, depending on the use to which they will be put. These instruments are ring-handled with a rachet lock to allow varying degrees of pressure to be applied. Other uses for artery forceps are blunt dissection, tape bearing and for tagging sutures or swab tails when used in large body cavities. Lahey swabs (also known as dissecting swab or peanuts) may be mounted on to artery forceps for blunt dissection. Examples of artery forceps in general use are Dunhill's, Mosquitos and Spencer–Wells (Fig. 5.5).

CLAMPS

Clamps are used for vascular, cardiac and general surgery. Vascular and cardiac clamps are curved or double-curved. Surgeons use atraumatic clamps which enable a firm hold on the adventitia of the vessel without causing damage to the intimal layer. They may be either fully or partially occlusive. Partial occlusion allows the vessel to be worked on while allowing blood through the remainder, e.g. the Cooley anastomosis clamp. Most are ring-handled with rachet locks, allowing a controlled degree of pressure to be applied. The most commonly used vascular clamps are the Cooley and DeBakey designs (Fig. 5.6).

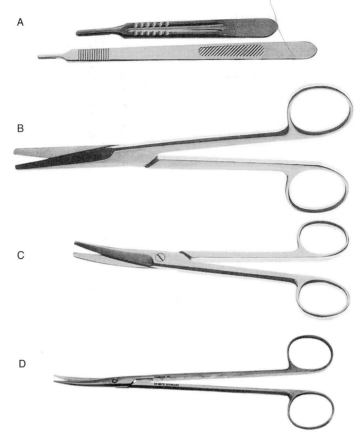

Figure 5.4 A. Bard Parker scalpel handles. B. Mayo scissors. C. Long curved dissecting scissors. D. Micro scissors.

Intestinal clamps can be subdivided into crushing or non-crushing (occlusion) types. This refers to whether the jaws are elastic or not, thus indicating the potential damage to the underlying tissues. Prior to bowel resection crushing and non-crushing clamps will be applied to the proximal and distal ends of the potential specimen, with the non-crushing clamps placed at the anastomosis sites. The bowel is then resected between the two clamps at either end of the specimen and the crushing clamps are removed with the specimen. Bowel clamps are used to prevent spillage of bowel contents into the peritoneum. Examples of non-crushing intestinal clamps are Doyen's, which are either straight or curved, and crushing intestinal clamps are Parker–Kerr's (Fig. 5.7).

GRASPING/HOLDING INSTRUMENTS

Grasping/holding instruments consist of tissue and dissecting forceps as well as needleholders, spongeholders and towel clips. Tissue forceps provide a secure grasp on tissues: they are usually ring-handled with a rachet lock. They have teeth or ridges in varying configurations which interlock and are therefore toothed or non-toothed. Examples are Babcock's and Allis tissue forceps (Fig. 5.8). These instruments are used to hold tissue for retraction or for dissection.

Dissecting forceps are used to grasp and hold tissues or for tying sutures. There are various designs. Smooth, serrated or atraumatic forceps are used to grasp delicate tissue. Toothed forceps are designed to grasp thicker tissue and are also used for skin approximation. Examples of non-

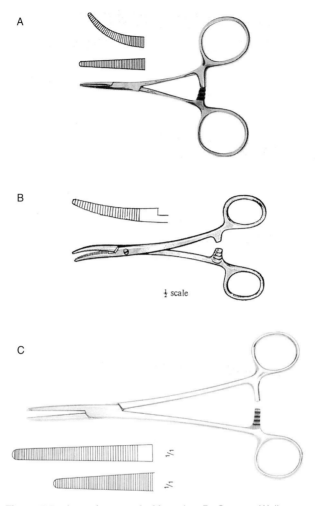

A

B

$\frac{1}{2}$ scale

C

Figure 5.5   Artery forceps. A. Mosquito. B. Spencer Wells.
C. Dunhill.

toothed forceps are DeBakey's and McIndoe's; toothed forceps in common use are Adson's and Bonney's (Fig. 5.9).

Needleholders are made in different shapes, sizes and styles, all designed to hold a needle securely when suturing tissue. Most are ring-handled but spring-handled types may be used for microsurgery. Needleholders are the most frequently abused instrument as they have constant metal-to-metal engagement. The jaws are short and most have tungsten carbide inserts to reduce wear from needles and prevent needles rotating in use. These can be replaced when worn. The inner surface of the jaws is composed of finely cross-serrated teeth. Needleholders need to be strong enough to allow the passage of a needle through relatively thick tissue but delicate enough to prevent damage to fine needles. The type of needleholder chosen depends on the size of needle required for a particular type of surgery. Examples are Crile–Wood's and Derf's (Fig. 5.10).

Spongeholders are available in various lengths. A swab is folded and placed within the jaws of the instrument and used for skin preparation prior to the commencement of surgery, as well as for tissue retraction and for the absorp-

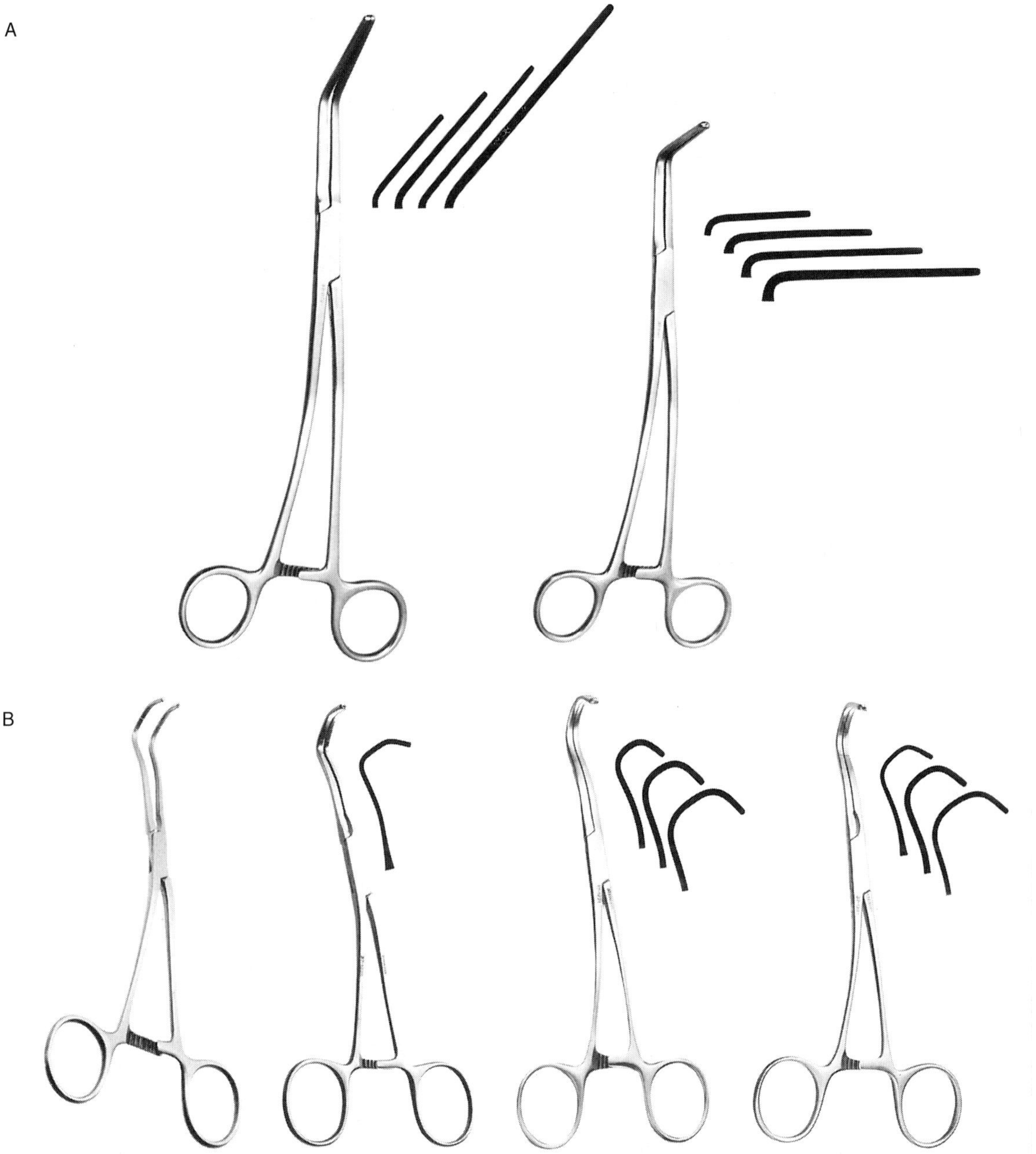

Figure 5.6 Multipurpose clamps. A. DeBakey aortic clamps. B. Cooley aortic clamps.

tion of blood in the surgical field, especially in the abdominal cavity. The holders may also be used to grasp or handle tissue.

Towel clips may be piercing or non-piercing and their use depends on the type of surgical drapes used. Non-piercing are now more commonly used as piercing clips cause damage to both drapes and underlying tissue.

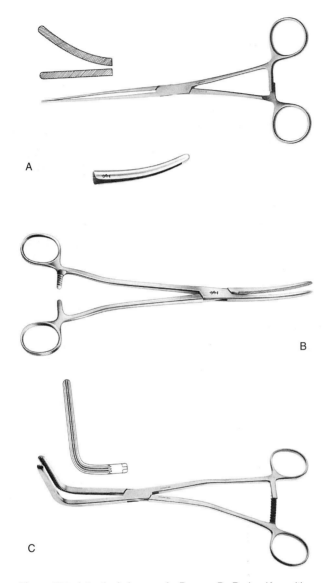

Figure 5.7 Intestinal clamps. A. Doyen. B. Parker Kerr with blade guard. C. Angled resection clamp.

RETRACTORS

Retractors are used to expose the surgical field and the size and type used depends on the site of surgery. There are two types: hand-held by a surgical assistant, and self-retaining, which are held open by their own action and are used to retract incisions for long periods. There are a variety of handles and blades available to suit the proce-dure. Examples of handheld retractors are Langenbeck's and Deaver's and self-retaining are Travers' and Balfour's (Fig. 5.11).

ACCESSORY INSTRUMENTS

Accessory instruments include suction, probes/dilators and dissectors. Suction instruments are available in various sizes and lengths:

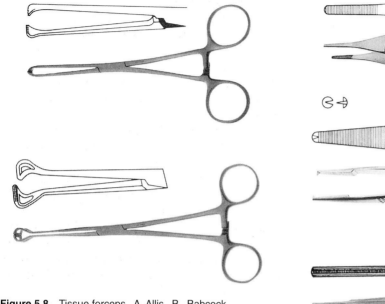

Figure 5.8 Tissue forceps. A Allis. B. Babcock.

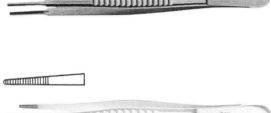

Figure 5.9 Dissecting forceps. A. Adson. B. Bonney. C. DeBakey. D. McIndoe.

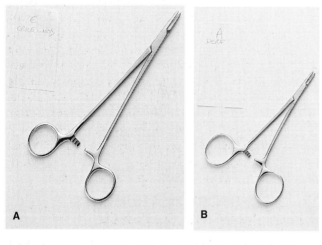

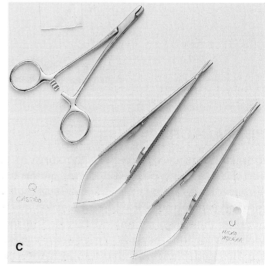

Figure 5.10 Needle holders. A. Derf. B. Crile–Wood. C. Micro.

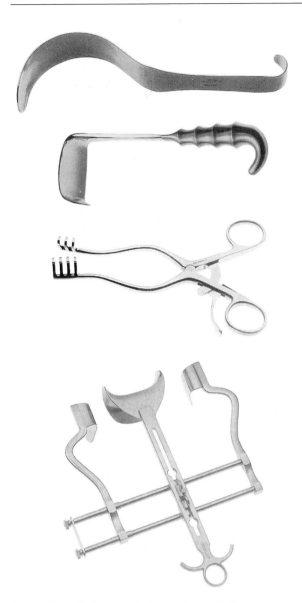

Figure 5.11 Retractors. A. Langenback. B. Deaver. C. Kelly. D. Travers. E. Balfour.

they may be manufactured from stainless steel or may be disposable. The choice of sucker depends on the surgical procedure. For abdominal, gynaecological and orthopaedic surgery a Yankauer sucker may be used; a Poole sucker may be used for abdominal surgery. Both are available in disposable form. Specialized types of suckers are available, for example, which have interchangeable inserts to prevent blockage during orthopaedic surgery.

For plastic, vascular and microsurgery a Zoellner sucker may be used. These have a stylet which allows the instrument to be unblocked during the procedure. Most suckers have a port which gives the surgeon fingertip control of the amount of suction pressure to a particular area of tissue (Fig. 5.12).

Probes are usually fine metal instruments designed to follow a tract or fistula to ascertain its direction. Dilators may be used in many areas of surgery; they are available in increasing sizes. Examples are Bake common duct dilators and Hegar uterine dilators.

Dissectors such as the McDonald allow the surgeon to perform blunt dissection of an area. A Watson–Cheyne dissector is an example of a double-ended instrument that is both a dissector and a probe (Fig. 5.13).

There are many other instruments available for use in various surgical specialties, examples of which can be found in manufacturers' catalogues. The theatre practitioner should be able to select the appropriate instrument set for a specific case. They must therefore be knowledgeable about the procedure to be undertaken, the relevant anatomy and surgical approach, the size of the patient and the surgeon's preference.

Most departments will have surgical instruments divided into sets, for example a basic set each for major, minor and plastic surgery. These sets can then be added to: for example, a laparotomy set may be added to a basic general set for any large abdominal procedure. Operating theatres will have instrument checklists for each type of set used within a department. These are usually packed into the set prior to sterilization, to enable the scrub practitioner to check that all instruments can be accounted for during a surgical procedure. Instrument lists can also be a useful teaching tool. It is important therefore that the theatre practitioner is knowledgeable about the design, use and type of instruments available in their department.

CARE OF INSTRUMENTS

To prevent damage to instruments they should only be used for the purpose for which they were

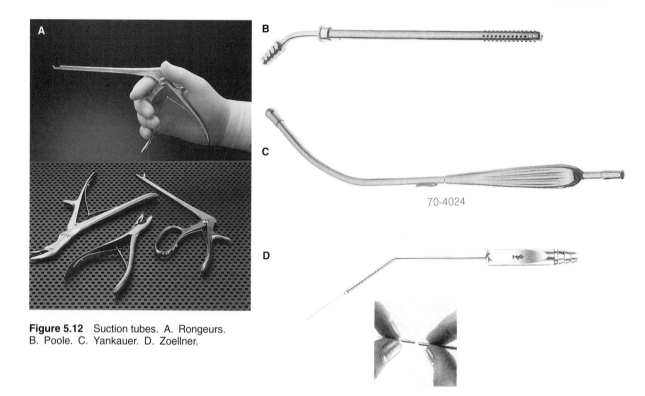

Figure 5.12 Suction tubes. A. Rongeurs. B. Poole. C. Yankauer. D. Zoellner.

designed. Contact, especially immersion, between stainless steel and corrosive substances should be avoided: this includes saline, hypochlorite and chemical disinfectants. All manufacturers advise that blood should never be allowed to dry on instruments and after each use they may be rinsed with sterile water. Delicate instruments such as micro instruments should be separated from others and handled with care. All instruments should be cleaned as soon as possible after use. Special care should be taken with instruments with lumina, for example suckers and hollow drills, as a build-up of debris can result in blockage. Decontamination can be achieved in a variety of ways:

1. **Hand washing**. The technique used should protect personnel handling the instruments from splashing, aerosolization and sharps injuries.[1] Local policies must be adhered to, with the use of adequate protective clothing for staff. Cool or warm water should be used as hot water causes coagulation of proteinaceous substances. A neutral-pH detergent should be used. Abrasive cleaners should not be used as these can cause scratches and scarring where debris can collect.[2]

Instruments with lumina should be irrigated thoroughly with cold water.

2. **Enzymatic products**. The rationale for detergenzyme products is that the enzymes will catalyse the decomposition process of organic debris while the detergent lifts the enzyme/debris complex off the instrument.[3] Research has shown that a 2-minute soak in an enzymatic solution provides an acceptable alternative to manual cleaning and decreases the risk of exposure of personnel to pathogens.[3] Enzymatic products may also be added to both washing machines and ultrasonic cleaners.

3. **Washing machines**. Automatic washer/dryer/sterilizers are ideal for cleaning soiled instruments. They will remove approximately 60% of blood and protein soil depending on the pH efficiency of the detergent used.

4. **Ultrasonic cleaners**. High-frequency sound waves are converted into mechanical vibrations, causing microscopic bubbles to form. These implode, causing minute vacuums which draw out debris. They are

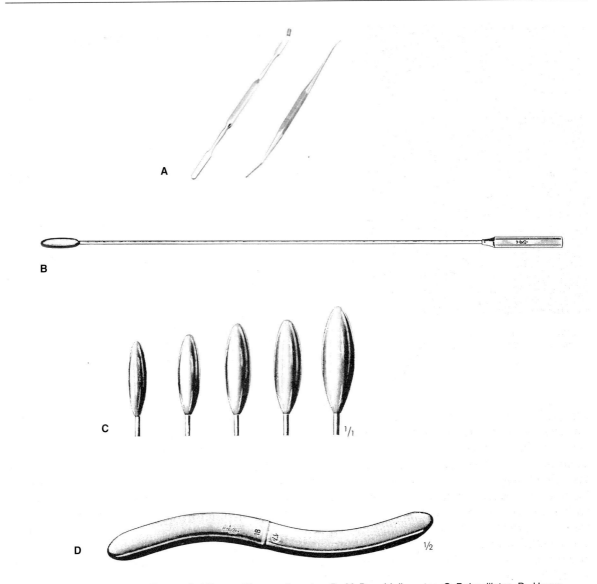

Figure 5.13 Dissectors and dilators. A. Watson–Cheyne dissector. B. McDonald dissector. C. Bake dilator. D. Hegar dilator.

very effective and remove 90% of debris soil, but they are not recommended for microinstruments as the vibrations cause weakness and damage.

Drying

All instruments must be dried thoroughly by hand or as part of the machine cycle, as water trapped in joints will contribute towards corrosion.

Lubrication

All manufacturers recommend lubrication prior to sterilization, especially after ultrasonic cleaning where all trace of lubricant is removed. Antibacterial lubricants should be used which contain rust-inhibiting agents, allow penetration of steam and lessen the growth of bacteria.

Once dried and lubricated, instruments are then sterilized. This is dealt with later in the chapter.

Handling

1. Instruments should be passed in a decisive manner, the handle of the instrument being placed directly and firmly into the surgeon's hand so that it is ready for immediate use. The practitioner should therefore be aware whether the surgeon is right- or left-handed.

2. Sharps should be passed in a receiver unless the surgeon is unable to look away from the surgical field, in which case they are passed so that the surgeon has control of the handle, and the blade edge is downwards.

3. Sharps and other instruments should never be allowed to rest directly on the patient, to prevent injury to the patient or damage to the drapes, which could lead to a subsequent loss of sterility. After use all instruments should be returned to the instrument trolley.

4. All curved instruments, e.g. clamps and scissors, are passed so that the curve of the instrument is in the same direction as the surgeon's palm.

5. Needles should be mounted on to the needleholder with the needle pointing in the direction of use.

6. Retractors are passed so that the surgeon or assistant can grasp the handle.

7. All instruments should be handled carefully, and heavy instruments should never be placed on top of fine ones. Dropping of instruments should be avoided. Instruments should never be heaped together at the end of a procedure: they should be placed in groups or handled individually. Sharps and fine delicate instruments should be handled separately.

8. Practitioners should be aware that surgeons may use hand signals to indicate the type of instrument required, and familiarize themselves with such signals.

GENERAL SAFEGUARDS

If there is any question regarding the sterility of an instrument it should be discarded immediately.

After each use, and prior to the start of any surgical procedure, all instruments should be checked for damage and stiffness. If any instrument is found to be faulty it should be discarded and repaired or replaced. Theatre practitioners should be aware of the repair procedure for instruments in their department. Assessment of individual instruments should determine whether they can be repaired or if they should be replaced.

- Forceps and hinged instruments should be checked for alignment of the teeth and jaws.
- If the instrument is held up to the light the tips of clamps must be closed, with no light visible between the jaws.
- Scissors should be checked to ensure sharpness. Heavy scissors should cut through four layers of a gauze swab at the tips; fine scissors should cut through two layers.
- Needleholders should hold the needle firmly, without allowing it to rotate easily.
- All instruments should be checked for cracks, chips and worn areas.

REFERENCES

1. AORN 1991 Proposed recommended practices – care of instruments, scopes, and powered surgical instruments. AORN Journal 54: 316, 318–320, 322–328
2. Underwood L 1983 The care and handling of instruments. Hospital Topics January/February 61: 46
3. Kneedler J, Darling M 1990 Using an enzymatic detergent to prerinse instruments. AORN Journal 51: 1326–1328, 1330–1332

Sutures

Sutures are used for almost every operative procedure, and the range available is increasing rapidly as manufacturers aim to improve their products and surgical teams require 'safer' sutures. The feelings of confusion on the first occasion a theatre practitioner or student is asked for a suture is undoubtedly universal. Staring in a bewildered way at the huge selection available on a suture rack is a distinct memory for many theatre staff (Fig. 5.14). However, it is a fairly straightforward topic and if it is clearly explained an understanding can quickly develop.

In order to assist fully in the surgical team all theatre practitioners, especially scrub and circulating personnel, should have a good understanding of the following areas:

- classification of suture materials
- strengths
- absorption rates
- needle types, sizes and shapes
- reading a suture packet
- selection of suture materials
- care, handling and storage of sutures.

First it is necessary to define exactly what a suture is, and its function. A suture may simply be defined as a length of material used to maintain approximation of body tissues until healing has occurred. The function of a suture in an operative procedure can be identified as one of the following:

- To approximate (hold together) body tissues or structures which have been divided or severed as part of the surgical intervention. This is necessary until the tissues have enough strength of their own to resume this function, that is, until healing has occurred.
- To approximate a body tissue or structure with an implant in order to keep the implant in the correct position. Examples of this are grafts used in arterial surgery, valves used in cardiac surgery, and lens implants used in ophthalmic

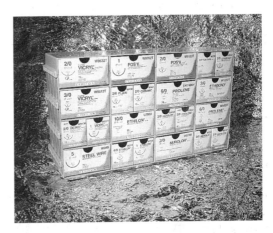

Figure 5.14 A suture rack.

surgery. In these instances healing will not take place owing to the presence of a non-living structure, and so the sutures must be permanent.

- To ligate (tie off) blood vessels in order to prevent bleeding. The correct term for this is a *ligature*, although the material used is the same as is used for sutures. The use of sutures for this purpose is generally decreasing, as electrosurgery (diathermy) is now available to seal blood vessels quickly and efficiently throughout surgery.
- To clearly identify and separate specific structures during surgery in order to assist with the surgical procedure by acting as a marker. An example of this is the identification of blood vessels in vascular surgery.
- To allow gentle retraction of a specific structure during surgery in order to improve vision and access for the surgeon. An example of this is gently holding open the dura during operations on the brain or spinal cord
- To identify the exact nature and orientation of a specimen of body tissue removed during surgery, in order to assist in the exact histology in the laboratory. An example of this is the identification of the posterior aspect of a breast

lump with a suture, in order to differentiate it from the anterior aspect.

Sutures are therefore used for a variety of purposes, and are required to join together a variety of body tissues: muscles, fat, fascia, nerves, blood vessels, cornea, bowel, tendons and skin. This is why the variety of suture materials is so great, in order to allow the most suitable to be used in each situation. The theatre practitioner must therefore develop a good understanding of the classification of suture materials.

CLASSIFICATION OF SUTURE MATERIALS

Suture materials can be described according to their fate within the body, that is, what happens to them following surgery. They can be identified as *absorbable* or *non-absorbable* (Fig. 5.15). (N.B. Suture materials and needles marked [a] are an Ethicon trademark; those marked [b] are a Davis and Geck trademark.)

Absorbable

This type of suture is absorbed by the body at varying durations following surgery, ranging from 7 days to 6 months. They are therefore used in areas of the body that will heal sufficiently to maintain tissue approximation within these time spans, once the suture has been absorbed. Examples are plain catgut, chromic catgut, Vicryl[a], Dexon[b], PDS[a] and Maxon[b].

Non-absorbable

These types of suture remain within the body unless removed intentionally. They are therefore used in areas that have poor healing, or where natural healing cannot occur owing to the presence of an implant, such as an arterial graft or heart valve. Examples are silk, Prolene[a], Novafil[b], Ethibond[a] and linen.

Sutures may also be classified according to the origin of the material used, as either *natural* or *synthetic* (Fig. 5.15).

Natural

Natural sutures are made from materials that originate from an animal or plant source. Although these are certainly the oldest suture materials their use is diminishing, with modern materials which produce less local tissue reac-

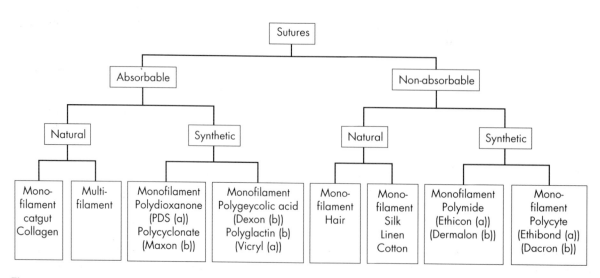

Figure 5.15 Suture materials.

tion being preferred.[1] Suture materials that originate from animals are generally termed 'catgut', which can be defined as 'a sterile strand prepared from collagen derived from healthy mammals'.[2] They are made from the submucosal layer of sheep's intestines, or the serosal layer of beef intestine, and are packaged in a spirit solution. Care should be taken when opening the packet to avoid splashes to the eye. Plant sources of suture materials include linen and cotton.

Synthetic

Synthetic sutures are made from a wide variety of polymers (complex molecules). They give a more uniform and predictable performance than natural materials and cause less reaction in surrounding tissues. Examples are Prolene[a], Maxon[b], Ethibond[a], Dexon[b] and PDS[a]. The advantages of synthetic materials include a more predictable absorption rate for absorbable sutures and, if non-absorbable, greater strength.[3]

Finally, sutures may be classified according to their structure, as either *monofilament* or *multifilament* (Fig. 5.15).

Monofilament

These sutures are made from a single strand or 'filament' of material. They are all synthetic materials, apart from catgut and collagen. Examples are Maxon[b], Novafil[b], PDS[a] and Prolene[a].

Multifilament or polyfilament

These sutures are made up of several strands or filaments of material, either braided or twisted together to form one thread. This is advantageous as it produces a more flexible thread which is easy to handle and use. Examples are Dexon[b], catgut, Vicryl[a], silk and Ethibond[a].

A disadvantage of multifilament sutures is the increased likelihood of bacteria being harboured within the braided material, potentially causing infection, and the material passing through the body tissues less easily, causing tis-

sue trauma, although this is reduced if the braid is coated.[3]

Each suture material therefore has three main characteristics. It is either:

- absorbable or non-absorbable
- natural or synthetic
- mono- or multifilament.

It is also necessary to consider further components of sutures, the strength of the suture material, the absorption rate, and the type (if any) of needle required.

STRENGTH AND SIZE OF SUTURE MATERIALS

The strength and size of the suture material is an important component in its description and is essential to consider when selecting particular sutures for use. The strength of a material denotes its tensile strength, which is measured on its knot-pull abilities, that is, the strength of the material when a knot in it is being pulled. Each suture size has specific knot-pull abilities and specific diameter limits. The gauge of a material is either a fraction number, ranging from 10/0 (very fine) to 2/0, a medium-diameter thread, or a whole number, from 0 (a thick thread) to 5, a very thick thread. The smaller the size of thread the less tensile strength the material has. Theatre practitioners should therefore be familiar with the material gauge of the sutures they use, either as described above or the now standardized metric gauge, and the uses of different-strength threads.

Each suture therefore has a further component to add to its three main characteristics:

- the strength or 'gauge' of the suture material.

ABSORPTION OF SUTURE MATERIALS
Non-absorbable sutures

These remain in the body until removed intentionally. They are not absorbed, as they are able to resist the enzymatic digestion of the body. Most of the natural non-absorbable materials such as silk and linen do, however, lose their strength within the body in a relatively short time.[1] Synthetic non-absorbable sutures generally both remain within the body and retain strength. Examples of these are polymer- and polythene-based sutures and steel, used for the approximation of bone.

Absorbable sutures

The absorption rate of suture materials varies greatly. Plain catgut is digested within 70 days, although strength loss occurs before this, in approximately 7–10 days. The synthetic monofilament Maxon is absorbed in approximately 6 months. The advantage of an absorbable suture is that the risk of residual suture material acting as a breeding site for infection is reduced.

It is important, however, for the surgical team to consider that a certain percentage of the materials strength is lost *well before* absorption actually occurs. The details for each material therefore need to be considered in relation to the nature of the wound to be closed and the estimated healing time. The period over which a suture material retains its full strength is known as tensile strength retention.

Sutures are absorbed in the body by one of two processes. Surgical gut (catgut), for example, is absorbed by enzymatic and phagocytic (white blood cell) action as the body attempts to rid itself of the foreign structure within it, i.e. the suture. Modern synthetic absorbable sutures are absorbed by a naturally occurring chemical process called hydrolysis. This involves the polymer reacting with water to cause the breakdown of the suture material. Manufacturers' product information should be studied to obtain the absorption rate of their suture materials.

Each suture therefore has two components to add to its three main characteristics:

- its strength or gauge
- its absorption rate.

NEEDLE TYPE, SIZE AND SHAPE

Modern suture materials are supplied as either non-needled or with an 'atraumatic' needle.

Non-needled sutures

These suture materials do not have a needle either attached to the thread or loose in the packet. They may therefore be used either as ligatures, with which to tie off blood vessels, or with an eyed needle.

Eyed needles

Eyed needles are not attached to a suture and hence need to be threaded with suture material by the scrub person, for use by the surgeon. These were the most commonly used needles until the development of atraumatic needles in the 1920s. Their use continued long after that, however, in many specialties such as neurosurgery and gynaecological surgery, owing to surgical preference.

Non-traumatic needles

Non-traumatic needles have sutures attached to them in such a way that only one thread is pulled through the tissue, as opposed to two threads with an eyed needle (Fig. 5.16). 'Non-traumatic' therefore refers to the minimization of trauma as a result of single thread use. The thread is fixed to the needle by being placed in a drill end or a flange end (as seen in Fig. 5.16), which is then crimped around the thread.

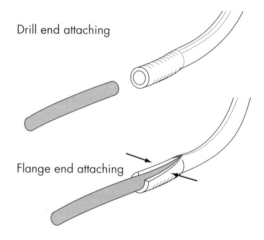

Drill end attaching

Flange end attaching

Figure 5.16 Non-traumatic needles.

Needle	Description
● **VISI-BLACK**	Designed to give outstanding visibility against tissue, and where blood is present, the slim taper point design of the VISI-BLACK needle brings improved penetration and minimises trauma.
● **INTESTINAL Needle**	In order to increase the control which the surgeon has available in placing intestinal sutures, the point profile of this range of needles has been altered to provide substantially improved penetration. In addition, an extra degree of flatting has been applied to increase stability in the needle holder and to permit accurate placement of the needle through the tissues.
● **HEAVY Needle**	In some situations where particularly strong needles are required a heavy wire diameter needle would be appropriate.
● **ETHIGUARD** **BLUNT TAPERPOINT Needle**	Where evidence of needle-stick-injuries is a major concern, particularly in the presence of blood borne viruses, the ETHIGUARD BLUNT TAPERPOINT needle virtually eliminates accidental surgical glove puncture.
● **BLUNT POINT Needle**	This needle has been designed for suturing extremely friable vascular tissue, such as the liver.
⊗ **CC Needle**	As a result of a unique point design the CC Needle provides significantly improved penetration. This is achieved with no increased tissue trauma compared to the conventional round bodied needle. The squared body geometry, in addition to providing a stronger fine vascular needle, also means this product is particularly secure in the needle holder.

Figure 5.17A Needle types.–Round bodied. (Reproduced with permission from Ethicon Ltd.)

Needle	Description
TAPERCUT Needle	This needle combines the initial penetration of a cutting needle with the minimised trauma of a round bodied needle. The cutting tip is limited to the point of the needle, which then tapers out to merge smoothly into a round cross section.
P Needle	Designed for use primarily in skin closure, the P range of needles has the point profile of conventional or reverse cutting needles but with exceptionally sharp cutting edges to offer ease of penetration in all skin types. The needle body is squared in cross section which significantly improves resistance to bending and ensures maximum stability in the needle holder.
SLIM BLADE Needle	Specifically designed as a delicate instrument for use in Plastic and Cosmetic Surgery, the geometry of the point design has been altered to provide clean and smooth penetration. A new design of forcep flats has also been incorporated to ensure maximum stability in all types of needle holder.
PRIME Needle	Specifically designed for surgeons seeking excellence in skin closure, the PRIME hollowform needle is manufactured to the highest specification to produce the sharpest needle in the ETHICON range.
CUTTING Needle	This needle has a triangular cross section with the apex on the inside of the needle curvature. The effective cutting edges are restricted to the front section of the needle and run into a triangulated body which continues for half the length of the needle.
REVERSE CUTTING Needle	The body of this needle is triangular in cross section having the apex cutting edge on the outside of the needle curvature. This improves the strength of the needle and particularly increases its resistance to bending.
TROCAR POINT Needle	Based on the traditional TROCAR POINT, this needle has a strong cutting head which then merges into a robust round body. The design of the cutting head has been improved to ensure powerful penetration, even when deep in dense tissue.

Figure 5.17B Needle types.–Cutting. (Reproduced with permission from Ethicon Ltd.)

The use of non-traumatic needles is now very widespread, and they are likely to be the needle of choice for many surgeons in most clinical situations. Within the operating theatre there can be found many different non-traumatic needles, which vary according to the type of needle point and the size and shape of the needle.

Common needle types

There are four main needle types, which have distinctive features in relation to the point and shaft of the needle (Fig. 5.17):

- round-bodied needles
- cutting needles
- reverse cutting needles
- blunt needles.

Round-bodied needles

These needles are used for the approximation of soft tissues, as they are designed to separate body tissues and fibres rather than cut them. The design allows for the point to penetrate the tissue followed by the shaft of the needle, which has a 'round body' giving the smallest possible hole size. This allows the tissue to close tightly around the suture material, forming a leakproof suture line. They are used in intestinal, cardiac and vascular surgery where a leakproof suture line is essential.

Cutting needles (standard or conventional cutting)

These needles are used for suturing tough or very dense body tissue. The needle has a triangular point, with the apex of the triangle on the inside of the needle's curvature and the effective cutting edges restricted to the front half of the needle. This merges with a flat body, which is easily held in the needleholder. Uses are the approximation of fascia and skin.

Reverse cutting needles

A reverse cutting needle is triangular in shape, with the apex of the triangle (the cutting edge) on the outside of the needle. The three cutting edges continue the whole length of the shaft. This needle is strong and resistant to bending. It is used for the approximation of heavy muscle and skin.

Blunt needles

These needles are completely blunt and thus simply pass through soft tissue. They are used for suturing the extremely friable tissue of the liver and other vascular soft organs of the body.

Suture companies have their own additions and variations to these four commonly used types, such as taper-cut needles and trocar-point needles. There have been many developments in needle manufacture aimed at producing a safer surgical environment:

- *Visi-black[a]*: a needle of excellent visibility against the body's tissues
- *Ethiguard[a]*: a blunt taper-point needle that will penetrate tissue but virtually eliminates glove puncture
- *Protect point[b]* have a point that will not pierce a gloved hand; these developments have become essential for the protection of the surgical team and the patient against bloodborne pathogens
- *CC needles[a]*: these have a minute penetrating tip which is 40% less in diameter than the round-bodied needle that follows it. This is advantageous when penetrating calcified vessels, grafts and fibrous tissues. It is designed for cardiac and vascular use.

Needle shape

The choice of needle shape will depend on the location and accessibility of the tissues to be sutured. The main shapes are described as:

- quarter-circle
- three-eighths-circle
- half-circle
- five-eighths-circle
- J-shaped
- straight.

Generally, a more confined suturing site will need a greater curved needle, such as a five-eighths-circle or a J-shaped needle. An easy-access superficial tissue such as the skin or subcutaneous fat can be easily sutured with a quarter-circle or a straight needle.

Each suture needle therefore has a particular *type* (point and shaft) and a particular *shape*. The final consideration is the needle's length and strength.

See Fig. 5.18.

Needle length and strength

The strength of a suture needle is mainly determined by the diameter of the wire from which it is made. The diameter and strength are usually closely related to the gauge of the suture material, with a heavy thread requiring a strong needle and a very fine thread needing a more delicate one.

The length of the needle used also depends on the location and accessibility of the tissue to be sutured. There is a huge variation in the size of needles, from a large 110 mm five-eighths-circle needle to a tiny 4 mm needle. Smaller needles are used on a needleholder, and larger ones may be hand-held.

Each suture needle therefore has a particular *type, shape* and *length*.

READING A SUTURE PACKET

All the information given in this section so far is clearly shown on the suture packet, making reading a suture packet an essential skill for all theatre practitioners. Manufacturers of sutures aim for their box and the suture packet to tell theatre practitioners exactly what is inside, usually with a diagram for ease of recognition; they are often colour-coded. Figure 5.19 shows suture packets from a manufacturer and indicates how practitioners can quickly read a packet to identify exactly what is inside.

Additional information on a suture packet includes:

- length of suture thread
- expiry date, sterility assurance
- manufacturer
- product number

- code number: this is specific to that suture material type, strength and needle combination. It is commonly used for identification of suture requirements on the surgeon's preference card, and by the scrub theatre practitioner when further sutures are required.

SELECTION OF SUTURES FOR SURGERY

The selection of a suture and needle for each stage of an operation is the surgeon's choice, but it is an area where the theatre practitioner can have great influence and input as they often have a wider range of experience and more up-to-date product information.

Factors that contribute towards an ideal suture include:

- comfortable and natural handling
- minimal tissue reaction
- not creating a situation ideal for bacterial growth
- secure knot holding
- ease of use
- safety for the surgical team.

Surgeons and theatre practitioners should have a good knowledge of a specific suture's properties in relation to the above.

The factors to consider when choosing a suture should include those discussed in this section:

- absorbable or non-absorbable
- natural or synthetic
- mono- or multifilament
- absorption rate
- needle point and type
- needle shape
- needle strength and length.

These factors must be considered in relation to each stage of the operation, with special consideration of:

- functions of sutures at each stage
- healing abilities
- healing rate
- strength of tissue to be approximated
- tension the sutures are likely to be under
- access to tissues.

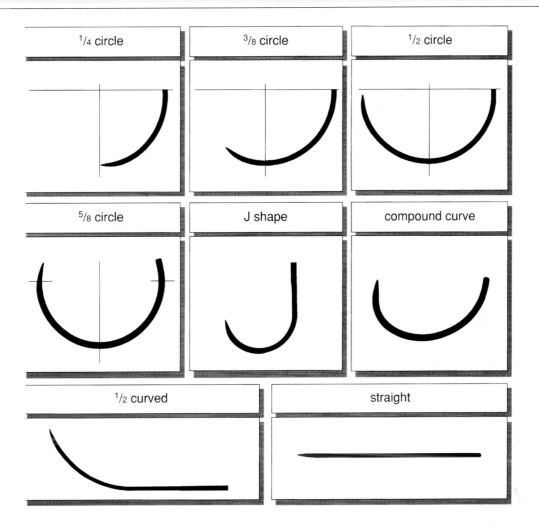

Figure 5.18 Needle shapes. Choice of needle is governed by the accessibility of the tissue to be sutured; normally, the more confined the operative site the greater the curvature required. (Reproduced with permission from Ethicon Ltd.)

The requirements of a suture material have not changed greatly since 1920 when Moynihan[4] identified his ideal requirements:

• it should achieve its purpose
• it should disappear as soon as its work is accomplished
• it should be free from infection
• it should be non-irritant.

The selection of sutures is therefore a complex process. It is further compounded by historical influences in many surgical specialties, and the 'role-model' influences of those who taught the surgeon.

It is helpful if the surgeon's choice of sutures for an operation are documented on their preference card, which should be kept in the theatre. This enables theatre practitioners to check surgeons' preferences for different stages in each operative procedure.

CARE, HANDLING AND STORAGE OF SUTURES

Suture materials should be kept dry and dust free in the clean area of the theatre. This prevents contamination of the suture packets from fluids which may potentially contaminate the contents, and also prevents the packet from becoming dust-laden. Information on the suture pack should be checked by the scrub person before it is opened by the circulating practitioner. This should include the type, expiry date and sterility assurance. The scrub person must be aware of sutures which are packaged in a spirit solution and open these carefully to avoid splashes to the eyes.

Manufacturers often provide operating theatres with racks designed to house boxes of suture materials (Fig. 5.14). These are very useful and sutures are therefore:

• easily visible
• dry and dust free
• easily transferable to other operating theatres
• stored efficiently
• specific to each operating theatre

• able to be kept in the way theatre practitioners choose, e.g. all skin sutures together, in groups for each type of surgery in the theatre, such as gynaecology and dental, or in groups of suture materials, easily identifiable by colour coding
• stored safely, and boxes are unlikely to fall from the rack
• easily identifiable when stocks need replacing.

Large operating departments can maximize efficiency by having a central store of sutures, which can be decanted to individual theatres as required. This allows good rotation of stock and decreases the likelihood of suture materials becoming out of date. It also avoids the practice of stockpiling in individual theatres, which often means large amounts of a department's budget may be held in stockrooms, a poor practice financially. Finally, it allows large orders to be placed with the suture companies rather than small orders from individual theatres, which often means financial benefits for the department.

It is very important, however, that a central store of sutures is efficiently managed and that a department does not run out of specific sutures. Indeed, theatre practitioners may well store sutures secretly, thereby minimizing the advantages of the system. There may be some exceptions to this, such as sutures that are only used in one theatre, or sutures that are expensive and whose use needs close monitoring. These arrangements need to be worked out locally. For a central storage system to work efficiently, a named person is needed with designated responsibility for ordering and supplies. This prevents over-ordering and ensures maximum benefits for the department. This person should also be aware of the system by which sutures may be obtained quickly from manufacturers in the event of a sudden change in the needs of the department or a particular surgeon, or indeed the unavailability of a particular suture. Each theatre practitioner should be aware of the supply mechanism within their department.

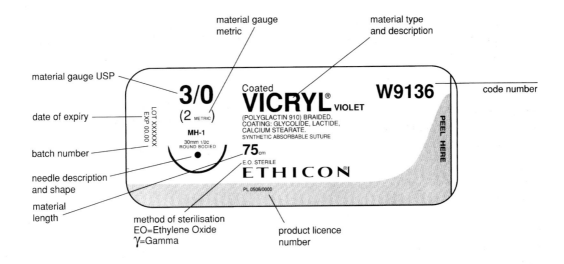

Carton Label

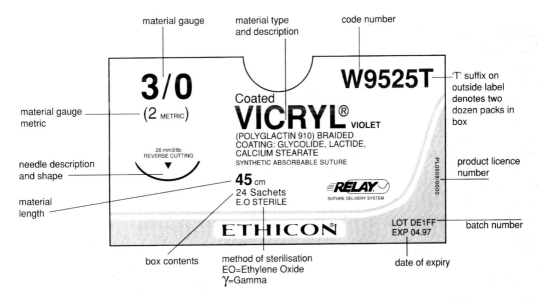

Figure 5.19   An explanation of package labelling. (Reproduced with permission from Ethicon Ltd.)

Storage and supplies are also important in the operating theatre itself, and issues relating to good storage practice have been discussed. It is important that theatre practitioners also follow certain guidelines:

• Keep an adequate supply of required suture materials within the theatre at all times. This should be checked before each operating list, and replacements obtained at this time.

• Check the expiry date and sterility assurance on each suture box before placing it in the rack.
• Do not overload suture boxes in an attempt to be well stocked up. This can cause trauma to the suture materials or the outer packet, and means the boxes become difficult to use. It also provides an inaccurate indication of supply needs.

REFERENCES

1. Davis and Geck 1990 Educational Fact Sheet No 3. Classification of sutures. Davis and Geck, Hampshire.
2. Ethicon 1993 Suture materials and surgical needles. Ethicon Ltd, Edinburgh

3. Eden C 1993 A classification of suture materials and needles. Surgical Nurse 6: 23
4. Moynihan B 1920 The ritual of a surgical operation. British Journal of Surgery 8: 27–35

FURTHER READING

Davis and Geck 1990 Educational fact sheets for theatre nursing staff 1–11. Davis and Geck, Hampshire
Ethicon (undated) Anatomical insights – the abdomen. Ethicon, Edinburgh
Leaper D, Lucarotti M 1992 Sutures and Staples. Journal of Wound Care 1: 27–30

Mackenzie D (undated) A short history of sutures. Ethicon, Edinburgh
Price V 1994 Wound closure. Technic Issue no 131: 6–7

Stapling systems

Stapling systems are used in many surgical specialties for a variety of operative procedures. Surgical staples are made from stainless steel or titanium and are used to approximate tissues, thus having a similar function to sutures. The stapling device can be either reusable or disposable.

Reusable staple applicators have been used for many years in thyroid and gynaecological surgery – Michel clips, for example. Their use is declining as disposable devices become more popular.

Disposable staple applicators are now used in many operations for both internal tissues and skin. They are preloaded, lightweight and easy to use. Figure 5.20 shows a selection of disposable stapling devices.

SKIN STAPLES

These are presented on a disposable applicator containing an identified number of staples (15, 25 or 35), in a regular or a wide width. They are quick and easy to use for both the surgeon and the theatre practitioner. Operating and anaesthetic time is therefore reduced when staples are used.[1-3] The use of staples also means that threading and mounting of needles is not required: handling of blood-contaminated sharps is thus reduced and the possibility of needlestick injury is also reduced.[4] This is an important development and is popular with operating department staff concerned about the transmission of bloodborne diseases such as hepatitis B and HIV.

Benefits for the patient (in addition to a shortened operation time) include a decreased inflammatory response due to the non-reactive nature of staple materials. This results in less tissue reaction than when conventional sutures are used.[5,6] Wound healing is also enhanced, as if skin staples are correctly placed they are at the correct tension and tissue strangulation will not occur.[7]

The use of skin staples is also associated with less risk of wound infection than with sutures,[5,8]

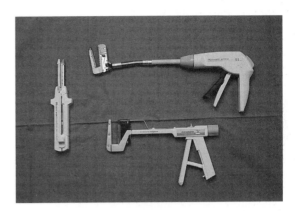

Figure 5.20 A selection of staple devices.

thereby providing a further benefit for both patient and hospital.

Postoperative skin staple removal is quick, easy to perform and relatively painless for the patient.[9] Each manufacturer provides a staple remover for use with its products.

Finally, staples have produced significantly better cosmetic results for the patient, owing to the staple's position *above* the wound edges; this is a further benefit.[6,10]

The advantages of skin staples must be considered in relation to their disadvantages, i.e. a higher cost than suture materials.

OTHER TYPES OF STAPLE

The use of staples in areas other than the skin has also increased rapidly, owing to technological advances and the availability of improved products.

Bowel resection and gastrointestinal surgery

Stapling devices are available for anastomosis of the bowel following resection of a diseased or damaged section (Fig. 5.20). They are also useful in difficult operative sites, such as an oesophageal transection for bleeding varices, or a lower anterior resection. The latter involves the use of an end-to-end stapling device. Linear stapling devices are also available and are useful for sealing off the bowel, such as for closing a stomach remnant in a partial gastrectomy.[9] These devices produce a good seal, an important factor in the prevention of postoperative infection. A study by Weil and Scherz[11] found a decreased incidence of leaks and fewer complications when staples were compared to sutures in a study of 585 patients who underwent a Billroth II gastrec-

tomy, and concluded that stapling is at least as safe as, if not safer than, conventional hand suture in this type of surgery.

Laparoscopic surgery

Stapling devices are also available for use in the rapidly expanding field of minimally invasive surgery. They have contributed greatly to surgical developments in this area, as suturing via an endoscope remains a difficult technique.

REFERENCES

1. Dehnel W 1973 Staple suturing vs conventional suturing. AORN Journal 18: 296–300
2. MacGregor F, McCombe A, King P, McLeod D 1989 Skin stapling of wounds in the accident department. Injury 20: 347–348
3. George T, Simpson D 1985 Skin wound closure with staples in the accident and emergency department. Journal of the Royal College of Surgeons of Edinburgh 30: 54–56
4. Ritchie A, Rocke L 1989 Staple versus sutures in the closure of scalp wounds: a prospective, double blind, randomized trial. Injury 20: 217
5. Stillman R, Marine C, Seligman S 1984 Skin staples in potentially contaminated wounds. Archives of Surgery 119: 821–822
6. Traub A et al 1981 Cutaneous wound closure: early

staple removal and replacement by skin tapes. Contemporary Surgery 18: 93–101
7. Davis and Geck Educational fact sheet no 7: Skin Stapling
8. Pickford I, Brennan S, Evans M, Pollock A 1983 Two methods of skin closure in abdominal operation: a controlled clinical trial. British Journal of Surgery 70: 226–228
9. Leaper D, Lucarotti M 1992 Sutures and staples. Journal of Wound Care. Nov/Dec 1: 27–30
10. Bucknall T, Ellis H 1982 Skin closure. Comparison of nylon, polyglycolic acid and staples. European Surgical Research 14: 96
11. Weil P, Scherz M 1981 Comparison of stapled and hand sutured gastrectomies. Archives of Surgery 116: 14–16

Surgical gowns and draping systems

DRAPING SYSTEMS

The use of surgical drapes is necessary to create an area known as the sterile field around the surgical wound. This is achieved by placing sterile drapes over the patient, leaving only the necessary area around the incision site exposed. All items used in the operation must remain within the sterile field, and it should not be breached by non-sterile items. Draping the patient is an essential aspect of aseptic technique in the operating department. It is the first part of the surgical procedure (following the administration of anaesthesia and skin preparation), and plays a vital role in the prevention of contamination of the surgical wound site.

Theatre practitioners, especially scrub and circulating personnel, play an important role in the draping procedure. In order to participate fully in the surgical team theatre practitioners should have a good understanding of the following areas:

- definition and function of surgical drapes
- requirements of a surgical drape
- definition and function of surgical gowns
- requirements of a surgical gown
- types of gown and draping systems available:
  - linen
  - disposable (single use)
  - reusable
  - plastic incisional drapes
- advantages and disadvantages of each system
- safe disposal of used surgical drapes
- storage of surgical gowns and gloves
- principles of draping the patient for surgery.

Definition of a surgical drape

A surgical drape is a sterilized piece of cloth or material used to maintain a sterile field during surgical intervention. The material should be resistant to blood and body fluids in order to provide an effective barrier between sterile and non-sterile areas.

Functions

A surgical drape can be used in the following ways:

- Placed in close proximity to the intended incision/operation site in order to create a sterile field. This is generally followed by the draping of all the patient (except the operation site) in order to create a wide sterile field. Any area needed for anaesthetic management must be within the access of the anaesthetist and assistant, for example the head (to manage the endotracheal tube or other assisted airway) and the arm, which is often needed for intravenous access. This therefore creates a sterile field on which gloved hands may be placed.
- To cover any surfaces used during the operative procedure, in order to extend the sterile field. This includes instrument trolleys, bowl stands and a Mayo table if used. This therefore creates a sterile field on which instruments may be placed.
- To cover any other items used during the operative procedure that cannot be sterilized by conventional methods. An example of this is using a sterile surgical drape to wrap tubing connected to an air cylinder when using power tools. This also includes covering items adjacent to the sterile field, such as a drip stand, in order to prevent potential contamination.

Requirements

In order to meet these functions a surgical drape must meet certain requirements.

1. **A barrier against fluids**. A surgical drape protects the surgical incision site (which has been prepared with a cleansing solution) and subse-

quent wound from the other areas of the patient's body (which have not been prepared). In order to be effective it must therefore be able to resist fluid absorption. Absorption of blood or other fluids through the drapes over a non-prepared area of the body will allow contamination to extend by a 'wicking' action towards the incision site, causing a primary wound infection.[1] Although several materials claim to act as a barrier against fluids, this is not necessarily enough information. Theatre practitioners need to establish how long the barrier is effective for, as some materials do not remain equally impermeable for long periods of time.

2. **A barrier to microorganisms**. A surgical drape is required to be a barrier against microorganisms in order to prevent contamination of the wound. It is necessary therefore for the weave or the 'mesh' of the fabric to be close enough to prevent the passage of microorganisms from the non-sterile environment (e.g. air and theatre personnel) to the sterile field.

3. **Sterility**. A surgical drape is used in very close proximity to the surgical wound, and can therefore itself be the source of possible contamination. All drapes used must be sterile and the packaging clearly able to demonstrate such sterility. Drapes must be wrapped so they are easy to open, with the packaging able to maintain sterility. Theatre practitioners must check the following when opening surgical drapes:

- sterility (by a recognized mark on the packaging)
- expiry date
- packaging is intact
- packaging is not wet or appears to have been wet (this may mean contamination of contents has occurred).

The material used must therefore be able to be sterilized by a recognized method such as steam, ethylene oxide or irradiation.

4. **Lint and particulate free**. A drape, even if sterile, may also contaminate a wound by the introduction of lint or particulates. Particulates can be fibres of any material that becomes free from the main drape itself. If undetected they can remain in the wound and cause problems as for-

eign bodies. This may include infection or delayed healing due to local tissue reaction.

5. **Easy to use**. Surgical drapes must be easy to use for both the surgeon and the theatre practitioners. This entails that they:

- unfold correctly
- are not too large to handle
- stay in their required position
- are soft enough to drape adequately
- do not tear during normal use
- are of an adequate size to cover the patient (and trolleys) without touching the floor.

6. **Maintain patients' body temperature and dignity**. Loss of body temperature is a potential problem for many patients in the operating theatre. This is due to many reasons (see Chapter 4), including the fact that they are usually unclothed (either partially or completely) and not moving at all. The surgical drape therefore has a further function: that of maintaining the patient's temperature and their dignity by keeping them covered.

7. **Fire safe**. Surgical drapes must meet fire protection standards, to ensure there is no risk from static electricity or from any other fire hazards.

The theatre practitioner and surgeon must therefore consider each type of drape available, in relation to the above requirements, before an accurate assessment and informed decision can be made.

Other considerations

A further consideration is of course the cost of the drapes, as this is one of the fundamental price considerations in a surgical procedure. This will therefore influence the cost of the patient's treatment and, whether in a private setting or in the internal market of today's NHS, will have some effect on purchasing arrangements and contracts.

However, the cost is more than financial. Many theatre practitioners, surgeons and others involved with hospital supplies are now also concerned with the cost to the environment. This entails the environmental concerns in the manufacture and source of the drape material, and the difficulties inherent in the disposal of non-linen drapes.

SURGICAL GOWNS

Definition

Surgical gowns are long-sleeved garments which tie up at the back and cover the wearer completely from the neck to the mid-calf. Sterile surgical gowns are an essential item of clothing for the surgical team. They are worn over theatre clothing by the operating surgeons, the scrub theatre practitioner, and any student, learner or visitor who wishes to have close observation of the surgery. They are put on following the scrubbing-up procedure and are worn with sterile surgical gloves.

Functions

Gowns and gloves prevent microorganisms from the hands and clothing of the surgical team being transferred to the wound, either by direct transmission or indirectly by the surgical instruments. Surgical gowns and gloves also protect the surgical team from any microorganism the patient may have, for example the bloodborne pathogens of hepatitis B and HIV.

Requirements of a surgical gown

In order to meet these functions a surgical gown must meet certain requirements.

1. **A barrier against fluids**. This needs to be a two-way barrier, first to protect the patient from microorganisms on the wearer's skin or clothes that may contaminate the wound via a wicking action if the gown becomes wet, and secondly to protect the wearer from any microorganisms present in the blood or body fluids of the patient. Although these would not generally be harmful to the surgical team (as intact skin is an effective barrier against them), they may be a hazard in one of two ways:

- if the patient's blood or body fluids come into contact with any open wound a person in the scrub team may have
- if the patient's blood or body fluids come into contact with the mucous membranes of a member of the scrub team.

The surgical gown therefore needs to be fluid repellent. Many gowns offer extra protection on the sleeves and front panel, where passage of fluids and microorganisms is most likely and most hazardous. Barrier Extra Protection (Johnson and Johnson), Reinforced Proguard Dermashield (Smith and Nephew) and Guardian/High Risk gowns from Molnlycke, are examples.

2. **A barrier against microorganisms**. As described in the section on drapes, the surgical gown must be a barrier against microorganisms. The make-up of the fabric must therefore be such that it prevents the passage of microorganisms from the patient to the wearer, and from the wearer to the patient.

3. **Sterility**. The surgical gown must be able to be sterilized by conventional methods, and the packaging must be clearly able to demonstrate the sterility of the contents. Further information on sterility is given in the section on surgical drapes.

4. **Lint and particulate free**. The surgical gown material must not allow lint or particulate to become free, as this can cause wound contamination, as described in the draping section.

5. **Comfortable to wear**. The surgical gown is likely to be worn for many hours, and must therefore be lightweight, comfortable and non-irritating to wear. It must be permeable to air in order to allow the skin to breathe and prevent heat build-up in the wearer.

The gown should fit the wearer and allow adequate freedom of movement. It should not reach the floor, as this is poor infection control practice and is a hazard for the wearer. Gowns should therefore be provided in different sizes and lengths – fine adjustment to the length may be made if the gown has a waist tie.

It is necessary for the gowns to be cuffed in order to keep the sleeves securely in the surgical gloves at the wearer's wrist. The cuff should be comfortable to the wearer.

6. **Resistant to tearing**. The gown must be resistant to tearing and puncture in order to provide an effective barrier. Gowns are susceptible to tearing in the arms and at the cuff attachment if handled roughly when donning surgical gloves.

7. **Maintain sterility when put on**. The outside of the gown will be in contact with the sterile field during surgery and therefore should not be touched until the wearer has sterile gloves on. The gown must be folded to allow the scrub person to handle it, and put it on holding the inside surfaces only. The wearer should be able to gently shake it for it to open fully. Vigorous shaking should be avoided as this creates air and dust movement. The technique is described more fully in Chapter 6.

The ties or fasteners of the gown should be easily identifiable and easy to use. Once tied they are not sterile and thus will need to be covered up. This can be achieved by having a wraparound back. This is necessary to prevent possible contamination if the surgeon or a member of the surgical team has to turn their back on the open wound during surgery.

8. **Antistatic and fire safe**. The same considerations apply as were discussed in relation to surgical drapes.

TYPES OF DRAPING SYSTEM AND GOWNS AVAILABLE

Draping systems and surgical gowns fall into three main categories:

- linen/woven
- disposable/non-woven
- reusable (non-linen).

These may be supplemented by the use of plastic incisional drapes.

Linen/woven

Linen gowns and drapes are the oldest type and continue to be used in many hospitals, despite some limitations. Indeed, the effectiveness of ordinary cotton surgical gowns has been demonstrated since 1948.[2] The term linen is used loosely, and may be somewhat misleading as many such drapes are cotton based.

Early linen materials aimed to provide the primary function of a drape – that of a barrier against infection. They certainly did so to some extent but how much they actually retarded the passage of fluids effectively is questionable: the sight of a surgeon's theatre clothes soaked with blood following removal of a linen gown after performing an abdominal operation is evidence that they were not very effective. This 'strikethrough' of blood is more likely in hand-deep wounds, with 88% of hand-deep operations demonstrating wet gowns.[3] Strikethrough of blood or fluids presents a twofold problem:

- The surgeon and others close to the operation site are not protected against the blood and body fluids of the patient.
- The patient is not adequately protected against contamination via the drapes – a 'wicking' process allows contamination of the operation site from a non-prepared area, either from the patient themselves or from the surgical team.

It has been noted that 'The most common source of surgical infections is the patient himself ...'.[4] More modern cottons/linens are tightly woven fabrics which can be chemically treated in order to improve barrier qualities by giving a moisture-repellent finish.

The theatre practitioner, if considering the use of linen/cotton surgical drapes and gowns, must question the attributes of the material in relation to the following questions:

- How tightly woven is the fabric? This can be measured in approximate thread count per square inch. An average thread count is 280 per square inch. Muslin, used for surgical drapes for many years, does not retard the passage of fluids effectively as it has a thread count of only 140 per square inch. It would not therefore be thought to be an effective barrier today.
- Has the material been chemically treated to improve its barrier qualities?
- Does the gown meet national requirements, e.g. Department of Health Performance Specification and DHSS guidelines?

These three factors may improve the performance of the drape in relation to infection control.

Care of linen drapes and gowns

Linen drapes are generally considered to be economical but the following points are essential to ensure their continued integrity:

- Drapes and gowns must be inspected regularly for holes, tears or wear and tear resulting in 'thinning'.
- A system must be in place to ensure that this inspection takes place regularly.
- Care must be taken to minimize holes caused by towel clips or other perforating instruments. Non-perforating towel clips must be used.
- The theatre practitioner should also consider for how long linen/cotton materials are effective. A review of infection control practices by AORN[5] suggests that cotton gowns and drapes lose their barrier properties after as few as 30 washings.

Advantages

- They are economical as they are reusable.
- Local control can be maintained as laundry can be dealt with in-house.
- They are environmentally friendly in terms of disposal.
- They provide excellent drapability.

Disadvantages

- Infection is reportedly higher in operations using linen/cotton. A review of infection control practices by AORN[5] quotes two studies in 1981 and 1984 which show that disposable gowns and drapes improve infection rates compared to cotton ones. The 1984 study enabled researchers to predict a 2.4:1 ratio of risk of infection when comparing cotton with disposables.[5]
- They may often shed lint/particulate into the wound.
- Fluid strikethrough is often immediate.
- Regular inspection may miss small areas of damage, meaning imperfect drapes can be used inadvertently.
- They are expensive in terms of inspection costs, a staff-intensive laundry, energy consumption for washing and drying, and water consumption.
- They are generally manufactured in a restricted range of sizes and designs.
- Quality of service will depend on the type and condition of laundry equipment and service.
- A large amount of linen is needed to cope with the lengthy 'turnaround' time.
- They are bulky to store.

Cotton is a comfortable fabric to wear but appears to be ineffective. Whyte[6] states that in other industries where airborne or contact contamination from staff is a problem, cotton is no longer used.

Theatre practitioners therefore need to consider all the above factors and obtain a financial analysis of local cost comparisons of linen with disposable or reusable fabrics. Recent research considering infection control issues and infection rates for differing systems must always be taken into account in order to obtain up-to-date information. Theatre practitioners must therefore be familiar with the research process, reading research, and how to do so with a critical questioning approach.

Disposable/non-woven

Synthetic non-woven materials are the basis of disposable drapes and gowns. They are made from processed cellulose fibres, used either alone or in combination with various reinforcing materials such as polymeric fibres. These are very effective in preventing bacterial migration – the fibres appear under the microscope as a random net and bacteria therefore have no direct route through the fabric. They are used in many operating theatres, and products are continually being developed by manufacturers in order to improve the materials and meet the needs of the surgical team.

Disposable materials have a reliable impermeability and are generally packaged to allow easy aseptic application. They are sterile, single-use items that are disposed of when used, usually by incineration.

Disposable drapes are available in a wide range of sizes and many have adhesive panels aimed to avoid the use of towel clips during surgery. They are also available in a wide range of designs, for example:

- drapes
- adhesive drapes
- table/trolley covers
- split sheets
- fenestrated sheets
- leggings
- aperture drapes
- isolation bags
- isolation drapes (orthopaedic)
- Mayo stand covers.

Drapes have also been specifically designed for many surgical approaches, for example arthroscopy, ophthalmology and abdominoperineal drapes. Disposable drapes are also available in preselected packs aimed at including all the draping requirements for a specific approach/operation. For example:

- basic surgical pack
- gynaecology pack
- cystoscopy pack
- ENT pack
- head and neck pack
- cardiac surgery pack
- ophthalmic pack
- orthopaedic pack
- neurosurgery pack.

They are generally packaged in such a way that, once opened, the contents of the pack are presented in the normal order of use. Advantages of this system are:

- ease of use for theatre practitioners
- quick and efficient to use for the surgical team, decreasing the length of operating time
- less packaging
- less opening of packages, thus less chance of contamination and less chance of infection for the patient.

The disadvantages are that the predetermined contents may be seen as restrictive, as well as expensive if all the drapes are not used, since unused drapes will have to be disposed of.

The use of disposable gowns and drapes is increasing in many operating departments, with many hospitals using them exclusively.

Advantages of disposable drapes and gowns

- Convenience
- Wide range of products
- Provide an effective barrier
- Packaging allows aseptic application
- Compact, thus easy to store
- Lint free
- Decreases cost of infection.

Various pieces of research[7] have shown that some non-woven fabrics can be about 10 times more effective in preventing bacteria dispersion than ordinary cotton. A 1980 study of 2000 wounds[8] demonstrated a substantial reduction in the amount of wound sepsis when disposable drapes and gowns were used – a rate of 6.4% with cotton and 2.3% with disposable fabrics. Similar results were obtained in another study in 1987.[9]

Disadvantages

- They can be expensive, as regular financial outlay is required.
- They are difficult to dispose of – incineration is required.
- A large amount of storage space needed for a large department (this difficulty can be overcome if the manufacturers are able to deliver frequently).
- There is concern regarding the ecological aspects of production.
- Drapability may have some limitations in surgical drapes.

Reusable gowns and drapes

In order to try and meet the needs of surgeons and theatre practitioners manufacturers have in recent years developed surgical drapes that are reusable, but for a limited number of occasions. They are aimed at those who do not wish to use disposable drapes, but require a higher-quality service than linen can provide. They are generally produced from tightly woven materials (such as polyester) that have been chemically treated to improve fluid repellence, or have a fluid repellent/non-linen lining.

Reusable gown and draping systems are managed in one of two ways; either the manufacturer provides the gowns and drapes to the hospital, and laundry, monitoring and quality control are managed 'in-house', or the manufacturer delivers the gowns and drapes to the hospital on a daily or weekly basis (as arranged), and collects soiled laundry at the same time. A designated delivery/collection area is therefore needed. Advantages of this arrangement are that the department can arrange for its required stock levels to be maintained, and that often the drapes and gowns are 'rented' rather than purchased. This allows the best use of a department's storage areas, and gives financial benefits for agreed requirements and prices.

Whichever system is used, an integral part of quality control is monitoring the number of uses of each item. Many manufacturers have identified 75 as the maximum number of times a drape or gown can be used. This can either be recorded by a bar-coding system, or by marking a grid on the drape with an indelible pen.

Advantages of reusable drapes and gowns

• There is less clinical waste produced than with disposables and so lower costs associated with the disposal of waste, both financial and environmental.
• There is less capital outlay if the system is managed by rental.
• A wide range of products is available.
• If the hospital laundry is used, more items can be included per load than with linen.

Disadvantages

• The use of strong detergents is required for washing, which raises some environmental concerns.
• Supplies are dependent on deliveries if in-house laundry is not used.
• Quality of drape is completely dependent on the efficiency of the monitoring of use system.
• Supplies may be difficult to regulate if the needs of the department change regularly.
• Specially designed or fully integral drapes are not possible.

The theatre practitioner and surgeon therefore need to consider many factors before deciding which drape system to use – linen, disposable or reusable. A key factor is likely to be the financial costs of the products. It is necessary to consider the hidden costs of a system as well as the obvious ones. Hidden costs of disposable drapes include the polythene bags, removal, transport and incineration or landfill costs, whereas the hidden costs of a reusable (non-linen) system include the regular telephone calls to place orders or amend requirements, and the cost of disposable drapes if the delivery system fails. Many research studies are available to support various draping materials – these must be incorporated into the cost analysis/decision-making process in any department.

Plastic incision drapes

There are now a wide range of plastic drapes available to supplement disposable or woven drapes. These incision drapes are placed over the incision site, in order to prevent bacteria from the patient's skin reaching the surgical wound, particularly in areas with many skin crevices, sebaceous glands and hair follicles. Their function therefore is to create a sterile working field immediately around the operation site, by immobilizing bacteria which could migrate towards the wound. The use of such drapes has two further advantages:

1. They keep the surgical drapes in the correct position and provide stability, thus eliminating the need for towel clips.
2. They keep the patient's skin clean, requiring minimal cleansing postoperatively. The ideal requirements of an incision drape are that it should be:

• impermeable to bacteria, yet allow the skin to breathe
• non-irritating
• transparent
• adhesive to the skin and conformable
• elastic
• allow for easy incisability.

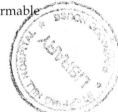

These requirements were identified as far back as 1942 by the surgeon Dr Michael DeBakey: '... If there could be applied to skin in the region in which the incision is to be made some impermeable substance which is sterile and which would adhere to the skin, the incision could be made through it and absolute protection from skin contamination would be afforded'.[10]

Manufacturers offer various types, sizes and designs of plastic incision drapes, and theatre practitioners must consider how they perform in relation to the above requirements. A further consideration is the action of the drape on bacteria, as some are identified as being 'antimicrobial' and provide a chemical as well as a physical barrier. For example, the 'Ioban 2 antimicrobial film' from 3M has iodophor incorporated into the adhesive coating of the film to provide a sustained release of iodine to the skin surface.

STORAGE OF SURGICAL GOWNS AND DRAPES

The exact nature of the storage arrangements used for gowns and drapes will depend on the type used, whether linen, disposable or reusable. The main factors to consider in relation to storage are as follows:

1. Gowns and drapes must be easily accessible to the theatre staff. The amount used by a large busy operating department is immense, and so turnover of supplies is rapid. Large storage facilities must therefore be available within the operating department itself, rather than within the hospital supplies department. A central store which can be decanted into individual theatres as required (at the beginning of each list for example) has many advantages:

- allows accurate ordering of supplies
- prevents stockpiling in individual theatres
- allows bulk orders to be placed, which generally has financial benefits.

2. Storage areas both within and outside the theatre itself must be clean, dry, tidy and well lit. Cleanliness is essential as the items are brought into the operating theatre, and so outer wrappers need to be clean and dust free. A dry environment is important, even though outer wrappers should be waterproof. Any moisture in contact with non-waterproof outer wrappers will facilitate contamination of the contents, thus destroying sterility.

Drapes are large, bulky and often heavy items, and need to be kept in large numbers. The storage area therefore needs to be tidy and well lit so that theatre practitioners can see easily and the drapes do not become a hazard by falling off shelves. A well-lit area, especially if well organized, will mean that gowns and drapes can be easily identified according to size and type. This should prevent the wrong drapes being opened by mistake, for example.

DISPOSAL

At the end of an operation all used gowns and drapes must be safely and correctly disposed of. It is essential that this does not happen until the operation is complete, and that swab, needle and instrument counts are correct. Nothing should leave the theatre until this has been established.

Gowns should be removed by the wearer while still wearing gloves. The correct procedure is as follows:

- Circulating theatre practitioner to undo neck and back ties or fastener.
- Scrub practitioner to remove gown by touching the outside only.
- Scrub practitioner to pull gown off over gloves (leaving gloves in place), fold or roll the gown up gently, and place in the correct disposal bag.
- Scrub practitioner to remove gloves.

This allows the gown (which is likely to be contaminated with the blood and body fluids of the patient) to be disposed of while the wearer is still adequately protected by their gloves.

It is poor practice for the scrub person to try and undo their own neck and back ties as this is likely to spread blood from their gloves to the back of their neck.

Once the wound has been cleaned and a sterile

dressing applied, the scrub practitioner can allow the careful removal of the surgical drapes. These must be gently rolled or folded to prevent any spillage or aerosol of blood occurring, and placed directly into the correct disposal bag.

Local policies must be adhered to regarding disposal of clinical waste or linen from the operating theatre. Theatre practitioners must be aware of these policies and ensure that all staff within the theatre are also familiar with correct procedures – this includes medical staff, all theatre practitioners, and any other members of staff such as healthcare assistants or orderlies. Most hospitals require that linen used in the operating theatre is double bagged, securely tied, and returned to the laundry as soon as possible. Linen should be washed within 11 hours in order to ensure that body protein is removed.[11] Similarly, disposable drapes and gowns should be double bagged in the correct bag for clinical waste, securely tied, and collected for disposal by incineration or landfill. Arrangements for the collection of reusable linen by the company must be clear to all theatre practitioners, and the collection point located within the operating department if possible.

It is good practice for all clinical waste and linen which leaves the operating theatre to be correctly labelled. This may help in the event of a lost item, from the patient or from a member of staff. Correct labelling includes:

- operating theatre number
- date
- morning or afternoon list
- number of the patient on the list.

This maintains confidentiality but allows easy retrieval of clinical waste if necessary.

PRINCIPLES OF DRAPING

Whichever type of drape is used the principles of draping remain the same. Draping is performed by the surgeon, the surgeon's assistant and the scrub practitioner. The ultimate responsibility for the correct preparation of the patient's skin and correct draping lies with the surgeon, who needs the help of the surgical team. Good teamwork is therefore essential. The theatre practitioner must take an active role in this, and have good knowledge and techniques. The aim of good draping technique is to place the sterile drapes on the patient in a way that does not contaminate either them or the surgical team. Draping is an essential component of good infection control and adequate time must be allowed. This is obviously a practical skill that can best be learnt by observing experienced theatre practitioners, by closely supervised practice and by experience. It is essential, however, that the theatre practitioner is aware of the principles of draping, and the reasoning behind them. The principles are provided here, with explanations, and are intended to enhance learning within the operating theatre.

1. Draping is performed after the surgeon has prepared the skin with an antiseptic solution. This reduces the numbers of microorganisms present[12] and thereby decreases the risk of wound infection. A wide area of the skin is prepared but only the area required for surgical access is left exposed during the draping procedure.

The area prepared with antiseptic must be allowed to dry before sterile drapes are applied: if drapes become wet, a wicking action may allow contamination from non-prepared areas to occur.

It is important that the surgeon has adequate access to the operation site, and that any necessary movements (such as the repositioning of a limb during orthopaedic surgery) do not expose any unprepared skin areas.

2. Drapes should not be shaken unnecessarily as any movement will disturb any dust or microorganisms within the environment. They should therefore be handled as little as possible (this also minimizes the problem of particulate becoming free from the drape), and placed gently on to the patient.

3. The scrub person should have the drapes prepared in the order of use for the operation to be performed. Prepackaged systems are usually presented in this way, but adaptation may be necessary in order to suit the needs of the surgeon, the patient and the specific operation to be

performed. If drapes are ready in the correct order, this means a minimum of movement once the patient is prepared. This is beneficial as increased air movement will disturb dust and microorganisms in the theatre.

The scrub practitioner must therefore have a good knowledge and understanding of:

- the surgery to be performed
- the relevant anatomy
- any specific surgeon's requirements, e.g. needs access to the pedal pulses during arterial surgery
- any specific patient care issues or relevant considerations, e.g. patient has had a previous leg amputation.

Knowledge of these will mean the theatre practitioner can plan the draping procedure accordingly, assist the surgeon fully, and prevent delays which lengthen the anaesthetic time.

4. Drapes should remain folded while being carried to the operating table and must be supported while being put in place, to avoid touching non-sterile areas. Large drapes which cover large areas of the patient and the operating table need at least two members of the scrub team to position them. The scrub practitioner should ensure that the drape is supported at all times in order to prevent contamination by allowing it to fall incorrectly, thus needing to be moved into the correct position.

5. Drapes must be placed directly into their required position, not positioned and then moved, as this allows contamination by the movement of microorganisms from the patient's skin. Even areas of prepared skin have been shown to have microorganisms left, although fewer than before.[12]

6. Drapes must not be allowed to touch non-sterile items or equipment in the operating theatre. Items that need to be close to the operative field should therefore be moved in after the sterile field has been created by the drapes. This includes items such as:

- operating lights
- electrosurgical (diathermy) units
- suction units

- stools if the surgical team will be sitting
- air cylinders.

The scrub practitioner should ensure that as wide an area as possible is free from equipment to allow draping to take place. The circulating practitioner should ensure that these vital items are moved in towards the sterile field after the application of drapes, in order to allow surgery to commence.

7. When being positioned, drapes must be held in such a way that the hands of the surgical team are protected from possible contamination. The corners of the drapes must be wrapped around the hand, so that the gloved hand will not come into contact with the non-sterile area being covered. Also, the drapes should be allowed to fall into position by gravity once correctly placed. The members of the scrub team must not allow their gloved hands to become close to non-sterile areas.

8. Sterile drapes should not be allowed to fall below waist level until in their correct position. This area is not considered sterile, as it may have been contaminated inadvertently. If a drape does fall below this level, or is contaminated in any other way, it must be discarded immediately.

9. Although the exact draping order will vary for each operative procedure, the overriding principle is that the area around the incision site should be draped first, followed by the rest of the patient.

10. Drapes should be held securely in place during surgery to maintain the sterile field and allow good surgical access. This can be achieved by the use of:

- non-perforating towel clips;
- plastic incision drapes;
- adhesive panels on the drapes themselves.

11. If the sterility of a drape is questioned in any way, it should be discarded immediately and new drapes obtained.

The above principles also apply to the draping of instrument trolleys, the Mayo table, and any other necessary items.

The scrub practitioner must ensure that all members of the team adhere to these guidelines, as some of them may be unfamiliar with acting as a member of the scrub team and with aseptic technique. The scrub practitioner and the circulating person must therefore closely observe the draping procedure at all times, and take immediate action if sterility is breached in any way.

REFERENCES

1. Beck W, Collette T 1952 False faith in surgeon's gown and drape. American Journal of Surgery 83: 125–126
2. Duguid J, Wallace A 1948 Air infection with dust liberated from clothing. Lancet ii: 845–849
3. Hoborn J 1984 In: Whyte W 1988 The role of clothing and drapes in the operating room. Journal of Hospital Infection II (Suppl C): 2–17
4. Drake C 1977 In: Aseptic principles and performance of draping materials. 3M Healthcare, Loughborough
5. AORN 1989 Operating room practices: myth or science? AORN Journal 49: 645–649
6. Whyte W 1988 The role of clothing and drapes in the operating room. Journal of Hospital Infection 11 (Suppl C): 2–17
7. Whyte et al 1983 A bacteriologically occlusive clothing system for use in the operating room. Journal of Bone and Joint Surgery 65B: 502–506
8. Moylan J, Kennedy B 1980 The importance of gown and drape barriers in the prevention of wound infection. Surgery, Gynaecology and Obstetrics 151: 465–470
9. Moylan J, Fitzpatrick K, Davenport K 1987 Reducing wound infection. Improved gown and drape barrier performances. Archives of Surgery 122: 152–157
10. DeBakey M, Giles E, Honold E 1942 The protection of the surgical field with an impermeable adhesive skin coating. Surgery, Gynaecology and Obstetrics 74: 499–504
11. Ryan P 1979 Reusables vs. disposables? Defending your position. AORN Journal 30: 419, 423
12. Ritter M et al 1980 In: Aseptic principles and performance of draping materials. 3M Healthcare, Loughborough

FURTHER READING

Barrie D 1994 How hospital linen and laundry services are provided. Journal of Hospital Infection 27: 219–235

Noriega L 1984 The OR nurse's view: sterile barriers. Surgical Rounds,. February: 117–121

Medical Devices Directorate Performance specification for cotton and polyester/cotton reusable operating theatre fabrics. DoH, London

USEFUL ADDRESSES

Amba Medical Ltd
Unit 5
Bonville Trading
Estate
Bonville Road
Brislington
Bristol
BS4 5QH

Angelica International Ltd
Ashton Road
Golborne
Warrington
WA3 3UL

Johnson and Johnson Medical
Coronation Road
Ascot
Berkshire
SL5 9YT

3M Health Care Ltd
3M House
Morley Street
Loughborough
Leicestershire
LE11 1CP

Molnlycke Ltd
Health Care Products
Southfields Road
Dunstable
Bedfordshire LU6 3ES

Rotenco
Lojigma International Ltd
Elgin Industrial Estate
Dunfermline
Fife
KY12 7SA

Smith and Nephew
PO Box 81
Hessle Road
Hull
HU3 2BN

Sterile Theatre Services Plc
Unit M
Harlow House
Shelton Road
Willowbrook Industrial Estate
Corby
Northants
NN17 1XH

Surgical gloves

Sterile surgical gloves are worn by the surgeon and assistant(s) and the scrub practitioner – the surgical scrub team. They are therefore one of the most commonly used 'tools of the trade' of the theatre practitioner. They are made from latex rubber or rubber sheets, and must be thin enough to allow good dexterity for all the members of the surgical team.

FUNCTIONS

The original use of surgical gloves, which were developed in the early years of this century, was to protect the hands of nurses and surgeons from the strong antiseptic chemicals used during surgery, such as carbolic acid. Such antiseptics are no longer used, but surgical gloves have two other important functions within the operating department:

1. To allow sterile instruments, swabs and sutures to be handled by the surgical team during the operation. Sterile surgical gloves, if correctly worn, mean that items used are not contaminated by microorganisms on the hands of the scrub team. The main function of the surgical glove is therefore to protect the patient.

2. Surgical gloves provide protection for the scrub team from the blood and body fluids of the patient. Intact gloves will prevent blood coming into contact with the skin of the wearer, which is potentially dangerous if they have an area of broken skin. There are many viral diseases with which the surgical team is threatened, for example viral hepatitis (especially B and C); herpes simplex viruses (types 1 and 2); cytomegalovirus; papillomavirus; and human immunodeficiency virus. Surgical gloves are therefore the first line of defence against infection for both the patient and the surgical team.

REQUIREMENTS

There are many types of surgical gloves available from various manufacturers. The theatre practi-tioner must be aware of what is required from a surgical glove, in order to assist in purchasing a range suitable for the operating department. The requirements of a surgical glove can be outlined as follows:

1. Sterile, and easy to identify as such from the packaging. This is necessary in order to fulfil the first function of a surgical glove.

2. [?]e protection against fluid and bloodborne [?]s. This is necessary in order to fulfil the [?] unction of a surgical glove. The gloves must therefore be waterproof and strong enough to prevent easy tearing or damage. Some gloves are designed to be especially tough, for orthopaedic and other rigorous surgery: Dextron from Becton Dickinson, and EP Extra Protection from Ansell, for example. Gloves are now available that are clearly able to indicate when a puncture has occurred – Biogel Reveal from Regent, for example, is a double-gloving system which turns green in the presence of blood or body fluids.

3. Sensitive, flexible and pliable, in order to allow the surgeon to feel the organs and tissues of the body. This is vital, as precise dexterity is necessary for the success of an operation. Some gloves are designed to be especially sensitive, and have a high level of grip to increase control over delicate instruments for use in ophthalmic and other microsurgery; Biogel M from Regent, is one such example.

4. Easy to don. Surgical gloves should be easy to don using a closed gloving technique which allows the wearer to put the gloves on in an aseptic manner, without touching the outside with a non-gloved hand (see Chapter 6). Surgical gloves must therefore be packaged in such a way as to facilitate this. Gloves should also be easy to don in other situations – when double gloving is required, or during a necessary mid-operation glove change, for example. A glove that is easy to don will glide on to the hand with a minimum of pulling.

5. Comfortable to wear and the correct size. Surgical gloves will be worn for many hours by

all members of the scrub team. They must therefore be comfortable and not cause cramp in the hand due to tightening. Gloves should be available in a range of sizes (5–9), including half sizes, in order to provide the wearer with a good fit. Fit and comfort are important in the following areas:

- Fingers – too long will hamper dexterity and get in the way; too short will be painful and may force the fingernail through the glove;
- Length – the glove should be long enough to allow the cuff of the gown to be completely enclosed within it;
- Cuff – should be tight enough to hold the gown cuff in place, but not so tight as to constrict circulation and cause cramp. The cuff must also be strong, as it is used to pull the glove on.
- Palm – if a glove is too tight over the palm the hand is forced into an unnatural position, causing cramp and a decrease in dexterity.

The theatre practitioner must assist new staff to choose the correct size of glove.

6. Hypoallergenic. Many people suffer from skin reactions to surgical gloves and so hypoallergenic properties may help to minimize this problem (see below).

7. Strong. Surgical gloves must be strong enough to withstand vigorous handling without tearing.

8. Financially economic. Gloves are used for all types of surgery, by all members of the surgical team, so the cost per pair is an important consideration. Cheap gloves, however, may be a false economy, necessitating frequent changes if they are damaged.

9. Meet required standards. In the UK, these include those laid down by the Department of Health and the British Standard Institute.[1] It is helpful for the theatre practitioner to be aware of whether the manufacturing company holds Department of Health accreditation. Theatre practitioners should also be aware of the quality control mechanism that manufacturers use: do they use an inflation test, water test and electronic inspection, for example? This should be included in the product information supplied by the manufacturer.

10. Readily available. Surgical gloves are used by the hundred each day in every operating department. Their supply must therefore be consistent and the ordering and delivery system failsafe.

All these requirements should be considered by the theatre practitioner, and manufacturers' literature studied to establish how a glove performs in relation to each. Surgical gloves with other features are now available from various manufacturers which aim to improve one or more aspects of glove requirements. For example:

- Reinforced cuff to enhance strength.
- Antimicrobial surface – the glove is coated with a compound that offers broad-spectrum antimicrobial activity against certain bacteria and thus protects both patient and surgeon; examples are Nutex by Ansell and Bioguard by Regent. These may be especially useful when the surgery involves the insertion of an implant, such as in orthopaedic, cardiac and vascular surgery. Infection in these cases is a particular problem in terms of mortality and implant acceptance.
- Brown-coloured gloves that reduce the glare from operating lights, e.g. Eudermic from Becton Dickinson.
- Gloves with a minimal level of pyrogens. Pyrogens can be released from the walls of dead bacteria, which were present on the surface of the glove during manufacture and killed during sterilization. These can give rise to various pathogenic reactions in humans.

Theatre practitioners and surgeons need to consider these additional features carefully, and determine whether they are beneficial within their surgical specialty, and any financial implications.

PROBLEMS WITH SURGICAL GLOVES

There are two main problems caused by the use of surgical gloves, which affect both the patient and the surgical team. The theatre practitioner should have a good understanding of these complex problems, and aim to keep up to date with manufacturing developments and clinical research.

Allergies

Glove allergies – correctly called contact dermatitis – mainly affect operating theatre staff and surgeons, but can also affect patients, especially those who have multiple operations (see Chapter 3).[2] There has been a growing demand for gloves for non-sterile procedures in recent years, which has been attributed to the growing awareness of HIV, hepatitis and other viral infections.[3] There has also been an increase in glove allergies, apparently reflecting this increase in the wearing of gloves.[4] These can range from redness, dryness and itching to blistered and broken skin which causes immense pain and suffering. The allergy is to one or more of the components of latex gloves, or the chemicals used in their manufacture, which are known as accelerators.

Glove allergies are a highly complex issue, with many factors to be considered. These are fully discussed elsewhere (see Chapter 3).[2,3,5–7] Any theatre practitioner who develops contact dermatitis will need the support and advice of their occupational health department, and should be referred to a dermatologist.

To assist in the choosing of a hypoallergenic glove the theatre practitioner can ask if the glove has passed the modified Shelanski test: this is a complex, internationally recognized test used to identify a hypoallergenic glove. Company representatives can supply up-to-date clinical research regarding the use of hypoallergenic gloves, and may be able to recommend the most suitable.

Puncture

Glove puncture is a hazard for both surgeons and patients, as the barrier between them is broken and so the gloves cannot carry out their protective function. The causes of glove puncture include trauma from surgical instruments and suture needles. Brookes[8] identifies a number of ways of reducing needlestick injury to less than 3%:

- using forceps rather than fingers during dissection or suturing
- using retractors rather than hands for retracting tissues
- careful handling of the diathermy point when not in use
- handling wires with forceps.

Further steps towards safer surgery include the use of staples rather than sutures, and the use of diathermy, ultrasonic dissectors or laser knives as an alternative to scalpels.

Many studies have identified glove punctures following surgery; for example, Cruse and Ford[9] and Church and Sanderson[10] found that 11.6% and 11.5% respectively of the gloves they studied were punctured following surgery.

Other studies identify differing puncture rates for different surgical specialties. Holborn,[11] for example, found a 48% puncture rate in orthopaedic surgery compared to 16% in soft tissue surgery. Townsend identifies the incidence in cardiac surgery as 41% and in ophthalmic surgery as 6%. A study by Fell[12] identifies the incidence of glove puncture in relation to the length of operation time, with the incidence of defective gloves increasing in longer operations. Gloves used in operations of less than 15 minutes had a 5.5% rate of defects, and more than 3 hours a rate of 27.1%. This study also considers the location of the glove perforation, with the surgeon's left hand having the highest incidence, suggesting a link with suturing technique.

A further study[13] considers who in the surgical team has the most glove punctures, and identifies that surgeons had the highest rate, which agree with a similar study by Bliss and Alexander.[14]

REFERENCES

1. Ansell (undated) Gloves: the facts. Ansell Medical, Surrey
2. Townsend M 1994 Just a glove? British Journal of Theatre Nursing 4: 7–10
3. Fay M 1991 Hand dermatitis: the role of gloves. AORN Journal 54: 451–467
4. Heese A et al 1991 Allergic and irritant reactions to rubber gloves in medical health services. Journal of the American Academy of Dermatology 5: 831–839
5. Waywell L 1993 Contact dermatitis due to surgical latex gloves. British Journal of Theatre Nursing 3: 18–21
6. Gutteridge P 1993 Dusting powder in surgeons' gloves: A historical review. British Journal of Theatre Nursing (Suppl) 2: S6–S10
7. Kelly K 1993 Latex sensitivity in the operating theatre. Surgery Barrier Breakdown – new issues. Ansell Medical, Surrey
8. Brookes A 1994 Surgical glove perforation. Nursing Times 90: 60–62
9. Cruse P, Ford R 1980 The epidemiology of wound infection. A 10-year prospective study of 62,939 wounds. Surgical Clinics of North America 60: 27–40
10. Church J, Sanderson P 1984 Surgical glove punctures. Journal of Hospital Infection 1: 84
11. Holborn J 1981 In: Whyte W 1988 The role of clothing and drapes in the operating room. Journal of Hospital Infection 11 (Suppl C): 2–17
12. Fell M 1987 Failure rates in surgical gloves .In: Risks and complications. The patient and surgeons in theatre. The Medicine Group (UK) Ltd, Oxford
13. Barrie W 1987 Surgical glove perforations Risks and complication. The patients and surgeons in theatre. The Medicine Group (UK) Ltd, Oxford
14. Bliss S, Alexander W J 1992 Surgical gloves – a comparative study of the incidence and site of puncture. British Journal of Theatre Nursing Febuary: 16–17
15. Ellis E 1990 The hazards of surgical glove dusting powders. Surgery 171: 531–537

FURTHER READING

A review – Risks and complications: The patient and surgeon in theatre. Symposium held at the Royal College of Surgeons, London, 25 November 1987

AORN Operating room practices: myth or science? AORN Journal 49: 645–649

PRODUCT AND EDUCATIONAL INFORMATION

Ansell Medical,
Ansell House,
119 Evell Road,
Surbiton,
Surrey KT6 6AY,
UK

Becton Dickinson UK Ltd,
Between Towns Road,
Cowley,
Oxford OX4 3LY,
UK

Regent Hospital Products,
London International House,
Turnford Place,
Broxbavine,
Herts EN10 6LN,
UK

Puritee Medical Company Ltd,
2 Mill Court,
51 Mill Street,
Slough, Berks SL2 5DA,
UK

Implants

There is a wide variety of surgical implants for a wide range of surgical disciplines.

ORTHOPAEDIC SURGERY

Orthopaedic surgery probably has the widest range of implants, ranging from extensive trauma implants for the fixation of fractures to finger joint replacements. No single material is ideal for all purposes; materials commonly used are:

- metals – stainless steel, colbalt chromium alloys and titanium alloys
- ultrahigh molecular weight polyethylene (UHMWPE)
- silicon compounds
- braided polypropylene
- acrylic cement (PMMA).

Various metals are used for large joint replacement components, usually articulating with a polyethylene component, for example in total hip and knee components. Colbalt chrome and titanium alloys are stronger, more rigid and less liable to corrosion than steel.

It should be noted that the articulating surfaces of all joint implants should be protected at all times. A protective cover is normally supplied by the manufacturer, and this should not be removed until the time of insertion, to avoid inadvertent damage to the smooth surface.

Stainless steel is used for a wide variety of components, including plates, screws and intramedullary nails for fracture fixation. Stainless steel has tensile plasticity, which makes it possible to bend plates to the required shape during an operation without disturbing their strength.

Silicone compounds are used in orthopaedic implants for finger, toe and wrist joint applications, as well as stents for tendon sheath reformation. Silicone rubbers have poor abrasion resistance and therefore should not be used in weight-bearing application unless they incorporate sheaths of a higher abrasion resistance.[1]

Braided polypropylene is used to augment autogenous grafts for disrupted anterior cruciate ligaments of the knee. This allows the patient to mobilize earlier owing to the initial strength provided at operation and the gain of functional strength with time.[2]

Acrylic cement or polymethyl methacrylate is used to fix joint replacements into bony cavities. The cement can be likened to a grouting material that holds the implant rigidly in place. Charnley[3] calculated that the addition of cement increased the load-bearing capacity of the femur by 200 times. There are, however, problems that arise with the use of cement, which may result from poor surgical technique, which include loosening of the implant resulting in infection. Cleaning of the bony bed prior to insertion of the cement, and pressurization of the cement into the bone by mechanical injection to ensure intrusion are considered good surgical techniques.[1]

VASCULAR AND THORACIC SURGERY

Grafts are used in vascular and thoracic surgery to replace vessels damaged by arteriosclerosis, which causes narrowing and ultimately occlusion, resulting in ischaemia of the tissues supplied. Two materials will be discussed, Dacron and PTFE (polytetrafluoroethylene).

Dacron is available either knitted or woven; it is made of polyethylene terephthalate and is kink resistant with an elastic property. Some Dacron grafts are available with gelatin or collagen impregnation, which seals the graft and acts in a similar way to fibrin. Knitted Dacron has a high patency and therefore requires to be preclotted with the patient's blood prior to use. Woven Dacron has a lower porosity; these and protein-impregnated grafts do not require preclotting.

PTFE consists of longitudinal fibres of Teflon linked with thinner fibres running transversely. It is strong and kink free but does not possess the elastic properties of Dacron. Newer versions of this material do possess some stretch characteristics, designed to provide forgiveness when cutting the graft to the correct length.

All grafts come in a variety of lengths and diameters. Bifurcated grafts are also available.

Soft tissue patches made from multiaxially expanded polytetrafluoroethylene (ePTFE) are used for many surgical applications, for the reconstruction of hernias and soft tissue deficiencies. It provides an open latticework structure for cellular penetration and collagen deposition. Its flexibility allows the material to be implanted laparoscopically.

OTHER TYPES OF IMPLANT

There are a wide variety of other implants available and the theatre practitioner should be familiar with those in use in individual departments. They may include:

- silicone breast implants
- silicone testicular implants
- grommets
- cochlear implants
- ventriculoperitoneal shunts
- aortic and mitral valves
- dental implants
- internal fixation for maxillofacial fractures – wiring/plates and screws
- intraocular lens implants.

Most implants will be packed sterile by the manufacturer; if an implant is opened inadvertently, the theatre practitioner should refer to the manufacturer's literature as to whether it can be resterilized safely using the methods available. If there is any doubt concerning the sterility of an item it should be referred back to the manufacturer.

For any implant surgery, aseptic technique must be rigorously adhered to. At operation sites with poor antimicrobial defences (e.g. total hip replacement) clinical infection may result from microorganisms with a weak pathogenicity.[4]

Most implant manufacturers will also provide specialist instrumentation or insertion devices if applicable. Operative technique manuals may also be available for the surgeon and theatre practitioners.

All implant packaging should have details of the following:

- manufacturer
- type
- size (if applicable)
- code number
- batch number
- sterilization date
- expiry date of sterilization.

This will aid the practitioner in documenting the item used, ensuring the sterility of an item, and providing information for reordering. Details of the implant used should always be documented in the operation notes: many companies now provide sticky labels for this purpose. This is an important aspect for the theatre practitioner to consider. The Consumer Protection Act (1987) requires that theatre personnel keep records of the source, serial number and batch code of all products used in the treatment and care of patients. Failure to provide this information will result in the organization becoming the supplier and therefore taking on liability under the Act.

The National Association of Theatre Nurses[5] recommends that the minimum information recorded should include details of all long-term implanted materials.

When any implant is to be inserted the theatre practitioner must take special note of any patient allergies: it is not uncommon for patients to be allergic to certain metals or rubber compounds and this would obviously have disastrous implications for them.

Implants should be stored in a dry, dust-free area. A variety of stock should be available, with a system for stock replacement. Theatre practitioners should be aware of the method of ordering stock, the stock levels required for individual implants and the variety of individual items available to the surgeon. Strict stock rotation should be practised to avoid wastage and expense caused by implants reaching their sterilization expiry dates.

REFERENCES

1. Black J 1988 Orthopaedic biomaterials in research and practice. Churchill Livingstone, London
2. Miles S 1988 The Kennedy LAD ligament augmentation device. British Journal of Theatre Nursing 25: 18–20
3. Charnley J 1970 Acrylic cement in orthopaedic surgery. Churchill Livingstone, Edinburgh
4. Ayliffe GRJ, Lowbury EJL, Geddes AM, Williams JD 1993 Control of hospital infection. A practical handbook. Chapman & Hall, London
5. National Association of Theatre Nurses 1989 The Consumer Protection Act 1987; Guidance document. NATN, London

Wound dressing

The final aseptic procedure in the operating theatre itself is the application of a sterile dressing to cover the surgical wound. The theatre practitioner must be familiar with the following:

- types of wound closure
- functions and requirements of wound dressings
- types of wound dressing
- application of wound dressings
- role of the theatre practitioner in relation to wound dressings.

TYPES OF WOUND CLOSURE

A surgical wound is a major break in the patient's skin integrity and hence a possible entry route for pathogenic organisms. The choice of dressing for the surgical wound will depend on the method of closure the surgeon uses.

Primary

Most surgical wounds will be closed by primary closure, in which the skin and underlying tissues are closely approximated. This gives a good cosmetic result, minimal scarring and good protection against infection (Fig. 5.21). The risk of postoperative infection is therefore minimal – the skin edges have been approximated to achieve maximum integrity and wound healing will be rapid. Scab formation will begin as early as 2 hours postoperatively and epithelialization will probably have occurred partially by 24 hours post-surgery, and completely by 48 hours post-surgery. Indeed, two studies have shown that epithelialization of a sutured wound is complete within 24–48 hours.[1,2] The dressing will therefore be necessary for only a short time, if at all.

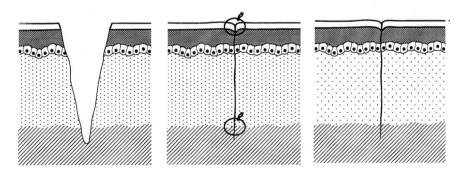

Figure 5.21   Primary closure.

Delayed primary

If primary closure is not possible because of the presence of infection or contamination by faeces, pus or foreign bodies – such as glass following a road traffic accident, for example – the surgeon may choose to leave the wound open for a short time. This is helpful as an obviously contaminated wound closed immediately is at considerable risk of infection and breakdown.[3] Delayed primary closure involves the superficial wound layers being left open once any body cavities that have been opened for the surgery have been closed. The open wound is then packed loosely with dressings. This allows the wound to develop resistance to infection over 4–5 days, when it can then be closed by primary closure. While still open the wound should be covered with a non-adherent dressing and disturbed as little as possible until primary closure is achieved (Fig. 5.22).

This method of delayed primary closure is most useful in traumatic wounds, and the choice of dressing will vary according to the individual situation. The surgeon, theatre practitioner and ward nurse can consider the choice of dressing in relation to the factors that constitute an optimum dressing[4] (Table 5.1). However, consideration must be given to the function of the dressing and pack used in delayed primary closure, which is to keep the wound open until it is appropriate to close it by primary closure.

Secondary intention

Wounds which have extensive tissue damage cannot be successfully closed by primary or delayed primary closure, as approximation of the skin edges is either impossible or undesirable. Such wounds are therefore allowed to heal by secondary intention. This involves the natural healing processes of inflammation, destruction, proliferation and maturation to occur from the base of the wound upwards, and thus is a slower method of healing (Fig. 5.23).

The choice of dressing for this type of wound will depend on a thorough assessment of the wound and its needs: the absorption of exudate and the formation of a moist environment, for example.

FUNCTIONS AND REQUIREMENTS OF A WOUND DRESSING

The function of a wound dressing is primarily to assist the body's natural healing processes by creating an optimum healing environment. Certain factors have been identified as features of a dressing that will contribute to such an optimum healing environment: these are identified in Box 5.1 and the rationale for each criterion is included.[4]

Most postoperative wounds will be healing by primary intention and will have skin sutures or staples present. The ideal postoperative dressing will therefore include factors identified by Turner[4] in addition to the following criteria:

- Protect skin sutures from catching on patient's clothing or bed clothing.
- Be able to stay securely in place when the patient is moving, thus needs to be adherent to surrounding skin, but not adherent to the wound itself.

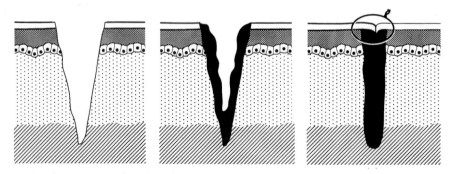

Figure 5.22 Delayed primary closure.

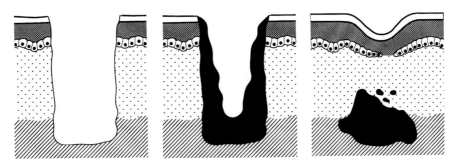

Figure 5.23 Secondary intention.

- Be comfortable for the patient.
- Be able to absorb blood.
- Protect the patient and others from the sight of the wound.

The final two criteria will now be briefly discussed.

Absorption of blood

The closure of a surgical wound requires effective haemostasis in the subcuticular and skin

> **Box 5.1** Criteria for an optimum dressing, with rationale (Adapted from Turner[4])
>
> To maintain high humidity between the wound and dressing (*to keep wound surface moist to promote rapid epidermal healing*)
>
> To remove excess exudate and toxic compounds (*to avoid tissue sloughing and minimize inflammatory phase*)
>
> To allow gaseous exchange (*to allow oxygen to the wound, thus accelerate epithelialization*)
>
> To provide thermal insulation to the wound surface (*to maintain wound at body temperature to allow high mitotic activity, rapid epithelialization, and improved granulation*)
>
> To be impermeable to bacteria (*to prevent contamination by airborne microorganisms which may infect the wound*)
>
> To be free from particles and toxic wound contaminants (*to avoid disrupted healing, granuloma and abnormal scarring*)
>
> To allow removal without causing trauma during dressing change (*to avoid stripping newly formed tissue on removal of dressing*)

layers, to prevent blood loss or the formation of a haematoma postoperatively. It is important, however, that haemostasis does not achieve a bloodless layer, as this is likely to be detrimental to healing. Furthermore, excessive use of diathermy leaves large amounts of dead tissue, thereby increasing the risk of clinical infection.[5] It is likely, therefore, that a patient will have some postoperative blood loss from the wound. A dressing serves to absorb blood from the wound site until effective natural coagulation takes place, probably within 24 hours. A wound dressing used in theatre should therefore be able to absorb blood, both in order to allow assessment of the amount of loss, and to prevent the patient's clothes and the bedclothes becoming badly soiled.

Protection from the sight of the wound

A surgical wound dressing provides a useful visual barrier to the wound in the immediate postoperative period, which provides many benefits for the patient's care. The formation of any surgical wound, however large or small, will have an effect on the patient's view of their own body image. Loss of self-esteem owing to altered body image is a major consideration when caring for a surgical patient. Adjustment to altered body image is often a long, slow and painful process during which the patient needs great support from nurses and other healthcare professionals. Acknowledgement and acceptance of their wound is an important part in this process, and the patient will need skilled care and support when viewing their wound for the first time. This will be especially important if the surgery has involved the removal of an external part of their body, such as a leg or breast, or involves a very visible part such as the face or head.

The patient also needs to be ready to view the wound, and to be conscious and rational. The immediate postoperative phase is therefore not an ideal time. Many factors contribute to this: the patient may be:

- drowsy and drifting in and out of sleep
- confused or disorientated
- unable to focus clearly
- unable to express themselves clearly.

They may therefore find the sight of the wound distressing but they may be unable to express their feelings, needs and questions, and so the distress and anxiety will increase. Furthermore, immediately postoperatively the surgical wound will have:

- blood loss/drains
- skin preparation fluids
- acute inflammation

and is thus not in an ideal state to be seen for the first time.

The dressing therefore provides an effective visual barrier for the immediate postoperative phase. This means the patient can view the wound for the first time when they are fully awake, orientated, able to express themselves clearly, and possibly with a family member or friend to support them. It also means the wound can be cleaned, the inflammation will have lessened, and drains may have been removed. The patient will also be in the ward, where a nurse can support them on a longer-term basis than can operating theatre staff.

TYPES OF WOUND DRESSING

The range of dressings available is increasing dramatically, and clinical research strives to prove the benefits of each. Modern dressings can be divided into categories, shown with their primary function in Box 5.2.

Box 5.2 Types of wound dressings and their primary function.

Semipermeable film dressings (wound protection, maintenance of moist environment, skin protection to prevent shearing)

Foam dressings (absorption of exudate in cavity or superficial wounds)

Alginate dressings (absorption of exudate and gel formation – improved healing environment)

Hydrogel dressings (provision of a moist environment)

Hydrocolloid dressings (gel forming to encourage autolysis and allow removal of devitalized tissue)

Polysaccharide pastes, granules and beads (absorption of exudate)

Odour-absorbing dressings (to absorb odour from a malodorous wound)

Traditional

Gauze

Woven gauze has been used as a wound dressing for many years, providing absorbent coverage which will protect the skin sutures and be a visual barrier for the postoperative phase. It does, however, have many limitations:

- It is likely to over-dry a wound.
- It can cause pain and trauma on removal, thus delaying healing.
- It is difficult to apply in a secure manner.
- It is not a barrier to infection.
- It sheds particulate into the wound.

It therefore achieves very few of the criteria of the optimum dressing, and its use is limited. Gauze is therefore only appropriate for clean wounds, closed by primary closure, for a short postoperative period.

Non-adherent dressings

Low-absorption pads such as Melonin can be used for postoperative wounds. These consist of a layer of polymeric film, which is placed in contact with the wound, backed with cotton/viscose fibre mixes. This allows the passage of exudate away from the wound and thus prevents sticking. They perform the functions of minimal blood absorption, protection of sutures, and a visual barrier for the postoperative wound. The non-adherent quality also means they should cause minimal trauma during removal. They are therefore suitable for fairly dry surgical wounds with minimal exudate, for a short postoperative period, and will need securing with tape or bandages.

Plaster-backed dressings

Many wound dressing products such as melonin are available with an adhesive backing. This avoids the use of tape and bandages and provides a non-adherent dressing with an adherent surround. Again, this provides some functions of a postoperative dressing (see above) but does not create an optimum healing environment.

Choosing a postoperative dressing therefore involves a thorough assessment of the patient, the wound and the products available.

Many traditional dressings meet very few of the criteria of an ideal dressing, and do not contribute to an optimum healing environment. Their use is therefore limited to the short term, mainly to achieve protection of the wound in the immediate postoperative period. They are not suitable for long-term use, when other products, which maximize the healing environment, are more suitable.

Many hospitals have a wound management protocol to promote continuity of care in relation to wound treatments and dressing products, which is based on clinical research.[6] Gourlay[7] questions why theatres are often not involved in using such protocols, relying on traditional dressings such as gauze and paraffin gauze, and identifies that the cost of traditional dressings is much less than modern products. However, Dealy[8] states that newer dressings need to be changed less frequently and enhance healing time. The surgical team must address this issue, which is no doubt compounded by separate budgets for operating theatres and surgical wards – meaning that an increased financial outlay for improved wound products for one budget (theatres) will result in financial savings for another budget (surgical wards) owing to the reduction in number of dressings, dressing packs and nurses' time required for dressing changes.

APPLICATION OF WOUND DRESSINGS

The wound dressing must be applied by the surgeon or scrub practitioner using aseptic technique. This is the final part of the operative procedure, and an important one. The scrub practitioner must not allow the removal of the surgical drapes until the dressing has been applied. Any movement of the drapes before this point may cause contamination of the wound by skin cells and particles from other areas of the patient's body. The wound and surrounding skin should be cleaned with normal saline (many antiseptics disrupt wound healing), dried and the dressing applied. The drapes can then be removed.

The patient should then be covered rapidly, to help their temperature (and the temperature of the wound) to return to normal as soon as possible. This is essential as wound healing processes occur at 37°C, and in a cold wound healing will be delayed.

ROLE OF THE THEATRE PRACTITIONER

The theatre practitioner should be involved in the following:

- Consideration, with the surgeon and ward staff, of the most appropriate choice of wound dressing products for routine immediate postoperative use. Wicker[9] states that nurses have a professional responsibility to ensure that there is a sound rationale underlying practice
- Documentation of selected products on surgeons' preference cards
- Supply and control of a stock of selected products in the operating theatre
- Understanding of the functions and limitations of both modern and traditional dressing products
- Application of wound dressings using aseptic technique

• Teaching new, junior staff and students in the operating theatre about wound healing and the requirements of dressings in the immediate postoperative phase.

REFERENCES

1. Ordman L, Gillman T 1966 Studies in the healing of cutaneous wounds. 1. The healing of incisions through the skin of pigs. Archives of Surgery 93: 857–882
2. Madden J 1976 Wound healing: the biological basis of hand surgery. Clinical Plastic Surgery 3: 3–11
3. Westaby S 1985 Wound closure and drainage. In: Wetsaby S (ed) Wound care. Heinemann, London, Chapter 5
4. Turner T 1985 Which dressing and why? In: Westaby S (ed) Wound care. Heinemann, London, Chapter 7
5. Westaby S, White S 1985 Wound infection. In: Westaby S (ed) Wound care. Heinemann, London, Chapter 8
6. Rodgers S 1991 Using proper protocol. Nursing Times 87: 43–45
7. Gourlay D 1994 Theatre practices. Nursing Times 90: 64–68
8. Dealy C 1990 The cost of wound care. Nursing 4: 14–16
9. Wicker P 1992 Wound dressings. British Journal of Theatre Nursing 2: 22–25

FURTHER READING

Bale S 1993 Wound assessment. Surgical Nurse 6: 11–14
Bale S 1993 Intervention in wound management. Surgical Nurse 6: 17–20
Cutting K 1990 Wound cleansing Surgical Nurse 3 : 4–8
Gibson C 1993 Cavity dressings ancient and modern – a little research. British Journal of Theatre Nursing 3: 8–10
Morgan D 1992 Formulary of wound management products, 5th edn. Media Medica Publications, Chichester
Rigby H 1992 Tissue healing: part 1. Surgery 10: 261
Rigby H 1992 Tissue healing: part 2. Surgery 10: 286–288
Thomas S 1990 Wound management and dressings. Pharmaceutical Press, London
Thomas S (ed) 1994 Handbook of wound dressings. Journal of Wound Care, London

Surgical swabs

Surgical swabs are one of the most commonly used items in the operating theatre, and the practitioner must be familiar with the following aspects:

- functions
- types
- requirements
- supply
- role of the theatre practitioner.

FUNCTIONS OF SURGICAL SWABS

The functions of surgical swabs are:

- blood absorption
- packing a cavity during surgery
- blunt dissection.

Blood absorption

The primary function of a surgical swab is absorption of blood during an operation. Almost all surgery involves blood loss, which must be controlled in order for the surgeon to have good access and vision at the operative site. This involves achieving haemostasis with either diathermy or ligatures, and using gauze swabs to absorb the remaining blood loss.

Packing a cavity

A second function of surgical swabs is to use them to pack an area or body cavity for a period of time during surgery. Swabs are used in this way in order to keep an area moist, such as the bowel during abdominal surgery, to keep an area separate from the operative field, thereby assisting exposure, and to achieve some degree of haemostasis by pressure. For example, large swabs (or packs) are usually used for packing the abdominal cavity; smaller cavities can also be packed, for example the use of mastoid (or tonsil) swabs to pack the tonsil bed.

The risk of a swab used for packing a cavity

during surgery being retained is obviously high. Swabs soaked in blood can be very difficult to locate within a body cavity and the scrub practitioner and surgeon must be vigilant about the removal of such packs (see section on swab counts).

Blunt dissection

Finally, surgical swabs may be used on an instrument to assist the surgeon with blunt dissection. Blunt dissection is the division of body tissues with blunt instruments such as sinus forceps, Watson–Cheyne dissectors, and McDonald dissectors. It is used in areas where sharp dissection (which uses scalpels, scissors and drills) would be potentially hazardous – in close proximity to nerves and blood vessels, for example. Blunt dissection therefore involves the gentle pushing and moving of structures with a blunt instrument, and small swabs can be helpful for this. For example, small Lahey swabs used on an artery forceps can be used to dissect around and locate blood vessels in arterial surgery; small swabs can be wrapped around spongeholders to gently dissect within the abdominal cavity during bowel surgery – often called a 'swab on a stick'. (Fig. 5.24).

TYPES OF SURGICAL SWABS

In the UK woven cotton swabs are most commonly used, to conform to the British Pharmaceutical Codex.[1] However, non-woven swabs are now available and research has shown that they have practical and economic advantages over traditional gauze swabs.[2]

The exact names of swabs used will vary in many operating theatres. The following is a general guide to the types of swab available, and in what circumstances they should be used.

Swabs are described either according to the type of surgery with which they are associated, or by their size. Each operating department

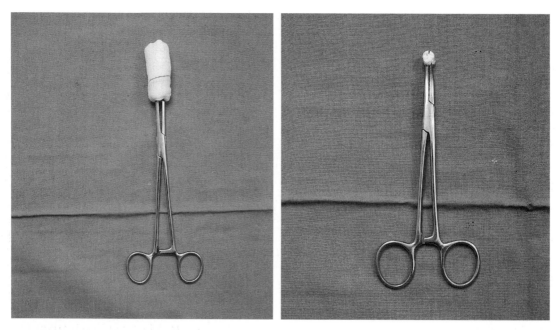

Figure 5.24 Mounted swabs. A. Small swab on sponge-holding forceps. B. Lahey swab mounted on artery forceps.

should have a clear policy in relation to the name used for each swab, and the use of various names within one department should not be allowed as this can lead to errors during surgery, and to ordering and supply problems.

- **Small swabs** Small swabs are often called 3 × 4s or 4 × 3s, referring to their measurement in inches, or general-purpose swabs. They are used for almost all types of surgery, especially operations with a small incision and limited surgical access. If used in the abdominal cavity they should be used on a sponge-holder, not loose.
- **Medium swabs** Medium swabs can also be called 5 × 7s, chest swabs, craniotomy swabs or rectangular swabs. They are used in areas of wider surgical access, where a greater blood loss is expected.
- **Abdominal swabs** These are large swabs, usually 18 × 18 inches in size, also called abdominal packs. They are used only in surgery with a large operative field and wide access. They have a fixation tape attached which is left outside the body cavity when the swab is used as

a pack, and a small artery forceps is attached in order to ensure that it is not retained at the end of surgery. The theatre practitioner must ensure that this tape is firmly attached when completing swab counts.

- **Tonsil swabs** These are small narrow swabs which are also called mastoid swabs because of their main areas of use, – i.e. the throat and tonsil bed, and the ear and mastoid areas. They are therefore mainly used in ENT and neurosurgery.
- **Lahey swabs** These are very small swabs used for blunt dissection rather than blood absorption. They have many other names in common usage: pledgets and peanut, for example. They are used in many types of surgery, especially vascular, and must always be used on an instrument.
- **Eye swabs** These are small pieces of lint used in ophthalmic surgery for blood absorption. They are usually used wet, and are always used on an artery forceps or on a special holding instrument.
- **Patties** These are small pieces of lint with a length of cotton firmly attached, used in neurosurgery. They are used to absorb blood and

to protect delicate tissues, and are usually used wet. They are used to cover and protect exposed areas of the brain during a craniotomy, for example.

- **Other types** There are a variety of other swabs which may be used in operating theatres – slightly smaller abdominal swabs, 10 × 10s for example. Figure 5.25 shows a variety of surgical swabs.

Requirements of surgical swabs

Surgical swabs must be manufactured to a high standard in order to achieve the functions previously discussed. They must therefore have the following characteristics:[2]

- highly absorbent (to absorb blood)
- X-ray detectable (Fig. 5.26) (to enable easy detection if retained)
- should not shed particulate or fibres (to prevent wound granulomas)
- high wet strength (to ensure it is not damaged by wringing)
- material should be soft and conforming (to assist with surgical access)
- should not form lumps when wet (to assist with surgical access).

Further important characteristics are:

- easily sterilizable by conventional methods
- provided in bundles of five with tie
- easily dispensed to the scrub person in a sterile manner, e.g. peel system packaging

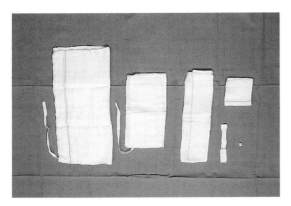

Figure 5.25   A selection of swabs.

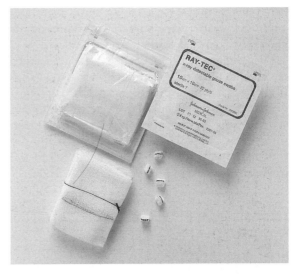

Figure 5.26   X-ray detectable swabs.

- provided in water-repellent protective packaging
- in packaging that is clearly labelled with contents
- conform to BP Codex
- free from linting, will not tear or shred.

Surgical swabs can be supplied in a predetermined type and number on instrument trays if a preset tray system is used, or as extra items to be used as required. They must always be supplied in fives in order to meet the requirements of *Theatre Safeguards*[3] and allow safe swab counts before and at the end of surgery.

ROLE OF THE THEATRE PRACTITIONER

The scrub practitioner must ensure that the surgeon has sufficient swabs to hand at all times, to use for blood absorption, and must be able to follow the surgical procedure and anticipate when additional swabs may be needed, and of what type. For example, when blood vessels are to be deliberately incised, and when there is a high possibility of accidental damage to a blood vessel, blood loss can be anticipated and additional swabs must be available immediately. The scrub practitioner must therefore have a good knowledge of the swabs required for each operation, and any particular surgeon's requirements should be recorded on their preference card.

The circulating practitioner must in turn ensure that the scrub practitioner has a good supply of swabs in order to meet the surgeon's needs. Good practice therefore involves having swabs ready in the operating theatre to open immediately as required, and ensuring the theatre is well stocked with swabs before the operating list begins.

Both scrub and circulating practitioners must conduct swab counts, as described in Chapter 6. The theatre practitioner should also ensure that new staff and students in the operating department are taught correct practices, have a good understanding of the use of swabs, and are aware of the correct terms used for each swab in the department.

REFERENCES

1. Norman A 1991 Swabs: the forgotten item of nursing care? British Journal of Theatre Nursing 1: 4
2. Burgess N, Moore H, Thomas S et al 1992 Evaluation of a new non-woven theatre swab. Journal of the Royal College of Surgeons of Edinburgh 37: 191–193
3. Medical Defence Union 1988 Theatre Safeguards. Medical Defence Union, Medical Protection Society, Medical Defence Union of Scotland, National Association of Theatre Nurses, Royal College of Nursing, London

PRODUCT INFORMATION

Vernon Carus Ltd,
Penwortham Mills,
Preston,
Lancashire PR1 9SN,
UK

Mölnlycke Ltd,
Health Care Products,
Southfields Rd.,
Dunstable,
Bedfordshire LU6 3EJ,
UK

Fluids and lotions

In this section the fluids used for skin preparation and wound irrigation will be described.

SURGICAL SCRUB SOLUTIONS

The two most commonly used surgical scrub solutions are povidone–iodine surgical scrub and chlorhexidine gluconate 4% in detergent. Both should be available as either can cause sensitivity reactions. They should be stored in a locked cupboard and contact with eyes should be avoided, as should ingestion.

SKIN PREPARATION SOLUTIONS

- Povidone–iodine alcoholic solution
- Povidone–iodine aqueous solution
- Chlorhexidine 0.5% in 70% industrial methylated spirits
- Iodine 1% in industrial methylated spirits 70% – iodine in spirit
- Chlorhexidine gluconate 0.015% and cetrimide 0.15% solution
- Industrial methylated spirit 70%.

The skin preparations used depend on surgeons' preferences and the area that requires cleaning. The general rule is that any solutions containing spirit should not be used on open wounds or mucous membranes. Spirit-based preparations should always be dried off prior to the use of diathermy, as severe burns may result.

Some surgeons prefer to use an iodine-based preparation as it stains the skin and the prepared site is therefore clearly delineated. Providone-iodine alcoholic has a quick-drying effect, but care should be exercised as it is also flammable and the area should be completely dry prior to the use of diathermy.

Chlorhexidine and cetrimide solutions are generally used for preparing the skin for gynaecological and rectal surgery as they are not so likely to cause skin irritation or allergy.

All flammable and volatile solutions should be stored in a locked cupboard owing to the risk of fire/explosion. A fire-resistant metal cabinet or box is normally used for this purpose within the theatre department. Quantities of flammable liquids for immediate use should be as small as is reasonably practicable, in relation to the usage required.[1] All other solutions should be stored in a locked cupboard. Contact with eyes should be avoided for all these solutions and they should not be ingested.

Iodine-based solutions should be used with caution on pregnant patients, as absorbed iodine can cross the placental barrier and be secreted in breast milk.

Prior to any skin preparation being used it should be ascertained whether the patient has any allergies, especially to iodine. Iodine-based solutions have a germicidal effect against fungi, spores, viruses and both Gram-positive and Gram-negative bacilli. The germicidal effect may last up to 8 hours as the iodine is released from the binding polymer.

Chlorhexidine-based solutions have a broad-spectrum bactericidal action which is effective against both Gram-positive and Gram-negative bacilli, yeasts and viruses. Its effects last up to 4 hours and there is no evidence of transdermal absorption.

OTHER SOLUTIONS

Other solutions that may be required include:

- sodium chloride 0.9%
- sterile water
- hydrogen peroxide
- methylene blue 1%.

Sodium chloride solution 0.9% may be used for wound irrigation, for example to remove any contaminated debris that may be in the wound following a compound fracture.

Sterile water may be used by the scrub practitioner to clean instruments, and may also be used in a splash bowl for surgeons to remove excess starch from their gloves before the start of surgery.

Hydrogen peroxide in a 3% solution (10 vol 3) may be used to clean dirty, infected wounds. It reacts with catalase in the wound, causing frothing which helps to lift out debris. It should not be used under pressure or in enclosed cavities from which the released oxygen cannot easily escape. Its use has resulted in serious consequences, such as oxygen embolus and surgical emphysema.[2] Stronger solutions than 10 vol should not be used as they may be caustic. It is not recommended for clean wounds.

Hydrogen peroxide should be stored in a cool place, protected from light. Theatre practitioners should wear gloves and eye protection when handling it to avoid eye and skin contact. Methylene blue 1% may be used as a staining agent. Its uses include gynaecological surgery to demonstrate fallopian tube patency and marking of skin for plastic surgery procedures.

Whichever solution is required in the sterile field, the principles remain the same:

- All fluids should be checked by the scrub and circulating practitioners, that they are in date and sterile if appropriate.
- Fluids should always be poured into a receptacle at the edge of the sterile field.
- Fluids should be poured from a height of approximately 10 cm into the receptacle, to avoid inadvertent contamination of the sterile field.
- Care should be taken to avoid spillage of fluids on to the trolley surface.
- Care should be taken to avoid pooling of any fluid on the drapes and under the patient, especially when diathermy is being used.
- Flammable skin preparations should be capped immediately after use and not left standing in direct sunlight.

All solutions are subject to COSHH regulations. Theatre practitioners should refer to the COSHH Data Sheets in their departments.

REFERENCES

1. Firecode 1987 Fire practice note No 2. Health Technical Memorandum 81

2. Sleigh JW, Linter S 1985 Hazards of hydrogen peroxide. British Medical Journal 291: 1706

Wound drains

Wound drains are used to drain fluid away from the operation site in the immediate postoperative period. The theatre practitioner must be familiar with the following aspects:

- definition and functions of wound drains
- types
- requirements
- problems
- role of the theatre practitioner.

DEFINITION OF A WOUND DRAIN

A wound drain is an item of material or equipment used to drain fluid from a body cavity.[1] They are either passive or active suction, with active suction systems being the most commonly used.

A passive drain allows fluid to drain via tubes into a bag, and works by either gravity or capillary action. If gravity is used careful positioning of the drain and consideration of the patient's postoperative position are essential. Capillary action drainage involves a gauze wick or pack being positioned to exit the wound to drain the fluid by a wicking action. Passive drains must therefore be inserted at an upward angle.

Active suction drains work by a vacuum mechanism, and so do not need to be inserted at an upward angle, although they must drain the most dependent part of the wound or cavity.[2] Suction is achieved by the negative pressure created when a vacuum is drawn in a closed drainage system (a container) attached to the wound drain.

FUNCTIONS

The function of a wound drain is to allow or encourage drainage of fluid away from the operative site in the postoperative period. Wound drainage may be either therapeutic or prophylactic.[3] Therapeutic drainage is used to drain an abscess of pus, bacteria and dead tissue, thus relieving local symptoms for the patient. Prophylactic drainage is used whenever it is anticipated that fluid may collect after surgery, and where leakage could occur from an anastomosis, for example. The type of fluid will vary according to the operation site, and includes bile, urine and various gastrointestinal juices, as well as blood. Preventing fluid accumulation can reduce the risk of infection and allow closer apposition of tissues, thereby improving wound healing.[2]

Apart from blood, fluids need to be removed as they may cause irritation for the patient. Also, removing them via a drain provides a clear indication to the surgeon of the state of internal healing in the postoperative period, and of any problems. Blood needs to be removed in order to prevent a haematoma forming, which can lead to postoperative wound breakdown. It also provides the surgeon with an accurate measurement of internal haemorrhage. One study[4] suggests a reduced occurrence of seroma in patients with a suction drain following axilla surgery.

TYPES OF WOUND DRAIN

Passive

A passive wound drain involves a piece of soft latex, PVC, corrugated plastic or rubber tubing draining fluid from the wound site into a bag or dressing. Alternatively, a piece of gauze or pack may be used to act as a wick, simply by creating an exit route from the wound.

Passive drains should be used with a drainage bag whenever possible, to prevent soiling of the dressing with body fluids and to establish a more accurate measurement of fluid loss from the wound site. Examples include a Yeats drain (made up of fine tubes), a corrugated drain, a Robinson drain and a Penrose or tube drain (Fig. 5.27).

Although passive drains are helpful for short-term use, active suction drainage systems have

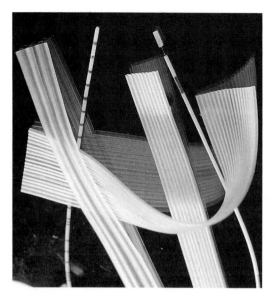

Figure 5.27 Yeats tissue and corrugated drains.

many advantages and should be used whenever possible.

Active suction drains

An active suction drain works by creating negative pressure in a container attached by tubing to the drain placed within the body cavity. This negative pressure creates 'suction' which drains the fluid away from the body cavity into the container (Fig. 5.28).

The vacuum is produced in various ways, for instance by squeezing a concertina, expelling air from a bulb, or using a pre-evacuated bottle, and manufacturers' guidelines must be followed to ensure correct usage.

The advantages of active suction wound drains are:

- reduced possibility of the patient developing a wound infection
- reduced handling of blood or body fluids for the healthcare professional
- accurate measurement of the amount and type of fluid loss from the wound
- avoids contamination of the wound dressing with drainage fluids.

REQUIREMENTS OF A WOUND DRAIN

The types of wound drain available must be carefully considered by the surgeon, the theatre practitioner and the ward nurse. Product information must be studied and company representatives should provide up-to-date clinical research in order to aid decision making. This type of information is essential in order for product selection to be based on sound scientific evidence and clinical information rather than cost.

A wound drain should meet the following requirements:

- sterility – the drain must be available in sterile form ready for insertion into the wound site
- easy to use in three key areas:
  — for the scrub theatre practitioner to obtain a vacuum
  — for the surgeon to insert
  — for the ward staff to change bottles as required
- provide accurate measurement of fluid drainage

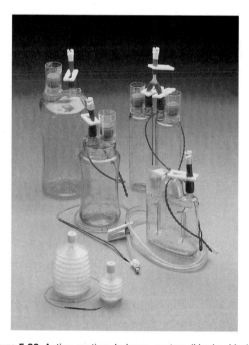

Figure 5.28 Active suction drainage system (Henley-Vac).

- drain material to be non-irritant to the patient
- lightweight for the patient to carry
- allow minimal contact with blood/body fluids for staff
- provide a clear indicator of vacuum, and when vacuum is lost.

Each product should therefore be considered in relation to these requirements, so that an informed choice may be made.

PROBLEMS OF WOUND DRAINAGE

The decision to insert a wound drain is not taken lightly by many surgeons, given that they are not without problems. Torrence[2] states that surgical drainage is associated with a number of risks, which increase if the wrong type of drain is used. The most common problems associated with wound drainage are:

- Infection – an additional potential route of entry is created by the use of a wound drain and the sutures used to secure it. Draining a wound with a gauze wick, for example, can cause ascending infection. This is less of a problem with active suction drains as the suction is away from the wound site, not towards it. The infection rates found in a large study of wound infection in relation to drains by Cruse and Frood[5] are shown in Table 5.1.

Both the type and the site of the wound drain are therefore important considerations in relation to infection. The surgeon, theatre practitioner and ward staff should always consider up-to-date research in order to assist their decision making.

- Blocking – the holes of a drain may become blocked with blood clot or debris. This can lead to the mistaken opinion that fluid loss has ceased and inappropriate drain removal.
- The drain can be accidentally removed by the patient or carers if it is not sufficiently secured.
- Dougherty and Simmons[6] identify further complications of surgical drainage in relation to the effects of a foreign body, mechanical effects/problems and physiological impairment.

Table 5.1 Wound infection in relation to drains[5]

Drain	Infection rate (%)
Clean wounds	1.53
Suction drain	1.8
Penrose drain via stab wound	2.4
Penrose drain via main incision	4.0

The benefits of wound drainage are therefore controversial, and relevant clinical research must always be considered. One study of thyroid surgery patients[7] showed that those with no drain had no more complications than those with a drain.

ROLE OF THE THEATRE PRACTITIONER

The theatre practitioner, surgeon and ward nurse should consider the range of drains available for both open and closed drainage of surgical wounds, and select the most appropriate for the types of surgery performed. This will ease the choice at the time of surgery, alleviate the storage problem (a smaller range of drains will be needed), and have financial benefits for the unit by allowing larger numbers of particular products to be ordered. The theatre practitioner should ensure an adequate supply of the chosen drains at all times. A surgeon's choice of drain should be recorded on their preference card for each operation, along with their choice of suture for securing the drain if required, and these must be available in the theatre. Not all drains are sutured – this is a matter of the surgeon's preference.

The scrub practitioner should check whether the surgeon does require a drain for each patient, and ask for the drain to be opened as required. It is prudent to check first, as opening and setting up drains is costly if they are not required.

The scrub practitioner should set up the drain in an aseptic manner as described by the manufacturer. Care should be taken when handling the drain trocar to avoid injury, and the trocar disposed of according to hospital policy.

The theatre practitioner should also be involved in teaching junior staff and students the principles of wound drainage, and correct technique. It is also helpful to communicate regularly with the ward staff in order to identify any problems with drains in the postoperative period, which may need to be discussed and referred to the manufacturers if necessary.

REFERENCES

1. Nightingale K 1989 Making sense of wound drainage. Nursing Times 85: 40–42
2. Torrance C 1993 Introduction to surgical drainage. Surgical Nurse 6: 19–23
3. Westaby S 1985 Wound closure and drainage. In: Westaby S (ed) Wound care. Heinemann Medical, London, Chapter 5
4. Cameron A et al 1988 Suction drainage of the axilla: a prospective randomized trial. British Journal of Surgery 75: 1211
5. Cruse P, Frood R 1973 A five-year prospective study of 23, 649 surgical wounds. Archives of Surgery 107: 206–210
6. Dougherty S, Simmons R 1992 The biology and practice of surgical drains Part 1. Current Problems in Surgery 29: 561–623
7. Wihlborg O et al 1988 To drain or not to drain in thyroid surgery. Archives of Surgery 123: 40–41

Suction

Suction apparatus is one of the most important pieces of equipment in the operating theatre. At least two suction units should be available, one for the anaesthetist, to assist in maintaining the patient's airway (see Chapter 4), and one for surgical use. If a large amount of blood loss is anticipated two suction units should be available for surgical use. Surgical suction should be available for all cases with a high blood loss or when large amounts of irrigation fluid are used. The scrub practitioner should set up sterile suction tubing, with an appropriate sterile suction end for the type of surgery performed. The distal end is handed away from the table to the circulating practitioner, taking care to maintain a sterile field. It is then attached to the suction apparatus and the unit switched on.

Surgical suction is used to remove blood and irrigation fluids to give the surgeon visual access to the operative site. If a haemorrhage does occur, it is important that the bleeding point can be found quickly and controlled.

It is important that the circulating practitioner records the amount of fluid loss collected in the suction bottles. This information may be required by the anaesthetist to maintain the patient's fluid balance, especially in cases with a large blood loss. Therefore all suction bottles have graduated markings for accurate recording, taking into account any irrigation fluids used.

Suction may be obtained with a mobile unit or from a pipeline supply to all theatre areas. Fluid collection is achieved by creating a vacuum in the collecting bottle. Most suction units will have a pressure gauge which allows the theatre practitioner to control the degree of vacuum, depending on the type of surgery.

There are various types of suction systems available, but all fall into one of two categories, either disposable or reusable. Disposable systems are usually closed units where the waste is contained in either disposable bottles or plastic liners within containers. Most disposable systems are disposed of by incineration. Many disposable systems may be fitted to standard suction machines and wall brackets. If plastic liners are used the theatre practitioner should ensure that they are correctly placed into the containers so that they remain upright during transportation to the incinerator.

Reusable systems involve glass bottles in which the blood and body fluids are collected and then disposed of in the sluice. The bottles are then washed prior to disinfection and autoclave sterilization. There are obviously more risks from splashing involved in the use of reusable systems, therefore protective waterproof aprons, gloves and goggles should be worn by all staff when undertaking this procedure. The cost implications of reusable and disposable systems have been estimated and were found to be equal.

Whichever type of suction system is used, disposable gloves should always be worn when disconnecting or emptying containers and the hands should be washed. Care should also be taken when disposing of suction tubing, to avoid splashing their contents.

General guidelines for the use of surgical suction

- A variety of sterile suction tubing and sucker ends should be available.
- Suction tubing should be available in a variety of bores to avoid blockage and collapse due to inappropriate use.
- The suction unit should be checked prior to the start of each operating list to ensure that it is in good working order.
- Following each case the suction bottle should be emptied, cleaned and dried (reusable systems) or the bottle/liner changed (disposable systems), taking the necessary precautions for staff protection.

Endoscopy

Rachael Hodson

Upper and lower gastrointestinal endoscopy is an expanding field in the diagnosis and management of gastroenterological problems. The use of endoscopic equipment and the management of patients undergoing these procedures has become highly specialized, and demands expertise from both nursing and medical standpoints.

Ideally, endoscopy should be performed in a specialized unit, with dedicated staff trained in endoscopy techniques and care. Endoscopy may be performed in the operating theatre as part of other procedures or in hospitals without a dedicated unit. The following chapter outlines the principles and practice of gastrointestinal endoscopy in this area.

PREPARATION OF THE ENDOSCOPY SUITE

The layout of the endoscopy suite is such that the patient remains the centre of attention for both the endoscopist and endoscopy assistant. The room needs to be large enough for a trolley to spin around on its axis, with sufficient space for all ancillary equipment and a minimum of three personnel. Geographical spheres of activity should be defined for doctors, nurses and trainees with the relevant equipment in the appropriate sector (Fig. 5.29). Care should be taken to avoid obstruction by leads and umbilical cords. There should be a separate room for clean-

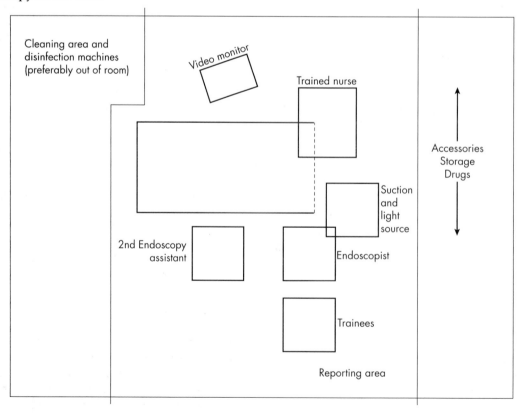

Figure 5.29 The layout of an endoscopy suite.

ing and disinfection of scopes, or an identified area of the suite for this purpose. Lights should be dimmable and there should be easy access to intercom, telephone and alarms. Oxygen and two suction system's (one for the scope, and one for the patient's airway) must be available.

Before any procedure, all instruments and electrical equipment must be checked to ensure they are in proper working order. There should be resuscitation equipment and drugs available within the area which should be checked daily. All staff and endoscopists must be trained in resuscitation methods and understand how to use the equipment available.

ENDOSCOPIC AND ANCILLARY EQUIPMENT

In order to provide a service for diagnostic endoscopy, a basic set of equipment is required.

Modern endoscopy uses flexible fibreoptic or video endoscopes (Fig. 5.30). Fibreoptic instruments utilize light transmission along glass bundles and video endoscopes are similar in design, but base their image transmission on a charged coupled device chip (CCD). An electrical charge is passed up the scope to a converting device, to generate a colour image on a screen. Light sources are required for both types of scope, and this is usually a high intensity xenon lamp. Both types of scope have an air-water feed device for insulation and irrigation (Fig. 5.31) and a suction facility. Modern scopes have two channels – one for air–water feed, and the second for passage of instruments. The working channel may vary in size or number, depending on the specialization of the scope. Most scopes utilize forward viewing, but duodenoscopes for endoscopic retrograde cholangiopancreatography (ERCP) are side viewing in order visualize the papilla.

When video endoscopes are used, a central processing unit (CPU) (Fig. 5.32) is required to convert the electrical signal into a visual image. Additionally, a variety of accessories are required, e.g. tissue sampling devices, irrigators, etc.

These instruments are delicate and expensive because of their electrical and fibreoptic components. When not in use, they should be stored

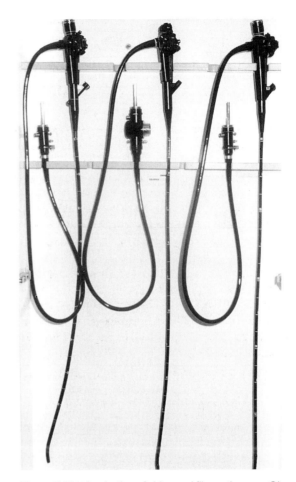

Figure 5.30   A selection of video and fibreoptic upper GI scopes.

hanging vertically in a locked cupboard, and for transportation outside the normal working environment, should be placed in a special endoscope transportation suitcase. When carried, the head, tip and umbilicus should be supported. They should be serviced according to the manufacturer's instructions.

CLEANING AND DISINFECTION

Endoscopic procedures carry a risk of infection – the most common being the transmission of Gram-negative bacilli in gastrointestinal (GI) endoscopy, and pseudomonas in ERCP. Bacterial colonization may occur within the mains water supply or washing machine. A scrupulous filtra-

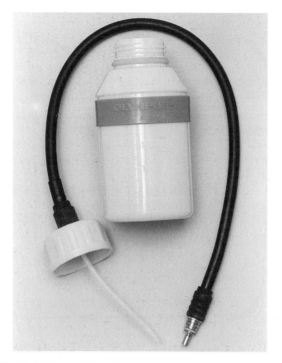

Figure 5.31 Water bottle.

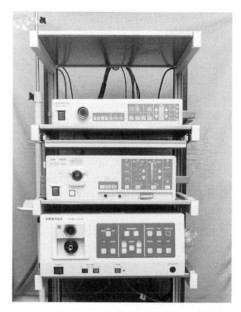

Figure 5.32 A stack system showing light source (top), video converter (middle) and central processing unit (bottom).

tion system, including a bacterial filter and culture swabs taken at regular intervals, will reduce contamination risks. Blood-borne viruses, especially hepatitis B and C and HIV, have the potential for transmission via endoscopes. Thorough cleaning and disinfection ensures decontamination. Particular risks may occur if biopsies are taken with inadequately sterilized forceps and each patient should be protected by consistently high standards as infected individuals cannot be readily identified.

Endoscopes must be cleaned prior to disinfection. Guidance is given in manufacturers' instructions; each channel must be brushed through in all directions and flushed with detergent prior to disinfection. Organic debris will prevent adequate penetration of the disinfectant, and fixing of this debris by aldehydes may cause channels to block and moving parts to stiffen. The use of automated washing machines does not preclude the first mechanical cleaning and brushing.

Flexible endoscopes are heat sensitive and are therefore not suitable for thermal disinfection or sterilization. Chemical methods must be used. The only currently recommended disinfectants are 2% glutaraldehyde or 10% gigasept. The British Society of Gastroenterology has recently reviewed contact times for 2% glutaraldehyde to bring its guidelines in line with manufacturers' and European recommendations. These are shown in Table 5.2.

Table 5.2 Recommended contact time for 2% glutaraldehyde

	Contact time
Before a list	20 min (to remove new vegetation)
Between patients	10 min (to destroy organisms which may be transmitted)
After a list	20 min (to reduce the likelihood of vegetation growing)
Scopes for use on pre- and post-known HIV or immunocompromised patients	60 min

CHOICE OF DISINFECTANT

The establishment of a disinfection policy is recommended, and once agreed and implemented deviations should not be permitted except by the agreement of the policy team. This will include choice of disinfectant, exposure time and rationale for cleaning. There is a new wave of chemical disinfectants and sterilants entering the market which are being heralded as alternatives to the present common methods. The following areas should be addressed satisfactorily prior to choosing any disinfection method:

- intended use of disinfectant
- microbicidal activity of the disinfectant and specific immersion/contact times
- pre- cleaning of equipment
- preparation for use
- compatibility with equipment/cleaning machines
- safety data and handling precautions
- shelf-life and stability/disposal methods.

Care of the endoscope is summarized in Table 5.3.

All endoscopic equipment should be thoroughly and mechanically cleaned with an enzymatic or neutral detergent, then sterilized before next use. This includes water bottles, valves or mouthguards. Any accessory with a metal or spiral component can only be effectively cleaned by dismantling and using an ultrasonic cleaner prior to sterilization or disinfection.

DISPOSABLE VERSUS REUSABLE EQUIPMENT

Most ancillary equipment, biopsy forceps or snares may be purchased as single use or reusable (Fig. 5.33). Some have a limited life expectancy, e.g. 5 uses. The advantages and disadvantages of both are summarised in Table 5.4.

STAFF PROTECTION AND ENVIRONMENTAL HAZARDS

All staff should be offered hepatitis B and tetanus vaccination and TB immunity should be main-

Table 5.3 Care of the endoscope

Pre-endoscopy	Post endoscopy
Clean and disinfect	Leak test Clean and disinfect Rinse and dry
Air, water and suction patent	Valves and O rings patent/oiled
Tip deflection accurate	Angulation check
Clear image	Secure ventilated hanging storage
Check ancillary equipment	Bacteriological test culture of scope Service according to contract

Table 5.4 Disposable versus reusable equipment

Disposable	Reusable
Lower cost/item	Higher initial cost
Throwaway	Require sterilization between uses – cost/COSHH considerations
Single use	Multiple use
Higher stock level	Repair costs
Frequent design change	Cleaning may damage or blunt delicate instruments
Optimal function each time	

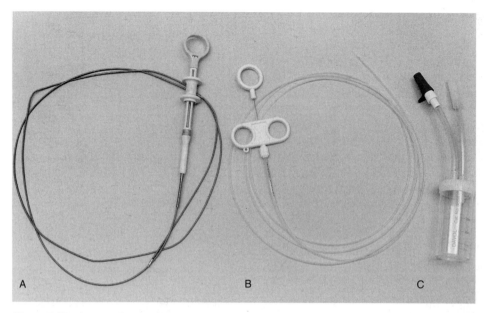

Figure 5.33 Accessories. A. Biopsy forceps. B. Brush. C. Suction trap.

tained. Routine barrier precautions to prevent contact with blood and body fluids should be observed. Gloves and disposable aprons should be worn and changed between patients, and goggles or glasses should be worn if eye splashes are likely. Care should be taken with sclerotherapy and intravenous needles and when handling spiked forceps. Common sense should be taken with the use of electrosurgery and body fluids. Staff working in rooms with X-rays should wear protective aprons and exposure badges. Thyroid shields and glasses are appropriate for those managing the 'head of the patient'. Smoke from laser plume is a hazard, and a radiation officer should supervise staff and practices when fluoroscopy or laser therapy are used.

The use of disinfectants, particularly the aldehydes, carry a risk of sensitivity and toxicity, and COSHH regulations and manufacturers' recommendations should be adhered to. Enclosed disinfectant units with facilities for the extraction of toxic fumes must be used (Fig. 5.34) (see Chapter 3).

SAFE ENDOSCOPY

Gastrointestinal endoscopy is a specialized field of practice and should no longer be undertaken

by inexperienced medical, nursing or ancillary staff on a part-time basis. The British Society of Gastroenterology's Endoscopy section represents the above staff by compiling guidelines on which to base safe practice in endoscopy. Working parties have produced a number of guidelines which can be used to form the basis of safe practice and develop standards of care relating to each area.

Any practitioner who is to undertake endoscopy should receive formal training. Current guidelines specify a minimum of 150 supervised procedures being undertaken, with documentation and review, prior to the endoscopist undertaking an unsupervised endoscopy. These guidelines are being amended to facilitate a national training schedule and skill maintenance programme for all endoscopists linked to professional registration. In-service experience should be supplemented by attendance at courses approved or organized by the endoscopy committee of the British Society of Gastroenterology to update endoscopists on newer equipment, techniques and management of patients. Such courses should include topics such as patient care, maintenance cleaning and disinfection of scopes and equipment, electro-

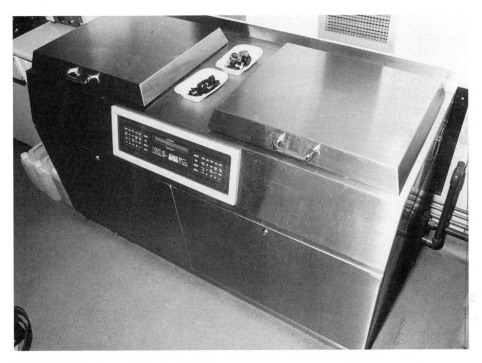

Figure 5.34 Enclosed automatic disinfector.

surgery, practice of safe sedation, recognition and management of complications, and therapeutic endoscopy.

There should be a core team responsible for the delivery of care during endoscopy and ensuring the maintenance of current and safe practice. There are a number of courses relating to the provision of endoscopic services, including the English National Board 906 Gastrointestinal Endoscopy and related procedures. This short course should be undertaken by at least one senior member of staff of the endoscopy team who can disseminate and facilitate good practice within the area. Training exists for non-nursing and nursing staff within the British Endoscopy Education Society and instrument manufacturers' training courses, allowing theory to be integrated into practice.

Staff of all grades and disciplines should be competent with basic resuscitation methods and first-line management of complications, and should undergo periodic retraining.

Staffing levels should reflect the workload and an endoscopy list is preferable to ad hoc procedures within an operating list. Staffing should include administrative support as well as staff within the room and recovery area. Each endoscopic procedure requires at least two endoscopy assistants, one of whom must be a qualified nurse or practitioner trained in endoscopy and dedicated to the care of the patient only. A second suitably trained person should also assist with the procedure. A registered nurse is required for patient preparation and recovery, to ensure the complete assessment, wellbeing and clinical observation of the patient.

GENERAL PATIENT CARE AND ASSESSMENT

Patient care and assessment should begin pre-endoscopy. A clear and concise appointment letter should be sent, with an explanatory leaflet, giving details of the nature and purpose of the proposed examination, preparation, dietary restrictions, possible risks to the patient, and any alternative to the procedure. Discharge restrictions and the requirement for an escort should also be included. A contact number should be available for patient information. Full information is essential for:

- informed consent
- reduction of pre-endoscopy anxiety
- toleration of procedure
- post procedure recovery and safe discharge
- post procedure education.

On arrival patients should be assessed by a qualified nurse. Inpatients still require assessment by an endoscopy trained nurse to ascertain special risk factors, drug contraindications, specialized care and reduce patient anxiety. This may be done on a pre-endoscopy visit.

Adverse risk factors should be identified pre-endoscopy. At-risk patients include those classified as American Society of Anesthesiologist grades III–V (Box 5.3).

The elderly, those with heart, lung or liver disease or failure, acute gastrointestinal bleed, anaemia, morbid obesity or shock may also be included in the at-risk category. A checklist may be used to identify these factors.

A drug history and allergy check should be taken to identify any concurrent problems which may cause an interaction with medications given during endoscopy. The nurse responsible for the patient should be familiar with drug interactions and effects of the drugs commonly used in endoscopy.

SEDATION, ANALGESIA AND MONITORING

Endoscopic procedures can be painful, and cause considerable anxiety to the patient. The nurse caring for the patient is best placed to ensure the dignity, privacy and high standard of care to the patient, reducing anxiety and discomfort. Diagnostic gastroscopy can be safely performed using pharyngeal anaesthesia (by spray or lozenge). It avoids the risks of sedation, yet suppresses the gag reflex to allow the passage of the scope. Patients may be reassured throughout the procedure, and be discharged quickly without any limitations on their daily activities. The absence of amnesia means full discharge instructions may be given, with patient information and education, possibly reducing follow-up visits.

Conscious sedation

Conscious sedation is a minimally depressed level of consciousness such that the patient is able to maintain a patent airway continuously and independently, and respond appropriately to external stimulation.

An indwelling cannula should be placed in a vein of all patients receiving intravenous drugs during endoscopy, and remain patent until the patient is recovered for discharge.

Benzodiazepines are used for sedation in endoscopy, with water-soluble midazolam being the drug of choice, due to its rapid action and short half-life of 1–4 hours. Diazemuls has a half-

Box 5.3	At-risk patients as classified by the American Society of Anesthesiologists
Grade III	Severe systemic disturbance or disease from whatever cause, even though it may not be possible to define the degree of disability with finality. Examples: severely limiting organic heart disease, severe diabetes with vascular complications, moderate to severe degree of pulmonary insufficiency, angina or healed myocardial infarction
Grade IV	Severe systemic disorders which are life threatening, not always correctable by operation, e.g. patient with organic heart disease showing marked signs of cardiac insufficiency, persistent angina, active myocarditis, advanced degrees of pulmonary, hepatic, renal or endocrine insufficiency
Grade V	Moribund patient who has little chance of survival, but is undergoing procedure in desperation

life of 24 hours with a breakdown to the active sedative desmethyldiazepam. Most endoscopy morbidity and mortality is related to sedation-induced adverse events, often caused by excessive amounts of sedation being given, or lack of patient monitoring. The manufacturer's schedule should be followed with particular attention being given to dose limits, especially in the at-risk groups. Dosages of all drugs should be kept to a minimum, with titration being undertaken to ensure the appropriate level of sedation is reached.

Opiates are used to produce analgesia during lung or painful procedures. It is recognized that the combination of an opiate and benzodiazepine is synergistic, i.e. produces a total effect greater than the sum of the two drugs. Smaller doses should be given to reach an end point of conscious sedation. When an opiate and sedation are required together, the opiate should be given first, followed by the sedative a few minutes later.

Children may require greater amounts of sedation for endoscopy, and should receive a planned anaesthetic assessment prior to the procedure. General anaesthesia may be preferable, particularly in young children. A Registered Sick Children's Nurse should be available to care for the patient with other members of the endoscopy team. Chronic alcohol abusers may require greater doses of benzodiazepines, as their increased levels of the liver enzyme cytochrome P450 destroy the drug. Patients on long-term benzodiazepines may not be amenable to sedation, as their system is already loaded with the drug, and sedation doses may not be effective.

Whenever benzodiazepines or opiates are used, their antagonists should be readily available in the department. Their availability should not preclude safe use of the smallest doses of the agonist. Flumazanil (antagonist of benzodiazepine) may take several minutes to completely reverse sedation-induced respiratory depression. The half-life of flumazanil is 50–60 min, resulting in a short-lived reversal. Its use should not be routine to preclude clinical monitoring or nursing care for patient safety.

Monitoring during endoscopy

Oxygen desaturation is common during sedation endoscopy, but may also occur with non-sedation gastroscopy. Pre-endoscopy pulse, blood pressure, respirations and SaO_2 allow a baseline for comparison during the procedure. The nurse should observe for clinical signs of hypoxia, respiratory depression or cardiovascular distress and alert the endoscopist to such. The use of pulse oximetry in the above patients is strongly recommended, as is carrying out endoscopy in normal lighting conditions for clinical observation of the patient. The provision of oxygen-enriched air before and during endoscopy has been shown to prevent and diminish hypoxaemia. Supplemental oxygen at 2–4 litres per minute via nasal cannula will not compromise patients, even those with chronic obstructive pulmonary disease. Continuous ECG monitoring is recommended in at-risk patients, those having opiates and benzodiazepines, and those having difficult or prolonged procedures.

The use of a sedation scoring system is recommended for monitoring patients peri- and post procedure. These measure the effect of sedative agents along a time scale from an affective, effective and physiological position. They can be used to determine when optimum sedation has been achieved, when adverse events are occurring and whether the patient is recovering from sedation in the expected manner (Fig. 5.35).

Care of the patient during the procedure

The endoscopist remains responsible for patient care throughout the procedure, but relies greatly on the observations and management of the patient by the nurse. The two endoscopy assistants within the room should be utilized as follows:

Trained nurse:
- assists with administration of drugs
- maintains patient's position
- clinically monitors patient and reports changes
- administers oxygen

AWAKE AND AWARE		REDUCED AWARENESS		CONFUSED	
Emotional affect	**Level of consciousness**	**Physical effect**		**Vital signs**	
Anxious 1	Fully Aware 1	Restless 1		Pulse ^ >10% 1	
Relaxed 2	Drowsy 2	Restful 2		Pulse change <10% 2	
Flat 3	Unrousable 3	Unresponsive 3		Pulse change >20% 3	
Responses	**Protective reflexes**	**Vocalisation**		**O$_2$ desaturation**	
Inappropriate 1	Present 1	Constant 1		No change 1	
Appropriate 2	Absent 2	Occasional 2		<5% 2	
Unresponsive 3		None 3		>5% 3	

Under sedated   -12   Optimally sedated   13–18   Over sedated   19–23

Figure 5.35 The Castle Hill conscious sedation scale.

- maintains airway and oropharyngeal aspiration
- maintains mouthguard
- provides verbal reassurance and encouragement to patient throughout the procedure.

Second assistant:
- responsible for equipment care
- assists with technical procedures
- correct labelling of specimens and visual records
- maintains ledger
- assists with emergencies.

Recovery

Clinical monitoring should be continued into the recovery period, and some patients may require supplemental oxygen and reversal agents. Written post-endoscopy instructions should be given by the endoscopist. Discharge criteria should be formed to establish standards for safe discharge of patients. The following should be considered mandatory prior to discharge:

- drink tolerated
- absence of pain and vomiting
- ability to walk without support
- stable vital signs and oximetry to pre-sedation
- flatus passed or bowels opened (lower GI endoscopy)

DISCHARGE OF THE PATIENT

All outpatients who have received sedation should be accompanied home by a responsible adult, who will have written instructions on what to do and who to contact if problems arise. As there is often post procedure amnesia with sedation, any discussion regarding the examination, advice or follow-up should also be in written form. Patients who have been sedated should not drive a vehicle, operate machinery, sign legally binding documents or drink alcohol for 24 hours post sedation. This is irrespective of whether a reversal agent has been given.

MANAGEMENT OF THE ILL PATIENT AND COMPLICATIONS

Major complications during routine diagnostic endoscopy are rare. The overall risks of all complications, minor and major, are approximately 0.5%. Complications may arise for a number of reasons, related to:

- intravenous cannulation
- sedative or other drugs
- procedural events
- patient-aided events – advertent or inadvertent.

Perforation and bleeding are the most serious complications of endoscopy, and are more common with therapeutic procedures. In many instances, the perforation may not be realised at the time of discharge, and the patient may present some hours later.

Patients with perforations of the upper GI tract may present with upper abdominal pain, vomiting, emphysema of the neck and subcutaneous tissues. These may be confirmed by chest X-ray and gastrograffin swallow.

Perforations of the lower GI tract may well cause the patient to complain of abdominal pain either during the procedure or in the early post procedure phase. They may complain of inability to pass flatus. On examination, they will have a distended abdomen. A plain abdominal X-ray will show free gas in the abdominal cavity, leading to the diagnosis. Patients who have undergone polypectomy may present at up to 10 days with a perforation caused by necrosis of the colonic wall. This may be accompanied by the passage of large, dark red clots or grey tissue from the rectum.

Bleeding may occur following endoscopy especially after therapeutic procedures such as polypectomy, sphincterotomy in ERCP, injection or banding of oesophageal varices or oesophageal dilatation. Patients rapidly become shocked and require urgent resuscitation, investigation and treatment, which may be performed by further endoscopic procedures.

Patient-aided events occur when undiagnosed or unknown disease processes come to the fore, or the patient has withheld vital information regarding their condition or lifestyle, e.g. alcohol or drug use. Each should be dealt with according to the presenting features, and appropriate medical advice sought.

DIAGNOSTIC AND THERAPEUTIC ENDOSCOPY

The development of flexible endoscopes has enabled clinicians to provide a wide variety of investigational and therapeutic procedures. Most routine diagnostic and therapeutic GI procedures can be performed using an end viewing scope with a single working channel suitable for biopsy, dilatation, polyp snaring and injection

therapy. Modern endoscopes have wide degrees of tip deflection and wide-angle lenses which allow a complete survey of the organ under examination. The increasing number and complexity of therapeutic procedures has led to the development of larger therapeutic endoscopes, with larger working channels, e.g. 4.2 mm channels versus 2.8 mm and multiple channels.

ERCP requires a specialized side viewing scope with an elevator lever (bridge) and the procedure is a combined endoscopic and radiological investigation, requiring fluoroscopy. In many instances, therapeutic procedures are required, and it is no longer acceptable for endoscopists to be trained in diagnostic endoscopy alone.

Any endoscopic unit wishing to provide a comprehensive range of diagnostic and therapeutic procedures should have a variety of endoscopes, and in sufficient quantities to allow for rapid patient turnover with complete disinfection schedules. In addition, there will be a need for a variety of accessory and specialist equipment. Endoscopic therapy is used in the management of gastrointestinal bleeding, oesophageal dilatation, insertion of oesophageal stents, extraction of foreign bodies, extraction of biliary stones, insertion of biliary stents, surveillance of inflammatory bowel disease and colonic polyp removal. In some units, laser therapy is available for tumour ablation. In addition, Argon Photocoagulation Therapy (APC) can be used for tumour ablation and control of bleeding.

THE FUTURE OF ENDOSCOPY

Endoscopy is becoming an increasingly specialized and rapidly expanding field, and clearly any hospital department wishing to provide this service should regularly update itself on new developments and techniques. Standards should be developed to maintain high quality care, incorporating clinical guidelines available from statutory organizations. Medical endoscopists should be trained to undertake therapeutic procedures at the time of initial endoscopy.

Nurses are currently developing skills in undertaking diagnostic upper and lower GI endoscopy and may provide a continuity of prac-

222 OPERATING DEPARTMENT PRACTICE

tice to patients and the endoscopy service. Nurses developing these roles should undertake an academic and practical, nationally recognized course in line with medical endoscopist training.

New procedures and investigations require a multidisciplinary approach to patient management, and new technological advances will see a decrease in simple, routine diagnostic endoscopy. There will be an increase in endoscopic investigations for other diseases, e.g. transoesophageal echocardiography for heart disease and endoscopic ultrasound for oesophageal, gastric and pancreatic cancers. Endoscopic therapy will increase as an adjuvant for other management techniques, e.g. minimal access surgery and trans/intra-hepatic portasystemic shunts

(TIPSS). Therapeutic endoscopy will increase, and become more complex and diverse. Because of these changes, endoscopy should be recognized as a specialty and increasingly endoscopy units will separate from theatre or day surgery units.

There will be further technological advances, with smaller diameter, double channel scopes becoming widely available for therapeutic work. 3D and computer-enhanced imaging is being developed. Virtual reality training will be available for endoscopic work.

Endoscopic practice will expand into the next millennium, but it will be the endoscopy team that ensures standards remain high to provide optimum quality care to patients.

FURTHER READING

British Society of Gastroenterology 1987 Report of a working party on staffing of endoscopy units. British Society of Gastroenterology
British Society of Gastroenterology 1990 Provision of GI endoscopy and related services for a district general hospital. British Society of Gastroenterology
British Society of Gastroenterology 1992 Recommendations for standards of sedation and patient monitoring during GI endoscopy. British Society of Gastroenterology
Cotton P, Williams C 1996 Practical gastrointestinal endoscopy, 4th edn. Blackwell Science, Oxford
Cotton PB, Tytgat GNJ, Williams CB 1994 Annual of gastrointestinal endoscopy. Current Science, London

Mason J, Shepherd M 1997 Practical endoscopy. Chapman & Hall, London
Medical Devices Agency 1996 Device bulletin – Decontamination of endoscopes (MDA DB 9607). Medical Devices Agency
Royal College of Surgeons of England 1993 Report of the working party on guidelines for sedation by non-anaesthetists. Royal College of Surgeons of England, London
Tytgat GNJ, Classen M 1994 The practice of therapeutic endoscopy. Churchill Livingstone, Edinburgh

Other endoscopic procedures

LAPAROSCOPIC SURGERY

Laparoscopic surgery has developed rapidly during the 1980s and 1990s and is now common in many operating departments. Nathanson and Wood[1] identify the reasons for this as:

- the development of laparoscopic instrumentation and the facility for the surgeon, assistant and theatre staff to see the laparoscopic image on the video screen
- the development of instruments to aid organ exposure by retraction and dissection
- the development of instruments for haemostasis by coagulation, clips or ligatures.

The use of the laparoscopic method for cholecystectomy has increased dramatically since its development by Mouret and Dubois in 1987,[2] and is now the chosen method of gallbladder removal for many surgeons and patients. It may involve the use of a laser, as described by Odlum,[3] or may not, as described by McKay[4] and Nathanson and Wood.[1] Other operations performed via this access route include appendectomy, hernia repair and bowel resection. It is likely that this type of surgery will increase in the future.

Each type of operation requires multiple access ports and specialized equipment and instruments (Fig. 5.36). Instrumentation has developed rapidly, and manufacturers provide excellent manuals and training related to the care of instruments. Instrumentation is either single use or reusable, and surgeons, theatre practitioners and theatre managers must consider the options available and the support and maintenance programmes offered by the company when purchasing decisions are made.

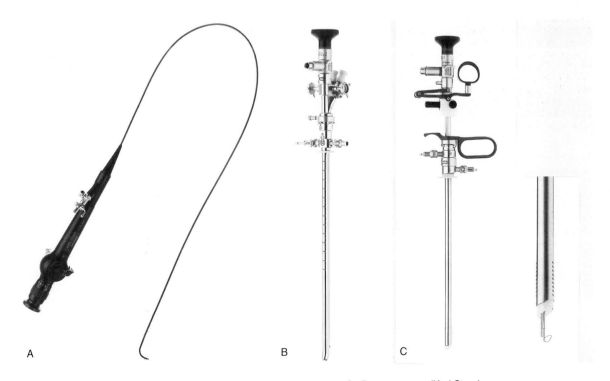

Figure 5.36   A. Flexible endoscope (choledoscope). B. Cystoscope. C. Resectoscope (Karl Storz).

The advantage of disposable laparoscopic instruments is that they do not become dull, do not stick, do not require difficult assembly procedures, and do not have missing parts, thus creating minimal frustration for the surgical team and minimal delay for the patient.[5] The cost issues must, however, be taken into account when deciding to use either disposable or reusable equipment. A full cost analysis, which includes the cost of maintenance, cleaning and sterilization of reusable equipment, should be undertaken: some guidelines for this are provided by Reichert[5] and Deloitte and Touche[6], based on American studies. These would therefore need adaptation for use in the UK. Further issues such as staff safety and training should also be considered.

Transcervical resection of the endometrium

This technique allows the removal of endometriosis transcervically and is used as an alternative to hysterectomy. It involves the use of a wire to cut away the endometriosis, in a similar way to transurethral removal of the prostate gland.

Other developments in minimally invasive surgery include nephrectomy, as described by Kidner,[7] hysterectomy, as described by Martin,[8,9] and lasertripsy as described by Pawlyn.[10]

REFERENCES

1. Nathanson L, Wood R 1991 Laparoscopy in the 1990s. In: Surgery. The Medicine Group, pp 2096–2100
2. Dubois 1989 La Presse Medicale 18: 980–982
3. Odlum M 1992 Laparoscopic laser cholecystectomy – a case study. British Journal of Theatre Nursing 1: 21–23
4. McKay M 1992 Laparoscopic cholecystectomy: theatre implications. British Journal of Theatre Nursing 1: 24–26
5. Reichert M 1993 Laparoscopic instruments. Patients care, cost issues. AORN Journal 57: 3
6. Deloitte and Touche 1993 Economic impact of laparoscopic surgery. Deloitte and Touche, Boston
7. Kidner M 1992 Laparoscopic surgery of the kidney and ureters. British Journal of Theatre Nursing (Suppl. – Urology) 1: S14–S15
8. Martin D 1992 Hysterscopy – a brief history. British Journal of Theatre Nursing 1: 9–11
9. Martin D 1992 Hysterscopy – operative procedure. British Journal of Theatre Nursing 1: 12–15
10. Pawlyn E 1992 Lasertripsy – the treatment of renal calculi. British Journal of Theatre Nursing (Suppl.–Urology) 1: S16–S17

Lasers

There are many different types of laser used in a wide range of surgical procedures, each with its own method of operation and associated hazards, therefore it is essential that the manufacturer's recommendations are adhered to at all times. It is possible to highlight hazards that are common to all laser types and the safety procedures that ensure all possibilities are covered.

The term laser is derived from *Light Amplification* by *Stimulated Emission of Radiation* (the term radiation applies to light energy only). Laser light is formed when an electron in a lasting medium (gas or crystal) is stimulated to produce two particles of light (photons). This stimulation is brought about by the application of energy. The stimulated light particles are produced in a mirrored chamber (oscillation cavity), where they bounce back and forth until the full power of the laser is obtained. The laser beam exits the chamber via a transparent window when required and is transported to the patient's tissue along a delivery device, which varies with the type of laser in use and the treatment required.

PROPERTIES OF LASERS

1. **Collimation** Laser light can be thought of as a highly directional parallel beam which makes lasers very accurate aiming devices; in theory the collimated laser light travels into infinity, which creates the need for safety precautions.

2. **Coherence** Light travels in waves. Ordinary light waves are random but laser light waves are in harmony (in phase). Therefore, particles of laser light travelling in these waveforms arrive at the target tissue at the same time. This produces a more concentrated form of light, creating a thermal effect.

3. **Monochromatic light** Most lasers produce light of one colour or wavelength. A KTP laser (see below) produces a single band of green colour; carbon dioxide lasers produce a band of invisible infrared light, which has implications

for safety. The exception to this rule is the argon laser, which may produce up to 11 different colours. In the surgical argon laser there are two bands of colour – green and blue.

The colour and wavelength of the laser light is important in respect of its absorption by tissues and the materials it can travel through. For example, the carbon dioxide laser beam cannot travel through glass and therefore cannot be used with flexible fibres. It is also highly absorbable in the presence of water and blood.

TYPES OF LASER

Lasers are usually distinguished by the colour of the light they produce. There are five main types:

- Argon (Ar^+)
- Carbon dioxide (CO_2^-)
- Neodymium-doped yttrium aluminium garnet (Nd: YAG)
- Potassium titanyl phosphate (KTP or KTP/532TM)
- Pulsed dye.

OPERATIVE USES

Lasers can be used in a wide variety of surgical specialties. The type used depends on what is available as well as the power limitations of each. The use of argon lasers is mainly for ophthalmic and ENT surgery. The carbon dioxide laser is used principally for cutting and vaporizing, mainly in ENT and gynaecological surgery. The Nd: YAG is mainly a coagulating laser and its uses are chiefly in gastroenterology and urology, for coagulating bleeding ulcers, debulking tumours and ablating local lesions. The KTP/532 TM laser produces all three surgical effects and therefore has a wide variety of surgical uses, including urology, ENT, gynaecology, orthopaedics, general surgery, neurosurgery, gastrointestinal and pulmonary surgery.

Pulsed dye lasers are used for stone fragmentation (lithotripsy) where it is convenient to deliver energy through a fine optical fibre. The photons are delivered to the tissues at a high rate so that the result is not a thermal effect but rather a shock-wave reaction.

EFFECTS OF LASERS

When the laser beam strikes tissue several inter-actions take place: the light is reflected, transmit-ted, absorbed and scattered within the tissue. It is the scattering of light that determines the surgi-cal effect. The heat produced at the site of impact will raise the temperature of the tissue, which passes through several stages: denaturation, coagulation, vacuolation, vaporization, car-bonization and incandescence. Of these effects the most significant are coagulation and vapor-ization, as these are what the surgeon uses. Cutting with a laser is basically a controlled, nar-row form of vaporization.

HAZARDS

Potential hazards fall into five main categories:

- electrical
- fire
- eye injury
- skin injury
- infective agents in smoke.

Electrical

All lasers use electricity, therefore there is the potential risk of electrocution if the instrument is installed or handled incorrectly.

All equipment should conform to British (European) safety standards and bear the BSI and CE marks. Inspection by the hospital elec-tronic/medical physics departments should be carried out at installation and at planned main-tenance intervals.

Fire

As thermal lasers use high temperatures to vaporize tissues there is a potential risk of fire. Precautions to prevent fire may include:

- a carbon dioxide fire extinguisher being available
- a bowl of sterile water for dousing the sterile field
- damp towels placed around the site of surgery (except when the laser is used in a contained area, as in endoscopic surgery)
- flammable skin preparations should be avoided; if used, the area should be thoroughly dried prior to activation of the laser
- an effective scavenging system for anaesthetic gases, as these support combustion in the event of an outbreak of fire
- non-flammable endotracheal tubes are recommended for head and neck surgery;
- avoidance of pooling of Providone-iodine solution, as this will give off toxic fumes if the laser is fired into it.

Eye injury

Eye damage can be caused by the laser light either striking the cornea and destroying it, or passing through the cornea and destroying the retina. Precautions to prevent this include:

- The use of safety eyewear, specific in appropriate optical density for the laser in use (except for carbon dioxide lasers, when ordinary spectacles will suffice).
- Knowledge of the nominal hazard zone. This is the distance, in the form of a circular area surrounding the source of laser light, within which eye damage may occur. It varies from laser to laser and should be taken into account when setting the local safety rules. In most cases the nominal hazard zone and appropriate precautions are applied to the whole of a particular operating theatre.
- Windows in the theatre should be screened to prevent the exit of laser light and reflection from the glass.
- The patient's eyes should always be protected, either with moistened pads taped over the eyelids for general anaesthesia or by safety eyewear for local anaesthesia.

Skin injury

Both patients and staff can suffer in this respect. Precautions include:

- use of damp towels, ensuring that the material does not get so hot that it scalds to the skin below if the laser is used for long periods of time. Frequent changing of the damp towels will therefore be necessary
- clear communication between the surgeon and the surgical team at all times
- careful use and placement of lasers with sapphire tips, which retain heat after the laser has been fired
- use of non-reflective surgical instruments to reduce the risk of reflection of the laser beam.

Infective agents in laser smoke

Lasers produce smoke, and it is possible that infective agents might be present in the smoke plume. This potential risk should therefore be avoided by the following measures:

- Biological smoke evacuation filters must be used to remove the smoke before it enters the hospital vacuum system. These should be changed regularly and checked for efficiency.
- The use of laser masks with smaller pore sizes than the standard theatre mask is recommended.

SAFETY STANDARDS
Patients

- Patients require careful preoperative explanation of laser procedures and safety precautions.
- Laser use should be documented in the patient's care plan.
- Details such as laser type, site, use, power settings/timings, patient details, operation performed, surgeon and laser operator should be recorded in the laser log.

- The surgeon should detail use of the laser in the patient's operating notes.

Staff

- All staff involved in using lasers for surgery should undertake a training programme and have been assessed as competent in the use of the equipment.
- Authorized laser operators and safety officers should be clearly identified for each individual laser in use in an operating department. These individuals carry total responsibility for safe practice in that area, and for the security of the laser keys.
- When the laser is in use the number of staff in the theatre should be kept to a minimum, with access to the theatre also restricted.
- Warning signs and lights should be visible as a deterrent to staff entering the area when the laser is fired (signs should not be a permanent fixture as this will lead to staff complacency).
- When not in use the laser must be kept in a secure place, with the keys in a locked cupboard.
- Any laser incident that occurs should be recorded on a special incident form and reported immediately to the Laser Safety Officer and Laser Protection Adviser.
- The laser must be placed in the standby or off mode when not in use, to prevent inadvertent firing.

All theatre practitioners should be aware of the training available in their department: the amount of training should reflect the amount of time the individual spends working with lasers. Each laser manufacturer also provides training programmes in the way of workshops and clinical training for all grades of theatre staff. All staff should be aware of the local rules and policies governing the use of lasers in their individual departments.

Principles, Uses and Hazards of Electrosurgery

P. Wicker

Electrosurgery, or surgical diathermy as it is often called, has been used in operating theatres for almost 100 years and in recent times there has even been an upsurge in interest, partly owing to new surgical techniques being introduced and partly because the equipment is more efficient and safer than ever before. This section will illustrate some of the basic principles of electrosurgery, the associated hazards to patients and some of the practices which can be used to overcome these problems.

PROPERTIES OF THE ELECTRIC CIRCUIT

Electrosurgery is the use of electric current to produce heat in human tissues. Electrosurgical current follows the same basic rules as applies to any electric circuit, and in order to understand electrosurgery the user must be aware of the basic principles governing an electric circuit.

Electric current flows when electrons pass from one atom to another. In order for this to happen, an electric circuit must be formed between the positive and the negative poles of an electrode. Voltage, measured in volts, is the force that enables electrons to move around a circuit. If electrons meet a resistance (impedance) to their flow, then heat is produced. This resistance is measured in ohms. The measurement of current, in amps, is an indication of the number of electrons which are flowing around the circuit. The power of an electric current is measured in watts and is an interaction between current, voltage, resistance and time. The same principles apply to an electrosurgical circuit, in which case the generator is the source of the electron flow (current) and voltage. The completed circuit is composed of the generator, the active electrode, the patient and the return electrode, with the connecting cables in between. The patient's tissues impede the flow of the current, leading to the production of heat. It is interesting to note that the electrode itself does not heat the tissues, as it would do in the case of cautery or electrocautery: rather, it is the flow of current which results in heat being generated within the tissues themselves.[1]

Another important principle applies to the frequency of the current. Mains electric current is alternating, in that it flows first in one direction and then reverses to flow in the opposite direction. Mains electric current oscillates like this at around 60 cycles per second, which is measured in Hertz (Hz). Electric current at this frequency interferes with the normal conduction of nerves and leads to the classic signs of electrocution: ventricular fibrillation, nerve stimulation and muscular seizures. Both nerve and muscle stimulation ceases at around 100 000 Hz. At this frequency it is possible to pass high-power electric current through a human body without causing electrocution.

Electric currents always return to the source where they were produced: this is called 'ground'. In the case of mains electricity the source is the power stations, which form part of a national grid to which all mains current returns. This ground is called the 'common earth' since it is the return point for all mains-powered electrical devices.[2]

ELECTROSURGICAL CIRCUITS

Electrosurgical generators are designed to increase the frequency of mains electricity to around 300 000 Hz in order to avoid electrocution while passing high levels of electric current through the patient's body. All varieties of electrosurgery rely on the principles of a circuit being formed, and there are currently two ways in which this can be set up – bipolar or monopolar circuits.

Bipolar electrosurgery (Fig. 5.37)

In bipolar electrosurgery both the active and the return electrodes are enclosed in one electrosurgical instrument, which is usually in the form of a pair of forceps. One tine of the forceps carries the current towards the patient (active electrode), while the other tine carries the current away from the patient (return electrode). The current enters the patient's body only in the tissues held between the tines. A patient return electrode is not required since the current is returned to the generator by one tine of the electrosurgical forceps. In most cases a patient return electrode should not be applied in any case, as this could potentially divert the current away from the second tine towards the patient return electrode, leading to a spreading out of the electrosurgical effect and, potentially, accidental patient burns.

Because such a small amount of tissue is exposed to the effects of the current, a relatively low-power current can be used and so bipolar electrosurgery is ideal in situations where high power might be dangerous, for example in neurosurgery or plastic surgery.[3] Bipolar circuits also avoid problems related to the use of pacemakers, since the current does not pass through the heart.

Monopolar electrosurgery

Monopolar electrosurgical circuits are most commonly used because of their effectiveness and versatility. In monopolar electrosurgery the active electrode and return electrode are separated, usually by a substantial amount of the patient's body. Normally the active electrode is in the form of an electrosurgical pencil or forceps, and the return electrode is in the form of a much larger, flat plate which is in contact with the patient's skin.

Grounded electrosurgical systems (Fig. 5.38)

When surgical diathermy machines were first introduced in the 1920s, grounded mains electricity was converted to grounded electrosurgical

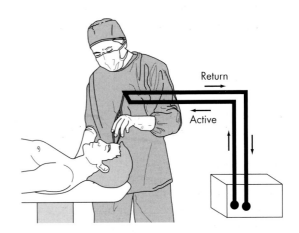

Figure 5.37   Bipolar electrosurgery.

current. In other words, the electrosurgical current tried to return to ground, which in this case was the common earth to which all other electrical devices were connected. It was assumed at this time that in order to provide a safe pathway for the current, the patient should be earthed with the return electrode.[3] However, electrical current always tries to return to ground by the path of least resistance, so if the return electrode failed to operate then the current would find an alternative way to earth via a contact between the patient and any other earthed object. This phenomenon is called current division, and under the right situations could lead to an accidental patient burn at the point of contact with the earthed object.

Isolated electrosurgical systems (Fig. 5.39)

As a result of these dangers, by 1968 improvements in technology had meant that isolated generator technology could be developed. The isolated generator works by creating a separate circuit which is not referenced to the common earth, but has its source within the circuitry of the generator itself. In other words, the current pathway in this situation is between the generator and the patient, rather than the common

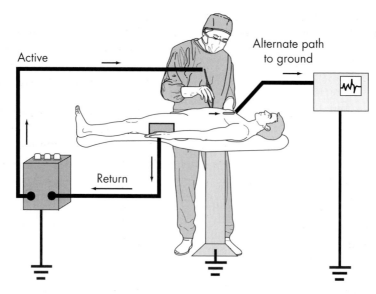

Figure 5.38 Grounded electrosurgical systems.

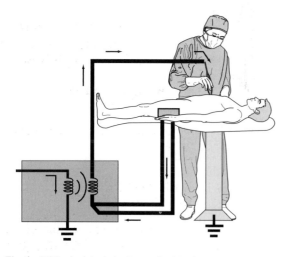

Figure 5.39 Isolated electrosurgical systems.

earth and the patient. As the current no longer needs to return to earth, other earthed objects present no difficulties, since the current does not recognize them as part of the circuit. Current division is therefore minimized and the potential for burns is reduced. Also, if the circuit between the generator and the patient is broken – for example if the patient plate falls off – current will cease to flow because it can no longer return to its

source, and the generator will be automatically deactivated.[4]

Both grounded and isolated systems are currently in use and both types are still being produced. It is advisable that the user checks to make sure that they know which type of system they are using in order to avoid potential complications.

Components of an electrosurgical system

Generators

The major manufacturers of electrosurgical generators include Valleylab, Eschmann, Erbe and 3M. All these manufacturers produce generators which fulfil certain criteria and reach or exceed certain specifications, which are stated in British Standard specifications produced by the Department of Health. For example, the generators must comply with a certain level of stray currents, use accepted symbols such as the outline man or heart symbols, and use standardized colours for active electrode switches and pedals.[3] Most of the generators produced today also have sophisticated monitoring systems which can check that the patient circuit has not been compromised. One generator, for example, monitors the voltage present over the patient: if this exceeds a certain level an alarm sounds and the current is deactivated.[3]

Active electrodes

This is the electrode where the electrosurgery is expected to happen. In most cases the active electrode is an instrument in the form of a pencil or forceps. They are usually fully insulated, apart from the distal tip which is exposed metal. In some cases the metal tip may be Teflon coated in order to prevent tissues sticking.[4] Modern minimally invasive active electrodes include extralong hooks and blades which are designed to be passed down cannulae. In endoscopic use the active electrodes are designed for various purposes, for example loops to snare polyps during polypectomy. Bipolar instruments are usually in the form of forceps, as this is the most effective way of providing a bipolar current.

With the increasing use of minimally invasive surgery it has become increasingly evident that there is a need to monitor the use of the active electrode. A device has been developed which does just this: it can monitor the active electrode for any insulation failure or signs of capacitive coupling with other instruments. At present this device is only available for use during minimally invasive surgery, where it takes the form of a plastic shield that covers the electrode and slips down the inside of the cannula.[4]

Patient return electrodes

These electrodes take the form of large plates which are attached to the patient's body. It is important to realize that the same current leaves the body at this point as entered it via the active electrode. On the basis of this fact, it can be assumed that the return electrode is capable of heating the tissues to the same extent as the active electrode. This is in fact true; however, the larger size of the return electrode causes the current density to fall, and the heating effect to be spread over a large area; therefore, burns do not normally occur. The patient return electrode is, however, a major area of concern and because of this its use has been closely monitored and covered by various areas of legislation related to the British Standards.[3]

Most electrosurgical generators have an alarm system which can detect whether or not the patient return electrode has been plugged in to the generator. The other major monitoring system which is present on some generators identifies whether the return electrode is in contact with the patient and whether the electrical contact is good enough to avoid accidental burning. One such system, the REM system from Valleylab, uses a dual-section plate.[5] A small current is passed through the plate and then the impedance on both sides of the plate is measured. This monitor can detect various possible error situations:

- one side of the plate becoming detached from the patient
- the plate not being attached to the patient at all
- one side of the plate conducting better than the other side
- the plate crumpling when the patient is moved.

The generator automatically deactivates if any of these situations arise.

SURGICAL EFFECTS OF ELECTROSURGERY

The only variable which determines the effect electrosurgical current has on tissues is the rate at which it produces heat. High levels of heat generated rapidly will cut tissues; low levels of heat generated slowly will coagulate tissue. The ability of the electrosurgical current to produce heat in the tissues can be changed by manipulating several factors: these include current density, power, time and waveform.

Current density is the ratio of the power of the current to the area of tissue it affects. Hence, for example, for a given power of current the tissue density will be high at the active electrode (because the current is concentrated over a small area). At the corresponding time the current density will be low at the return electrode, because it has been spread over a relatively large area of the plate.[6]

The power of the electrosurgical current can affect the surgical effects it produces. For example, a high-power COAG waveform can be used to cut tissue; similarly a low-power CUT waveform can be used very effectively to desicate tissue.

The time factor is also an important consideration, since a low-power current can lead to burns if applied over a long period of time and may be a factor in accidental burning caused by the formation of alternative pathways.

One of the facilities present in an electrosurgical generator is the ability to alter the waveform of the electrosurgical current. As the waveform changes, the effects on the tissues alter and a different surgical effect is produced. The three waveforms are traditionally called CUT, COAG and BLEND, and cause the surgical effects of cutting, fulguration and desiccation (Fig. 5.40).

CUT waveform

This is a high-current low-voltage waveform. The high current helps it to heat tissues quickly and the low voltage prevents the formation of sparks, which would tend to dissipate the heat being produced. Because the tissues heat quickly they swell and explode, leaving behind a hole in the cell matrix. The effect can be very clean, with the electrode acting very much like a scalpel.

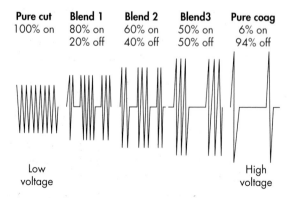

Pure cut	Blend 1	Blend 2	Blend3	Pure coag
100% on	80% on	60% on	50% on	6% on
	20% off	40% off	50% off	94% off

Low voltage   High voltage

Figure 5.40 Tissue effects change as the waveform is modified.

COAG waveform

COAG is a low-current high-voltage waveform. The low current causes a slow heating effect and the high voltage causes the production of sparks, which help to dissipate the heating effect over a larger area. The result is a slow heating of the tissues. At low power this leads to desiccation or drying out of the tissues, which causes coagulation of bleeding vessels. At higher powers the sparks cause a burning effect wherever they land, leading to necrosis and fulguration of tissues. This effect is sometimes called the 'spray' waveform. The technique is used in, for example, fulguration of the gallbladder bed during cholecystectomy, or fulguration of the cervix. At even higher power (around 120 W or so) the COAG waveform produces enough current density for the electrode to cut tissues. This technique is not advisable because of the tissue damage it causes, and also because the high power is not really necessary since a lower-power CUT waveform would achieve the same result.[7]

BLEND waveform

This combines the effect of COAG and CUT by altering the parameters of the waveform. BLEND 1 tends to be higher current and lower voltage than BLEND 3, so a move from BLEND 1 to BLEND 3 gives an increasing coagulation effect and a relative reduction in the cutting effect.

USES OF ELECTROSURGERY
Traditional uses

Traditionally, electrosurgery has been used in all settings where coagulation or cutting of tissues is required. Specialized uses have also been developed which have made procedures easier or more effective, and include, for example:

- bipolar coagulation of the fallopian tubes during sterilization
- polypectomy via flexible colonoscopy[8]
- papillotomy (widening of the papilla of Vater) via a gastroscope
- dissection of the gallbladder during minimally invasive procedures
- transurethral resection of the prostate

- endometrial ablation in gynaecological conditions.

Electrosurgery has come to the fore again with the recent increase of minimally invasive and endoscopic surgery. New techniques, instrumentation and technological developments have proved that electrosurgery still has significant advantages over laser surgery in many situations.

HAZARDS OF ELECTROSURGERY

Thermoelectric burns (Fig. 5.41)

These burns constitute the main danger to patients from electrosurgery.[3] The burns are always accidental, very rarely the result of faulty equipment and most often the result of the misunderstanding of the practitioner in the use of the equipment.

Inappropriate use

The process of electrosurgery is very simple and easily learned. That said, it is also the simplest of applications to get wrong, and is fraught with dangers. Common mistakes include:

- touching the side of the wound with unprotected forceps
- activating the current at the wrong time
- applying current to the wrong area
- using too much power.

One common mistake is to assume that insulation is intact without checking it first. For example, a burn to the side of a patient's mouth was caused when bipolar forceps were used during a tonsillectomy. The insulation along the length of the forceps had broken down and a pathway had formed in contact with the side of the patient's mouth.[9] The patient had to undergo major surgery and a long convalescence as a result.

In order to avoid keying the electrosurgery at the wrong time, the control pedal or switch should be in the control of the operating surgeon alone.

Using a high-power waveform is inherently more dangerous because any stray currents which are formed also have relatively higher power. Also, the increase in voltage makes inadvertent arcing to nearby tissues more likely. In

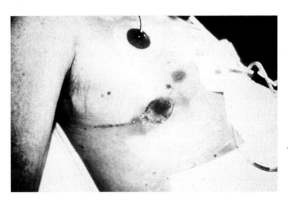

Figure 5.41 Thermoelectric burns.

most situations a lower-power waveform with the most appropriate characteristics would achieve the same results.

Current division

Current division occurs when an alternative pathway exists for the current to return to ground. This is most likely to occur with earthed electrosurgical generators, rather than with isolated generators, because in the earthed system contact with any other earthed object (such as a metal trolley) could provide a pathway to earth.[10]

Current division can occur when, for example:

- the patient return electrode is faulty, has not been placed on the patient or is not making good contact
- the patient return electrode is at a greater distance from the operative site and an earthed object lies between the active and the return electrodes
- a low-impedance alternative pathway exists
- a high-voltage high-power waveform is used.

Current division relies on there being an alternative pathway for the current to take, so the main principles to follow are that the correct return pathway should be as close as possible to the site of surgery, and all alternative grounded sites should be eliminated. The possible grounded sites include:

- Mayo stands coming into contact with legs
- ECG electrodes connected to a monitor

- metal-tipped rectal thermometers
- metal infusion stands touching the patient
- exposed metal armrests in contact with the patient.

The generator may incorporate a monitoring circuit for alternative current pathways. The presence of these pathways is assessed by monitoring the difference between the current leaving the generator and that leaving the patient return electrode. If the current leaving the return electrode is less than the overall current being used, then another pathway must be involved. It is important to realize, however, that monitoring systems are never foolproof and the patient should be visually assessed all the time for the presence of alternative sites.

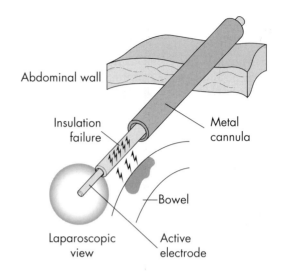

Figure 5.42 Insulation failure.

Minimally invasive surgery (MIS)

Although MIS has revolutionized surgery, it has brought with it a new set of concerns related to the use of electrosurgical current.[4,11,12]

- **Insulation failure** (Fig. 5.42) This is most likely to show itself with a high-voltage waveform, such as COAG, because the high voltage is able to break through the insulation or pass through already compromised insulation. Breaks in the insulation lead to current leaking out of the electrode at a site other than the intended one. In the case of MIS this site could be behind the surgeon's scope of vision, which is limited to around 180°. In order to reduce this possibility a low-power CUT waveform can be used, with the electrode in direct and full contact with the tissue. This waveform has a lower voltage and is therefore less likely to break down insulation. High-power COAG waveforms should be avoided wherever possible.

- **Direct coupling** (Fig. 5.43) Direct coupling occurs when an active instrument activates an adjacent inactive instrument. The phenomenon is called inductance and occurs because of the electrical field which surrounds any activated object. This situation is much more likely to occur during MIS because of the close proximity of several metal instruments. Once activated, the current in the secondary instrument tries to return to the patient return electrode, and in doing so may

cause an accidental internal burn to the patient. In order to avoid this situation the generator should not be activated while the electrode is in close proximity to another metal instrument.

- **Capacitance** (Fig. 5.44) A capacitor is formed whenever a non-conductor separates two conductors. This effect can occur when, for example, a metal electrode is separated from a metal cannula by plastic insulation. An electrostatic field is produced which induces a current in the second conductor. This current tries to return to the

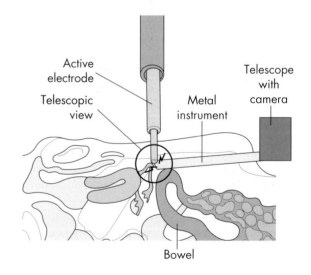

Figure 5.43 Direct coupling.

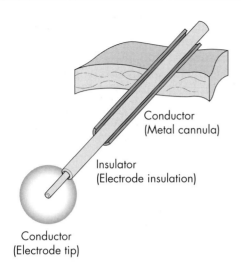

Figure 5.44 Instrument/cannula configuration creating a capacitor.

patient return electrode and in so doing may lead to accidental burns.

The worst situation occurs when a metal cannula is used with an outside plastic sleeve or collar. In this scenario the capacitively coupled current cannot leak through to the abdominal wall and must instead look for an alternative site, which might be tissue adjacent to the metal part of the cannula, for example bowel, fallopian tube, uterus, liver or stomach. Severe accidental burns can occur to these organs, in many cases without the surgeon's knowledge.[4]

Another example of capacitive coupling is when the surgeon attempts to coagulate a bleeding vessel by applying current to the non-insulated forceps which he is holding. The capacitor is created between his hand, the glove and the metal forceps. This may result in the surgeon receiving a small, but often painful burn to his hand.

In order to reduce the effects of capacitance an all-metal cannula (which allows the capacitive current to dissipate safely through the abdominal wall) should be used. Hybrid systems should be avoided and, if possible, an active electrode monitoring system as described earlier should be used.

Smoke inhalation

Smoke inhalation has recently been identified as a major problem because electrosurgical smoke

has been proven to contain carcinogens, toxins, viral DNA, bacteria and respiratory irritants.[13–15] Although there has been no legislation introduced to date in this country, in the USA the Association of Operating Room Nurses has recommended the evacuation of all surgical smoke, as all patients and perioperative personnel should be protected from inhaling it.[16] Several manufacturers have developed equipment which can be used to evacuate smoke using filters to clear particles from the suctioned air.

Ignition of alcohol-based substances

Alcohol-based skin preparation solutions are often used in the operating theatre. This can lead to problems when combined with diathermy, especially when waterproof drapes are being used, as solutions can pool on the surface of the table, the mattress and in the folds of the patient's skin. If the solution is not allowed to dry before draping the alcohol vapour becomes trapped and concentrations increase. This vapour can be ignited with a spark from the electrosurgery. Since alcohol burns at a very high temperature with a bright light, it is impossible to see the flame under the operating lights. Often damage is only evident when the patient's tissues or the drapes themselves start to burn. Serious injury with permanent scarring can be the result. In order to avoid this situation, alcoholic skin preparation solutions should be avoided or, if used, should be allowed to dry before draping.[1]

Interference with medical devices

Pacemakers and ECG monitors are highly susceptible to interference from electrosurgical current. When activated by electrosurgical current pacemakers tend to switch off, returning the patient into heart block. This can be avoided by employing a short return pathway which does not pass through the heart, or by using bipolar electrosurgery where the current only passes through the tissues between the tines of the forceps.

ECG screen interference tends to be a problem only from the point of view of reading the screen, since the heart itself is not stimulated by normal electrosurgical current. However, the fact that the screen is picking up electrosurgical waveforms implies that some current must be travelling down the ECG electrodes and leads, and this can cause burns under the ECG electrodes. In order to avoid this, the return electrode should be placed close to the site of surgery and the ECG electrodes kept out of the direct pathway between the active and the return electrodes.

A recent problem which has increased in significance is interference with VDU screens during minimally invasive procedures. This is caused by harmonics, or aberrant waveforms, outside the normal range for electrosurgery. Although not directly harmful, visibility is compromised and so this effect should be minimized if possible. This can be achieved by using generators which have been optimized for MIS; an example includes the Force F/X from Valleylab, which produces a waveform which is well within the acceptable limits.[7]

Another way in which interference can arise is if the insulation on the active electrode breaks down. This may happen with disposable devices which have been reused outside the manufacturer's guidelines.

PRINCIPLES OF SAFE PRACTICE

The effective use of electrosurgical equipment and the avoidance of accidental patient injury must be at the root of any discussion of electrosurgery. There are many instances where there are two ways of approaching a subject and neither way is necessarily the best; however, it is important for practitioners to know what alternatives are available and then be able to choose the most appropriate. A knowledge of the basic principles of electrosurgery will prepare the practitioner for delivering sound, knowledgeable practice. This may help to avoid problems and to ensure that the best care is offered to the patient.

Policies

The use of electrosurgery should be encapsulated within a formal and comprehensive policy and practice document.[10] The document should cover:

- the maintenance of equipment
- the minimum grade of staff able to use the electrosurgical equipment
- the documentation involved, including manuals, hazard notices and information
- the preparation and use of the equipment, before, during and after surgery
- patient care associated with the use of the equipment.

Education

An education programme is essential to ensure that patient care in relation to the use of electrosurgery is maintained at a high level. Very often the companies that supply the equipment are able to provide in-house lectures on its use. This can be a very cost-effective and efficient way of providing information. Various videos and computerized teaching aids are often available, along with practical hands-on experience.[12]

There are also books, documents and articles available from the National Association of Theatre Nurses (NATN). *Principles of Safe Practice in the Operating Theatre* is an example of a document which has been used as a standard against which all practice could be measured during litigation.[17] NATN has also produced a multimedia teaching aid which can be used alongside written information in order to aid learning.[18]

Safety checks

Safety checks should be carried out according to the manufacturer's recommendations. In most cases instruction will be offered along with the purchase of the equipment. Each generator or item of equipment will have a specific set of instructions; however, as a minimum, safety checks should include the following:

- Check all electrical cables and the general condition of the control panel, plug and switches before each use.
- Ensure that the equipment is clean and has no obvious faults or damage.
- Check that the generator is functioning correctly.

• Check that the alarm system is functioning prior to the patient's arrival in theatre.
• Check the insulation on the cables and take out of use if damaged.
• Ensure that the plate is clean and in working order.
• Ensure good contact between the patient and the plate, over an area of good muscle mass.
• Avoid shaving excess hair prior to applying the plate – choose another site if possible.
• Ensure that all connections for the active and return electrode are made prior to switching it on.
• Isolate the patient from any earthed metal objects.
• Check the plate site if the patient is moved during surgery.
• Place the plate as close as possible to the operative site.
• Check all connections with the patient and between components of the circuit if a power increase is requested.
• Check the patient for contact with earth if a power increase is requested.
• Keep the active electrode blade clean during use.
• Always use an insulated quiver to store the active electrode.
• Never coil the return electrode cable when it is in use.
• Beware of any modification to existing equipment.
• Make yourself familiar with the equipment in use.
• Always check the patient's skin at the site of the return electrode for signs of damage.
• Wipe foot pedals with warm water and detergent without immersing them fully in water.
• Keep the active electrode in the quiver until the generator is switched off. (Never lie the active electrode on an earthed surface (for example a metal trolley) while the generator is switched on as this can lead to patient burns.)
• Never reuse a single-use return electrode.

Quality assurance

Regular reviews can highlight poor practice before it has time to become established, and it can also help to establish and enforce good practice. This can be developed through a quality assurance system which looks at standards relating to such areas as education, preparation of equipment, use of equipment and patient care outcomes.[3]

RECENT DEVELOPMENTS

The development of electrosurgery has received a boost from the recent increases in the number of patients undergoing minimally invasive surgery. Many of the improvements have come along as a result of improvements in technology. In other areas a greater understanding of the needs of the surgeon in relation to surgery, and a greater awareness of the dangers associated with electrosurgery, have led to a change in the technology.

Bipolar cutting

Although this facility has been available for some time, it has only recently become practical because of the lack of suitable instrumentation. A pair of bipolar scissors has recently become available from Ethicon Ltd. These have the obvious advantages of bipolar technology and therefore are proving to be excellent for use during minimally invasive procedures.

Argon-enhanced electrosurgery

The active electrode, usually an electrosurgical pencil electrode, incorporates a device which passes a stream of argon gas around the electrode tip in order to improve the surgical effectiveness of the current. Argon is an inert, non-combustible gas which easily ionizes in the presence of electricity. This highly conductive stream of gas provides an efficient pathway for the current to pass to the tissues. The advantages of using this gas include reduced smoke and odour, reduced drag and tissue adhesion in CUT mode, reduced tissue damage and a flexible eschar which makes the tissues less prone to rebleeding.[4]

Tissue density feedback

The more exacting control requirements of laparoscopic and endoscopic procedures and techniques has encouraged the development of new surgical waveforms. Tissue density feedback refers to the ability of a generator to provide instant responses to the change in tissue resistance in order to produce a more consistent surgical effect. The effect is achieved by monitoring electrosurgical dosage and matching it to the preferred clinical effect on a wide range of tissue types and resistances. For example, the power of a particular waveform in a conventional generator alters as the tissue impedance changes during the electrosurgical process – the tissue dries out and impedance increases. A tissue density feedback-enabled generator is able to match its output to the change in impedance in order to give an enhanced electrosurgical effect. The advantages of this technology are said to be improved tissue cutting, reduced capacitive coupling and reduced interference with VDU displays.[7]

Dipolar electrosurgery

This innovation uses a high-power electrosurgical unit which operates without a traditional return 'plate' electrode, but which is in effect a newly configured bipolar current. Nuvotek, the inventors of dipolar electrosurgery, claim that their technology can give similar or better results than traditional monopolar electrosurgery using significantly lower power levels and that leakage currents, capacitive coupling, video interference and the possibility of return electrode burns are eliminated. The output is further enhanced by using clinical algorithms and 'tissue impedance detection' techniques, which ensure optimum power is delivered to the tissues with minimal tissue damage.

Bipolar techniques offer an alternative to monopolar electrosurgery, but the current tends to be low power and have limited cutting capabilities. The dipolar arrangement involves using two conductors, as in bipolar electrosurgery, but the current split between them is dependent on the impedance of the electrode in contact with the tissues. Current is alternatively switched between the conductors changing resistance of the active and return pathways. The overall clinical effect is that one electrode acts as both the active and return electrode.[18]

CONCLUSION

Electrosurgical technology is constantly improving to such an extent that the equipment is now capable of producing efficient current, specifically tailored to tissues and provided in a safety conscious environment. However, because of the features of electricity it is obvious that there is still room for fatal error. Qualified, competent and experienced use of this equipment by skilled and knowledgeable practitioners remains the main factor in providing the patient with the best and safest possible care.

ACKNOWLEDGEMENT

The figures in this section are published with the permission of Valleylab Inc., Boulder, Colorado, USA.

REFERENCES

1. Wicker CP 1992 Making sense of electrosurgery. Nursing Times 88: 31–33
2. Gruendemann J, Fernsebner B 1995 Technology management: electrosurgery. In: Gruendemann BJ, Fernsebner B (eds) Comprehensive perioperative nursing, Vol. 1 Principles. Jones and Bartlett, London
3. Wicker CP 1991 Working with electrosurgery. National Association of Theatre Nurses, Harrogate
4. Valleylab 1995 Principles of electrosurgery. Valleylab Inc., Boulder, Colorado
5. Valleylab 1996 REM polyhesive patient return electrodes. Valleylab Inc., Boulder, Colorado

6. Atkinson LJ 1992 Biotechnology: specialized surgical tools. In: Berry EC, Kohn ML (eds) Operating Room Technique, 7th edn. Mosby-Yearbook, London
7. Taylor DT 1995 Computer controlled instant response high frequency electrosurgery system that minimises tissue damage. Valleylab Inc., Boulder, Colorado
8. Wicker CP 1993 Electrosurgery. Scope, Pentax Medical, Harrow
9. Zinder DJ, Parker GS 1996 Electrocautery burns and operator ignorance. Otolaryngology – Head and Neck Surgery 115: 145–149
10. Wicker CP 1997 Electrosurgery. In: Principles of safe practice in the operating theatre (in press). National Association of Theatre Nurses, Harrogate
11. Tucker RD, Voyles CR 1995 Laparoscopic electrosurgery: complications and prevention. Association of Operating Room Nurses Journal 62: 49–78
12. Wicker CP 1997 Tissue density feedback (multimedia training pack) (in press). Valleylab UK, London
13. Hirschfeld JJ, Niloff PH 1992 Electrocautery smoke elimination. American Journal of Cosmetic Surgery 9: 305–307
14. Gatti JE, Bryant CJ, Noone RB, Murphy JB 1992 The mutagenicity of electrocautery smoke. Journal of Plastic and Reconstructive Surgery 89: 781–784
15. Patterson P 1993 OR exposure to electrosurgery smoke a concern. OR Manager 9: 6, 1, 21, 22
16. AORN 1995 Recommended practices for electrosurgery, AORN standards and recommended practices for perioperative nursing. Association of Operating Room Nurses, Denver, Colorado 155–161
17. NATN 1995 Principles of safe practice in the operating theatre. National Association of Theatre Nurses, Harrogate
18. Wicker CP 1996 Working with electrosurgery (multimedia edition). National Association of Theatre Nurses, Harrogate
19. Cobb GV 1996 Tissue cutting and coagulation by computerised dipolar electrosurgery. Nuvotek, Leeds

Powered tools

Powered instruments are used for orthopaedic, neurosurgical, dental, plastic and reconstructive surgery. They can be divided into two categories, air powered and electrically powered.

AIR-POWERED TOOLS

Air-powered tools include a variety of saws and drills used to resect, sculpture and repair bone. Most power tools are operated with compressed air or nitrogen, but never oxygen owing to the risk of explosion or fire. They are controlled by a hand switch or foot pedal. The compressed air or nitrogen may be delivered via cylinders or by a piped supply, and should be at a constant specific pressure in pounds per square inch (psi). Therefore, theatre practitioners should adhere to the manufacturer's recommendations for a particular tool. When cylinders are used it should be checked that there is sufficient air in the cylinder to complete the procedure (Fig. 5.45).

Air-powered tools are precision instruments and should be treated accordingly. Before the start of a procedure the instrument should be checked to ensure that all attachments are available and in working order. The scrub practitioner should be familiar with the use and assembly of each power tool and be able to connect attachments securely. All drill bits, saw blades and burrs should be checked for damage: damaged and blunt instruments prevent accurate use and risk danger to the patient from heat necrosis and metallic particles in the tissues.

The instruments have rotary, reciprocating or oscillating actions. The rotary action is used to drill holes, ream cavities and insert screws, wires or pins. Reciprocating cutting action is from front to back and the oscillating action is from side to side; both are used to cut, shape and remove bone (Fig. 5.46).

Attachments, drills and saw blades should be seated firmly and in accordance with the manufacturer's instructions before use. Prior to use the power tool should be tested once it is attached to the air/nitrogen supply: the surgeon should be warned so as to avoid inadvertent damage being caused to the patient.

When powered instruments are used on bone the surgical assistant should drip saline solution from a bulb syringe to cool the bone and remove debris, so that the operation site does not become

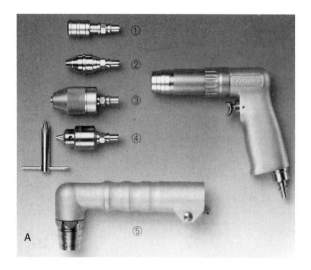

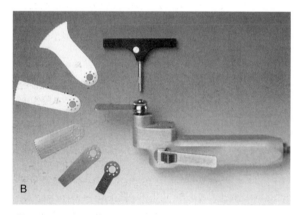

Figure 5.45 A. Universal air drill designed for reaming, drilling and wire insertion. B. Oscillating bone saw.

clogged with bone and the saw/drill bit hot. The surgeon and assistants should wear goggles to prevent water and bone debris entering the eye. Before the power tool is handed to the surgeon it should be ascertained as to whether the safety catch should be on or off, as some surgeons prefer the tool ready for immediate use and others do not, so individual preferences should be taken into account. The surgeon should switch the safety catch on before returning the tool to the scrub practitioner. When the tool is not in use the safety catch should always be on: this will avoid inadvertent damage or injury caused by the instrument.

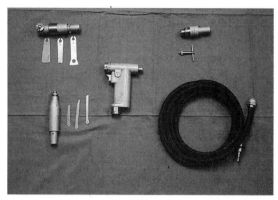

Figure 5.46 Air-powered hand piece with hose and attachments.

Care and maintenance of air-powered tools

The following are guidelines, but specific instructions from manufacturers should also be followed.

• After use the instrument should be cleaned immediately by hand.
• Power tools should never be cleaned in instrument washers or immersed in water, as this will cause the motor to rust and make expensive repairs inevitable.
• All attachments, adaptors and instruments should be removed from the handpiece.
• The handpiece and attachments can be washed under running water with a soft brush or cloth, taking care to prevent water entering the air inlet. To avoid this the hose may be left attached with its end out of the water.
• The drills and saw blades should be cleaned of all residue and checked for damage and wear. Any damaged instruments should be discarded and replaced.
• Air hoses should be cleaned, ensuring that no fluid enters them. Some hoses can have both ends coupled together to avoid this. If this is not possible the ends of the hose should be left out of the water.
• All parts of the power tool should be dried carefully.
• The turbines or handpieces must be lubricated after each use. Most manufacturers provide a resin-free oil for this purpose.

• Using the specified oil for a particular tool, the recommended amount of oil should be placed into the hose attachment. The power tool should then be reconnected to the air or nitrogen supply and the tool run at full speed for 5–10 seconds to disperse the lubricant.

• Most power tools can be autoclaved at temperatures up to 134°C. Sterilization using ethylene oxide is not recommended by most manufacturers except in special circumstances, and then proper exposure and aeration times must be established.

• Prior to sterilization all attachments should be dismantled and left unconnected. Hose contact with hot metal should be avoided and no pressure should be placed on the hose. The hose should not be coupled during autoclaving. Most manufacturers provide cases for sterilization to protect the power tool.

• Following sterilization, power tools should not be used until they have cooled to room temperature. The cooling process should not be accelerated, but in an emergency they can be cooled by blowing air through them.

ELECTRICALLY POWERED TOOLS

Drills, saws and dermatomes may also be electrically powered. These are mainly used in dental, plastic and ENT surgery. Most electric drill motors do not have sufficient power for major bone surgery and should not be used for this purpose. Their motors must be designed to be explosion proof, with sparkproof connectors. Flammable anaesthetic gases should not be used while these tools are in use. Prior to their initial use they should always be checked by the hospital electrician and labelled to this effect, with the date.

Electrically powered tools should be cleaned according to the manufacturer's instructions. Most control units should be kept clean by wiping with a damp cloth, without allowing any fluid to contact the working parts of the unit or the plug itself. The foot control should be kept clean in the same way. The control unit should be placed on a large solid surface, to avoid accidental dropping.

Cleaning and maintenance of the handpiece is again according to the manufacturer's instructions. Many are sealed units, with only the blade or drill attachments able to be removed. The handpiece should be cleaned with a damp cloth and then dried, or washed under running water with the attachment left in place, to prevent water entering the handpiece. They should never be immersed in water, and if this occurs accidentally the handpiece should be returned immediately to the manufacturer for repair. Lubrication of the handpiece depends on whether or not it is fitted with sealed bearings, which eliminate the need for lubrication.

Attachments should be cared for in the same way as for air-powered tools. Any damaged drills, burrs or blades should be discarded as their use can result in overloading of the motor performance. Dermatome blades are designed for single use only and should be disposed of safely in a sharps container.

Sterilization of the handpieces should follow manufacturers' instructions, but a general principle is that they should be steam sterilized at the same or slightly higher temperatures than air-powered tools. Ethylene oxide sterilization may also be used for some units.

A planned maintenance programme should be agreed with the manufacturer at the time of purchase of these power tools. The theatre practitioner should always follow the manufacturer's instructions for each individual tool, as different tools will have different care and maintenance instructions, which may result in inadvertent damage if the wrong instructions are followed.

Ultrasound

Ultrasound can be used for the removal or debulking of tumours. The Cusa system works by moving a titanium tip 23 000 times per second at an amplitude of 356 μm at maximum power. This causes cavitational bubbles to appear in the saline irrigation, which is delivered via the silastic flue that surrounds the tip. The bubbles implode, disrupting the cell structure; intracellular cavitation also takes place and the cells are destroyed by the implosion of the intracellular cavitational bubbles. Denatured cells are emulsified with the irrigant and are sucked away from the operative site via the hollow vibrating tip. Pressures in excess of 10 000 g and temperatures in excess of 5000°C are caused by the implosion, but they are produced at a microscopic level and only affect the cells in which implosion occurs.

The Cusa has an ability to cause efficient cavitation in high- or low-water content tissues, i.e. in both normal and tumour cells and in bone. High elastic/collagen content tissues such as vessels and nerve sheaths do not allow cavitation to occur readily, as this tissue resonates in time with the vibration and is therefore left intact.

Many surgical disciplines currently use the Cusa system:

- neurosurgery
- general surgery
- ENT
- maxillofacial surgery
- gynaecology
- cardiothoracic surgery
- urology
- breast surgery
- minimally invasive surgery.

With the advent of the CUSALap™ ultrasound can now be used in a wide variety of general and gynaecological minimally invasive procedures.

Many other uses are being investigated. With the addition of the Cem® system Cusa is now more versatile. This can be used to introduce electrosurgical cut or coagulation directly on to the tissue, either independently or simultaneously with ultrasonic vibration. This is particularly useful in the removal of vascular tumours and vascular organ surgery.

Operating microscopes

Operating microscopes are now used in a wide range of surgical specialties, including:

- ophthalmic surgery
- ear surgery
- plastic surgery
- neurological surgery
- microsurgery/hand surgery.

There is a wide range available and the type chosen will depend on its future use.

Microscopes may have a floorstand or a stationary or track ceiling mount. There are advantages and disadvantages to both. The floorstand type takes up valuable floor space and, as microscopic surgery involves a number of surgeons around a relatively small area, this constraint should be taken into consideration. Stationary or ceiling-track mounted microscopes obviously reduce the crowding of floor space, but can only be used in the operating theatre in which they are mounted, and cannot be removed at the end of the operation. Therefore, a corner of valuable theatre space will be taken up at all times.

Some microscopes have a video system or an assistant's eyepiece built in, which is useful for the surgeon's assistant and the scrub practitioner to watch the surgery and hence assist the surgeon (Fig. 5.47).

CARE AND MAINTENANCE

- The manufacturer's instruction manual should be available at all times.
- Designated practitioners should be given the responsibility for checking, setting up and storing the microscope.
- The designated practitioners should be given instruction from the manufacturer.
- Theatre practitioners should be aware of what maintenance they may be responsible for and when it is necessary to call the appropriate service engineer.
- Supplies of spare parts such as bulbs and fuses should be readily available.

- Care should be taken when moving the microscope, to ensure that it is not damaged and that staff are safe from injury.
- Microscopes are carefully balanced and should not be rolled across uneven flooring because of the danger of overbalancing.
- When not in use the microscope should be covered with a dustsheet to prevent dust accumulating on the lens.
- Care should be taken to avoid touching the microscope lens so as not to smudge it.
- The lens should be cleaned with the manufacturer's recommended solution and a lint-free cloth.
- Lenses not in use should be stored safely in a padded box to avoid breakage or damage.
- There should be a manufacturer's maintenance contract, with a yearly complete service carried out by a trained specialist engineer.
- Following surgery any contamination should be cleaned off immediately.

PREPARATION OF THE MICROSCOPE FOR SURGERY

- The microscope should be positioned for the comfort of the surgeon, taking into consideration the space requirements of other surgical and anaesthetic staff and their equipment.
- Care should be taken with the placement of the electrical lead, so that the microscope cannot be inadvertently switched off and it does not constitute a hazard to the theatre staff.
- The microscope should be switched on in the following sequence:
    — at the wall socket
    — at the stand
    — switch on the lights.

To switch off the microscope, reverse the sequence. This will avoid shortening the life of the lamps owing to sudden power surges.

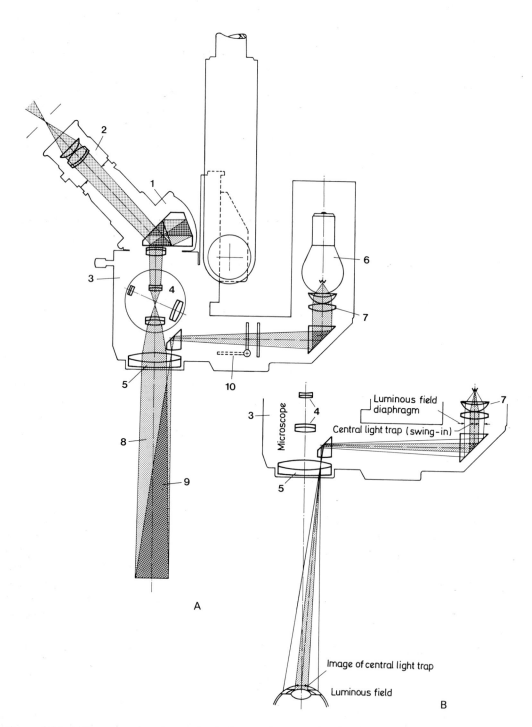

Figure 5.47 A. The component parts and optical paths of an operating microscope: 1. binocular tube; 2. eyepieces; 3. body; 4. magnification changer; 5. objective; 6. illumination; 7. collector lens system for illumination; 8. observation beam path; 9. illumination beam path; 10. swing-in filters. B. The principle of the swing-in pupil eclipsing device for ophthalmology, which protects the patient's macula from excessive radiation during long surgical operations.

- Cleanliness of the microscope should always be checked prior to its use.
- The microscope should be checked to ensure that:
  — all lamps are working
  — all functions are working, including, focus, zoom and magnification change
  — full smooth movement of the microscope arms is attainable.
- Prepacked sterilizable microscope caps or sterile microscope drapes should be available and in adequate supply. These will allow scrubbed personnel to control the movements of the microscope.

It should be stressed that only practitioners who have received adequate training and instruction should prepare and maintain surgical microscopes, owing to the precise nature of the equipment and its cost.

Tourniquets

A tourniquet is an instrument or device for temporarily constricting an artery of the arm or leg to control bleeding. Operations on the extremities can be made easier by the use of a tourniquet because of the resulting bloodless field, which allows the surgeon to perform accurate dissection without damaging vital structures and eliminates the delay and injury caused by excessive use of swabs. To provide a bloodless field, blood must be removed from the limb and then prevented from re-entering.

TYPES OF TOURNIQUET

- **Non-pneumatic** These are only used in exceptional circumstances, as the amount of pressure on the underlying tissues is unknown and therefore tourniquet time should be kept to a minimum.
- **Digital** A rubber catheter is secured around the base of a digit with an artery clamp.
- **Pneumatic** These work on the same principle as a blood pressure cuff, but are stronger and more secure. Most control units are designed to operate from a piped air supply or cylinder. The normal working pressure is within a range of 80–100 psi (7 bar). The pressure control enables the cuff pressure to be set at different ranges. Some control units have a warning indicator that will alert theatre staff in the event of total piped air failure. Most control units have clamps attached that enable them to be secured to a dripstand, at eye level.

The dimension of cuff used should be 20% greater than the diameter of the upper limb and 40% greater than the circumference of the thigh. When the correct size of cuff is used the pressure required to maintain a bloodless field is 50 mmHg higher than the systolic pressure for an upper limb and 100 mmHg for the lower limb (Fig. 5.48).

TOURNIQUET TIME

Tourniquet inflation times should be kept to a minimum. The time at which the tourniquet was inflated should be recorded and the theatre practitioner should inform the surgeon after an hour has expired, and at 15-minute intervals after this. There is no rule as to how long a tourniquet may be left inflated but the usual limit is 1–1.5 hours. If the time exceeds this the tourniquet should be deflated for 20 minutes or more and then reinflated. However, safe limits after reinflation are unknown.

After 2 hours of inflation critical levels of acidosis are reached owing to ischaemia. Tissues distal to the cuff become anoxic and recovery time is extended.[1] It has been shown that it takes 20 minutes following an hour of ischaemia for a limb to return to normal perfusion, therefore the

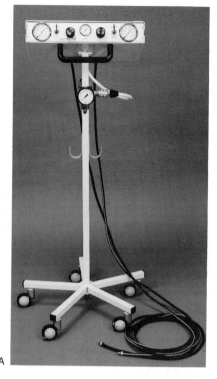
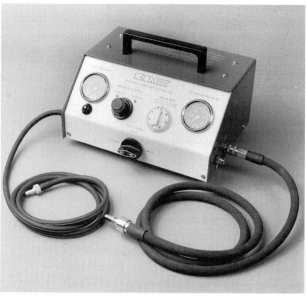

A

B

Figure 5.48 A. A single cuff pneumatic tourniquet control unit operated from a Froen gas cartridge or pipeline/cylinder compressed air supply. (Model 855A, Mk 2, Biomet Ltd.) B. A double cuff pneumatic tourniquet control unit operated from a pipeline/cylinder compressed air supply. (Model SCT, Braun & Co. Ltd.)

practice of briefly deflating the tourniquet and then reinflating it is doubtful in its advantages.

CONTRAINDICATIONS TO TOURNIQUET USE

- Peripheral vascular disease
- Severe crushing injuries
- Sickle-cell disease (although it may be used with care on patients with sickle-cell trait).

TOURNIQUET PARALYSIS SYNDROME

This is caused by pressure, not ischaemia, and is manifested by motor paralysis and sensory dissociation. It occurs when the pressure has been held above systolic blood pressure in an unanaesthetized patient for half an hour. Recovery can take up to 3 months.

POST-TOURNIQUET SYNDROME

Following the release of a tourniquet there is an immediate swelling of tissues due to hyperaemia and capillary permeability to proteins and fluids. This is manifested by:

- puffiness of hands and fingers
- stiffness of joints
- numbness
- colour change
- muscle weakness.

EXSANGUINATION

There are various methods of exsanguination: elevation and expressive exsanguination, which includes Esmarch bandages and Rhys–Davies exsanguinators.

- **Elevation** The limb is elevated for 4 minutes, allowing blood to drain through gravity. This is followed by reflex arteriolar constriction, which completes emptying. The tourniquet is then inflated.

• **Esmarch bandage** The bandage is applied from the distal end of the limb, with the bandage fully stretched on each turn and overlapping by half an inch. Once the bandage reaches the tourniquet cuff the tourniquet is inflated.

• **Rhys–Davies exsanguinator** (Fig. 5.49) This is an inflated rubber sleeve which, when rolled on to a limb, produces exsanguination without subjecting the limb to high pressure. It is simple to apply and requires very little maintenance. One module suffices for adults and children, and for both upper and lower limbs, except for extremes of sizes. The pressures applied are approximately 60–150 mmHg. The sleeve applies more pressure to the thicker, more fleshy part of the limb, and less to the bony parts, thereby reducing the risk of trauma around body prominences. It may be used on compound fractures or soft tissue injuries. The degree of inflation is checked by measuring the sleeve's circumference, and a device is included to reinflate the sleeve as slow air loss occurs with time. The exsanguinator can be cleaned easily with detergent. Application is as follows.

— The limb is elevated for 1 minute; the sleeve is rolled on to the operator's arm until the hand protrudes from the end.
— The patient's hand or foot is grasped, and with gentle pulling the cylinder is rolled on to the limb.
— The cylinder is rolled up to the tourniquet cuff, which is then inflated and the exsanguinator rolled off the limb.

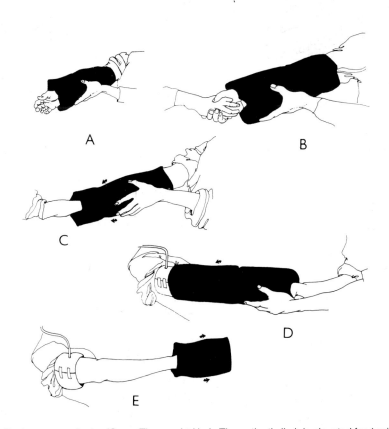

Figure 5.49 Rhys-Davies exsanguinator (Camp Therapy Ltd.). A. The patient's limb is elevated for 1 min and then the sleeve is rolled onto the operator's arm until the hand protrudes from the end. B. The operator grasps the patient's hand or foot. C. The limb is gently pulled and the cylinder rolled onto it. D. The cylinder is rolled up to the tourniquet cuff. E. The tourniquet cull is inflated and the exsanguinator is rolled off the limb.

Expressive exsanguination should not be used in patients with severe infection, tumours or deep vein thrombosis, proven or suspected.

There are dangers to exsanguination: Esmarch bandages may cause frictional shearing of the skin if tightly applied. Care must be taken if there are fractures, or foreign bodies superficial to the skin. A tourniquet should only be applied to one limb at a time, as overloading of the heart may occur in the elderly or unfit patient.

CARE OF TOURNIQUETS

- The tourniquet cuff, tubing, connectors, ties and closures should be checked before each use.
- The cuff should be placed as far from the incision site as possible to avoid interference with the operation.
- Before application of the cuff the limb should be padded with cotton wadding, applied carefully and smoothly, as the the smallest wrinkle may pinch or blister the skin.
- When applying tourniquets to the lower limbs of male patients care should be taken to ensure that the genitalia are not caught in the cuff.
- All pneumatic cuff pressure gauges and monitors should be checked regularly by qualified personnel, following the manufacturer's and departmental guidelines. Records should be kept of the maintenance of individual pieces of equipment.

- Cuff size and width should be appropriate for the individual: as wide a cuff as possible should be used.
- The tourniquet cuff should be placed at the point of maximum circumference of the limb, e.g. upper thigh and arm, not on areas where there is only a thin layer of tissue covering the bone.
- Once applied, the tourniquet cuff should not be rotated to a new position as this may damage underlying tissues.
- When preparing the skin, preparation solution should not be allowed to run under the tourniquet cuff on to the underlying padding as this may cause skin necrosis. The cuff should be protected to avoid this.
- The theatre practitioner should constantly observe the pressure gauge and equipment for signs of fluctuations and failure.
- Inflation pressure depends on the age of the patient, systolic blood pressure, the width of the tourniquet and the circumference of limb.
- Tourniquet inflation time should be kept to a minimum.
- The location of the cuff, personnel applying the cuff, cuff pressure, duration of inflation time and identification of the type of tourniquet used should be documented.
- After use the tourniquet equipment should be cleaned and stored according to departmental policy.

REFERENCE

1. Wilgis ESF 1971 Observations on the effects of tourniquet ischaemia. Journal of Bone and Joint Surgery 53-A: 1343

PREPARATION OF STAFF

The aim is to provide a clean and safe environment as regards dress and hygiene and to minimize the risk of infection to the patient.

Personal hygiene

All theatre personnel should shower or bath daily, although this should be done a few hours before changing into theatre clothes as skin shedding is at its highest rate at this time.[2] Hands should be washed frequently, especially after each episode of patient contact, and the nails cut short. Any instances of ill health and infections should be reported to a senior member of staff and a referral made to occupational health departments as necessary.

Operating theatre clothing

Theatre clothing acts as a barrier to prevent the dissemination of microorganisms to the patient and, conversely, protects the wearer. Theatre clothing consists of a trouser suit or dress, head covering, mask and shoes. Garments should be made of closely woven fabric that is easily washed at high temperatures without shrinking, such as 50% cotton with 50% polyester. Head coverings, either cap or hood, should be comfortable and allow for ventilation. Whichever style is chosen should contain and cover all hair and should be lint free. Theatre head coverings are disposable.

Disposable masks of high filtration efficiency should be worn in the theatre clinical areas where surgical practice is taking place, but should not be worn in other areas, including rest rooms, offices or store areas. Masks should be worn in the correct manner covering the nose, and should not be left hanging around the neck. The strings should be tied snugly and not crossed, as this prevents the mask conforming to the face. Most masks have a pliable strip on the top hem to provide a firm contoured fit over the bridge of the nose; this also prevents fogging of spectacles. Face masks should not be handled except to put them on or remove them. They should be handled by the ties only as the face

piece is highly contaminated and should not come into direct contact with the hands. After removal they should be discarded directly into clinical waste bags and good handwashing technique carried out. A fresh mask should be worn for each operation, and whenever possible damp masks should be changed.[2]

Orr[3] studied the effect of wearing masks on postoperative infection rates and found that it had no effect on the sepsis rate in general surgery. Davies[4] showed that even when adequate filtration is achieved by the mask, bacteria-laden air may escape from around the sides. Another study[5] showed that there is significantly higher bacterial shedding on to the operative field when no mask is worn than when a full mask is used. A relationship between density of contaminant and wound infection rate was not established. Although current research questions the need to wear masks, the authors would advise staff to wear them for personal protection.

All theatre staff should wear protective footwear and in areas where volatile or explosive gases are used antistatic shoes must be worn. Protective footwear should be provided for transient staff, including students and visitors.

Instruction should be given to all theatre staff on the correct manner of dress and the frequency of changing clothes within the department.

A designated changing area should be available, with secure storage facilities for outdoor clothes. Theatre clothing should be stored in a clean area, with a supply of all sizes available at all times. Staff should change in the following sequence:

- Remove all outer clothes and jewellery (except plain wedding rings) and wash hands.
- A theatre hat or hood is put on before donning theatre clothing: all the hair should be covered. Hoods should be worn by personnel with beards or long hair.
- Clean, laundered theatre clothes are worn daily, unless they become soiled, in which case they must be changed immediately or as soon as is practical.
- Clean protective theatre footwear is put on.
- The hands are then washed.

Theatre clothing should not be worn outside the department, although in emergencies staff may don their own shoes, remove headgear and wear a gown tied at the rear. On return to the department a clean set of clothes should be worn.

After a spell of duty theatre staff should change in the following manner:

- Theatre shoes are removed and stored in a clean area.
- Theatre clothing is removed and put into linen receptacles.

The surgical team

This consists of scrub and circulating personnel. Scrub personnel don sterile gowns and gloves and are directly involved with the surgical procedure. Circulating personnel supply the needs of the scrub team and coordinate other activities.

Universal precautions should be used for dealing with blood and body fluids and all personnel should use methods that avoid exposing the skin and mucous membranes. These include the following:

- Gloves should be worn for handling blood or body fluids, or open wounds and mucous membranes, and any material contaminated by blood or body fluids. Spillages should be covered with disposable towels to soak up the excess and cleaned up with gloved hands. The area should then be cleaned with a disinfectant appropriate for the surface.
- Masks and protective eyewear or face shields should be worn during procedures when aerosolization or splashing of blood and body fluids is likely.
- Hands and skin should be washed immediately following contamination with blood or body fluids. The wearing of gloves does not preclude the necessity for thorough handwashing between procedures.
- Impervious scrub gowns or plastic aprons should be worn during procedures likely to cause splashing of blood or body fluids.
- Any abrasions or cuts on the hands should be covered with a waterproof dressing.

Surgical scrubbing

The surgical hand scrub is performed prior to donning a sterile gown and gloves. This does not render the hands sterile but simply clean, reducing the numbers of microorganisms and therefore reducing the risk to the patient if the gloves are perforated during surgery.

The scrub room is usually separate from the operating room; it should be kept adequately stocked with sterile gowns, gloves and scrub brushes. Stock should be rotated so that none is past its expiry date. Sterile equipment should be stored away from the sink to avoid water contamination and provision for the disposal of waste paper and used brushes should be made.

Each operating department should have a policy for scrubbing to which staff must adhere. The procedure should include the following:

- Staff with upper respiratory infections or broken areas of skin on the hands and forearms should not scrub.
- All jewellery should be removed.
- Theatre hat and mask should be checked for comfort and adjusted to cover hair and face correctly.
- Theatre clothing should be secured with the top tucked into the trousers and the sleeves rolled above the elbows.
- Nails should be clean before commencing scrub techniques.
- Water temperature and rate should be selected for comfort.
- Wet hands and forearms.
- Dispense antibacterial soap or detergent into the palm using elbow or foot dispenser (Fig. 6.1A). Around 5 ml of scrub solution is sufficient for each application.
- Lather hands and arms to 2 inches above the elbow crease.
- Rinse with the hands flexed upwards so that the water flows downwards off the elbows.
- Use a nailbrush to work solution under the nails (Fig. 6.1B), either a prepacked disposable type or a reusable autoclavable type. The brush should be used only on the nails and not the skin, as this may cause abrasions.

- Hands and forearms should be washed and rinsed at least twice more, the whole procedure taking a minimum of 2 minutes (Fig. 6.1C). These further washes need not reach as far as the elbows – two-thirds of the forearm is considered sufficient.
- Following the final rinse the hands and arms should be elevated away from the body, allowing water to drop from the elbows (Fig. 6.1D).
- The hands and arms should be dried using a sterile towel for each side. Drying should start at the fingertips, using a corkscrew movement, discarding the towel on reaching the elbow crease. The towel should be folded to avoid making contact with uncleaned skin.

Research into scrubbing techniques has produced some surprising and cost-reducing outcomes. Babb et al,[6] in comparisons of soap-based scrubs and alcohol rubs, showed that 70% isopropyl alcohol was the most effective treatment. Ross[7] states that previous research findings show that the recommended preoperative hand disinfecting method is a traditional soap and water scrub for the initial case on each list, and a subsequent second-phase hand disinfection should be achieved with 70% isopropyl hand rub. Ross estimates the cost saving, using this method for second-phase disinfection, to be £300,000 in the UK.

Following this procedure a sterile gown and gloves are donned.

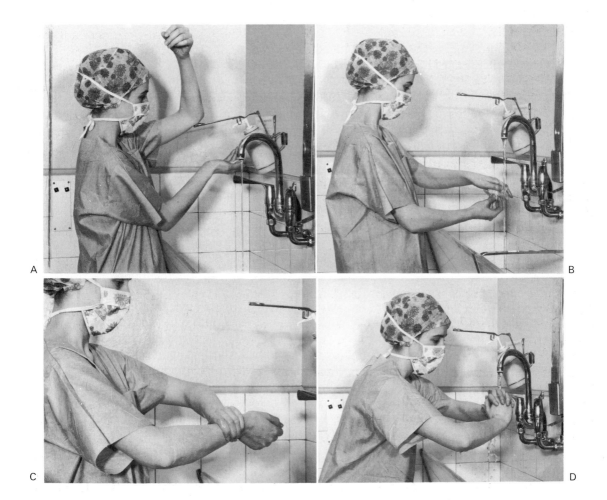

Figure 6.1 Scrubbing technique. See text for detailed description.

Gowning

- The gown should be checked to ensure that it is in a good state of repair and discarded if there is any doubt.
- The folded gown is lifted upwards and away from the table or shelf.
- The gown is grasped firmly at the neckline and allowed to unfold completely, with the inside facing the wearer.
- The arms are inserted into the armholes simultaneously, holding the arms at shoulder level and away from the body (Fig. 6.2A&B).
- The front of the gown is never touched with ungloved hands.
- Hands should not be passed through the cuffs if a closed gloving technique is to be used.
- The gown should not be shaken to aid unfolding as this risks contamination.
- While donning the gown care should be taken to ensure that it does not come in contact with unsterile areas.
- The circulating practitioner should secure the gown at the neck and waist, touching only the ties at the back of the wearer (Fig. 6.2C).
- If a wraparound type of gown is worn, once gloves are donned the front ties are untied by the wearer and the gown may be wrapped in one of various ways (Fig. 6.2D&E):
  — If another member of the team is gowned and gloved they may take this tie and the wearer turns, allowing the gown to wrap around themselves; the tie is tied at the front.
  — Some disposable gowns have a strip of paper on the end of the tie; this is passed to the circulator, the wearer turns to wrap the gown around themselves, and the tie is then pulled from the paper and tied at the front.
  — The inner wrapper of the sterile gloves may be wrapped around the tie, which is passed to the circulator and tied in the same way as above.

Scrub practitioners should not attach the tie to the instrument trolley to help in wrapping the gown, as this may cause the instrument trolley to become unsterile.

Gloving

The closed gloving technique is preferred (Fig. 6.3):

- The hands are advanced into the sleeves of the gown until its cuff seam is reached (Fig. 6.3A).
- The enclosed hand grasps the folded cuff of the glove of the opposite hand and the glove is placed on the upturned gown-enclosed hand, with the glove fingers extending towards the body and the thumb underneath (Fig. 6.3B&C).
- The glove cuff and the sleeve cuff are held together; the glove is then stretched over the hand and cuff by the other enclosed hand (Fig. 6.3D&E).
- The hand is then advanced into the glove, ensuring that the sleeve cuff remains inside the glove (Fig. 6.3F).
- The other hand is then gloved with the assistance of the already gloved hand (Fig. 6.3G).

A considerable number of surgical gloves become punctured during surgery. Hoborn[8] confirmed a high level of glove punctures and found that this was higher in orthopaedic procedures (48%) than soft tissue procedures (16%). The wearing of double gloves for orthopaedic implant surgery therefore appears to be a sensible precaution in reducing the risk of wound infection. The wearing of double gloves is also advised when undertaking procedures on patients who are known or potential infection risks to theatre staff safety.

Once the scrub practitioner is gowned and gloved they should understand the areas of sterility. These are from the fingertips to the elbows and from the below the chin line to the waist only at the front of the gown. Once scrubbed, the practitioner's hands must remain above waist level at all times, and when not involved in a sterile procedure the hands should be held together at chest height.

If a member of the surgical team perforates or contaminates a glove during surgery, the scrub practitioner may reglove them using the following method:

- The circulator grasps the outside of the glove and pulls it off inside out.

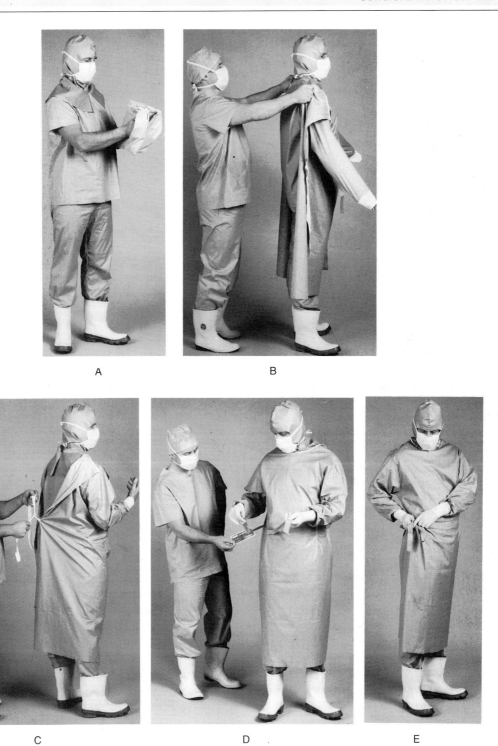

Figure 6.2 Gowning technique. See text for detailed description.

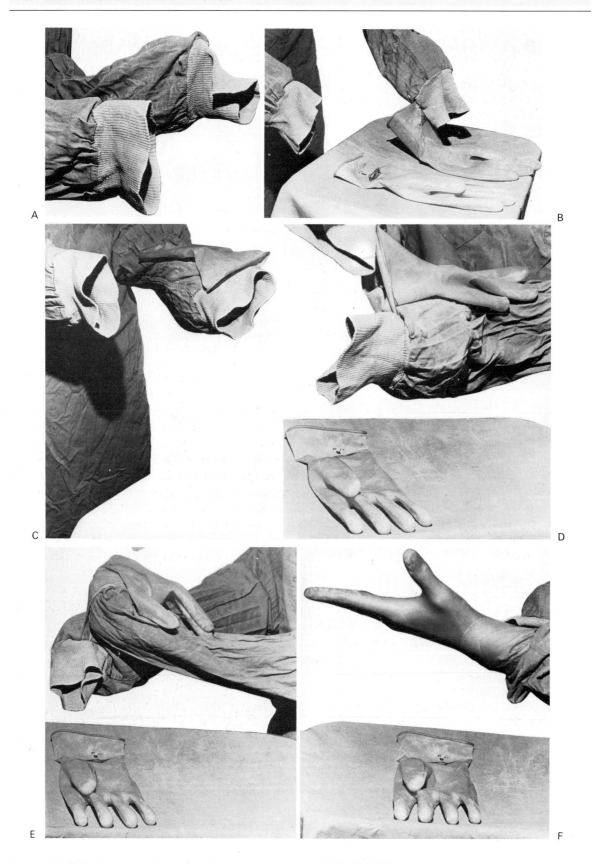

A

B

C

D

E

F

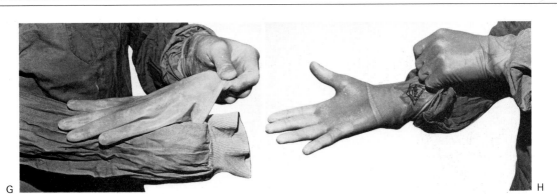

G   H

Figure 6.3 Gloving technique (closed donning). (Reproduced with permission from Pioneer Rubber Co. Ltd, USA.)

• The scrub practitioner holds the new glove with the fingers pointing downwards and the thumb towards the wearer.

• The glove is held open on the outer cuff.

• The team member slides the hand down into the glove, with the scrub practitioner exerting a firm upwards pressure.

The scrub practitioner may now prepare the instrument trolleys, which are covered with sterile drapes to establish a sterile field. The drapes should be large enough to cover the trolley adequately without trailing on the floor. Only the horizontal surface of the trolley should be considered sterile once draped. If a preset tray system is in use the trolley drapes may be included around the instruments. Whichever system is used the trolley is covered in the same way:

• Trolleys should only be prepared immediately before each surgical procedure.

• The drape pack or instrument set should be checked to ensure it is sterile and free from damage.

• The outer paper layer is opened by the circulator, taking care not to touch the inner layer.

• The scrub practitioner opens the side folds and allows them to fall on to the trolley, taking care not to touch the unsterile front of the trolley with their sterile gown.

• The front fold of the trolley cover is opened towards the scrub practitioner.

• The practitioner can now step nearer the trolley to open the rear fold without fear of contamination.

Instrument sets can now be arranged if using a preset system, or placed on to the trolley if not. Most departments will have a standard trolley set-up, which will ensure safety in the event of a change of scrub practitioner during an operation (Fig. 6.4). However, a standard trolley set-up cannot always be achieved for all types of surgery. For example, when setting up for a hip screw the scrub practitioner will have to stand behind the surgeons, owing to the confinement caused by using an isolation-type drape.

Instrument, swab and needle counts should be an integral part of the trolley preparation, which should be undertaken according to theatre policy

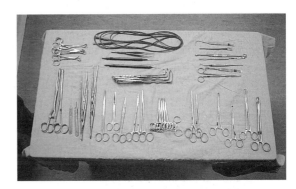

Figure 6.4 Trolley set-up.

and the Theatre Safeguards published by the Medical Defence Union.[9] During the preparation of trolleys the following practices should be observed:

- Two members of staff are required, the scrub and circulating practitioners.
- Aseptic principles should be observed.
- Sterile sundries should be passed to the scrub practitioner from the edge of the sterile field, thereby reducing the risk of trolley contamination.
- Sterile sundries should be taken from the circulator with a spongeholder, or a needleholder for blades and sharps, to prevent hand contamination or sharps injury.
- Containers for skin preparation or irrigation solutions should be placed near the edge of the trolley; the solutions should be checked for expiry date and then poured from above without contaminating the container or the trolley.
- Minimal movement of staff within this area is essential during trolley preparation.
- Swabs or sponges should be mounted to facilitate skin preparation by the surgical team.

PREPARATION OF THE PATIENT

The patient is positioned on the operating table, the operative site exposed, and the area prepared for surgery.

Skin preparation

Preparation of the patient's skin starts before transfer to the operating theatre. Before changing into a gown many patients will have had a shower or bath, using an antiseptic-based soap and taking particular care to scrub the operative site. Obviously this will not be the case with emergency or trauma surgery, when speed of transfer to the operating theatre is the priority.

Hair removal at the operative site is usually carried out according to the surgeon's preferences. Research has shown that it is preferable to remove hair as near as possible to the time of operation, as the greater the time between shaving and surgery the greater the potential for bac-

terial growth and the potential for postoperative wound infection.[10] Close skin shaving can result in soft tissue abrasions and small cuts which can encourage the growth of bacteria.[11] Other methods of removing hair are the use of depilatory creams and electric hair clippers. Depilatory creams should only be used if skin testing is carried out beforehand:[12] adverse skin reactions are the main reason why depilatory creams are not widely used. Electric hair clippers are recommended in preference to razors as they cause less trauma to the skin.[13] A comparison of hair clipping versus shaving found that clipping also carried a lower risk of infection.[14] Kovach[15] stresses that although they leave the skin intact, clippers are expensive and inconvenient as they need to be disassembled, cleaned, oiled and sterilized between patients.

The operative site is prepared with an antibacterial solution. The area prepared depends on the type of surgery performed, the site, hospital policy and the surgeon's preference. The incision site and the area around it is prepared, working from the site outwards. Once a swab has cleaned the outer aspect of the site it should never be returned to the operative site but is discarded and a clean swab used. For orthopaedic surgery the joint above and below the operative site should be cleaned. Skin preparation should be modified when dealing with contaminated areas for surgery, which should be prepared last; this applies to open wounds and stomas. For gynaecological surgery cleaning should proceed from the mons to the perineum to the vagina, with the anus cleaned last. Swabs used for skin preparation are part of the swab count and should be retained for counting at a later stage. The surgical team involved in skin preparation should change their gloves prior to draping.

Once the operative site has been prepared the drapes are placed to establish a sterile field and prevent contamination from unprepared areas of skin.

GUIDELINES FOR SCRUB PRACTITIONERS

- Instrument trolleys should be placed around the operating table. They must not come into contact with the patient to avoid causing pressure injury.

- Trolleys should be placed as near to the surgical field as possible to facilitate handing instruments to the surgeon.
- If a laminar air flow system is in use trolleys should be kept within its confines to maintain sterility.
- The scrub practitioner should never lean over the trolley or sterile field because of the risk of shedding skin particles or hairs.
- The integrity of the sterile field must be maintained at all times by all members of the scrub team.
- Any suspected or true break in aseptic technique should be dealt with immediately. Contaminated equipment should be removed from the sterile field and the area redraped.
- The scrub practitioner should always face the operative site so that they can observe the operation and anticipate the surgeon's needs.
- The scrub practitioner should have a knowledge of the anatomy involved and of the surgical procedure being performed.
- Instruments should always be passed in front of the surgeon and assistants, never behind them.
- Instruments should not be passed so that the surgeon's field of vision is blocked.
- Instruments should be passed in an ergonomic manner, allowing their immediate use (see Chapter 5).
- If the scrub practitioner has to leave the operating table to collect instruments, a suitable moment should be chosen and the surgeon's permission sought.
- If the scrub practitioner is unsure which instrument the surgeon requires the surgeon should be informed verbally of the instrument being passed.
- Scrub personnel should pass each other back to back.
- Movement, talking and disturbance of drapes should be kept to a minimum.
- All members of the surgical team must avoid leaning on the patient to prevent unnecessary pressure.

- Instruments should always be returned to the trolley immediately after use, to ensure patient safety.
- During an operation, nothing should be removed from the theatre without the permission of the scrub practitioner.
- There should be no unnecessary change of scrub practitioner during an operation. If this is necessary because of illness a full swab, needle and instrument count should take place.
- The instrument trolleys are the responsibility of the scrub practitioner: they should be removed at the end of the operation by this person, and all sharps safely disposed of.
- The scrub practitioner should inform the surgeon verbally that the swab, needle and instrument count is correct prior to closure of the surgical wound.
- The scrub practitioner should not leave the theatre until the patient has been transferred from the operating table.
- The scrub practitioner should inform the circulator of the operation performed, the type of wound closure material used, e.g. staples, non-absorbable or absorbable sutures, wound drains *in situ* and type of dressing applied, so that this information can be recorded accurately in the operating theatre records and the patient's care plan.
- The scrub practitioner should ensure that this information is given to the recovery room staff.

At the end of the operation the disposal of all instruments, drapes and sharps should be carried out in accordance with departmental policy. The scrub practitioner is considered to be the person of choice to dispose of contaminated materials while still protected by a gown and gloves.[16]

Soiled gowns and gloves should be removed without contaminating the arms, hands and theatre clothes:

- The front tie is undone by the scrub practitioner.
- The neck and waist ties at the back are untied by the circulator.
- The gown is grasped at the shoulders and pulled off over the gloved hands, turning it inside out without touching the theatre clothes.

• The gown is folded so that the contaminated side is inside, and is then deposited in the relevant linen or rubbish bag, according to departmental policy.

• Gloves are removed by pulling on the rolled cuff with the opposite gloved hand and inserting the gloveless hand inside the cuff of the other hand. Gloves should invert using this method; they are then disposed of in the clinical waste bag.

Theatre gowns and gloves should never be worn outside the operating theatre.

THE CIRCULATING PRACTITIONER

The circulating practitioner's first duty is to ensure that the theatre is clean and prepared with the relevant equipment. Other duties include:

• selection of sterile gown pack and size and type of sterile gloves;

• assisting the scrub team with gowning and gloving;

• opening packs and instruments for the scrub practitioner, using aseptic principles;

• remaining vigilant for any break in aseptic technique and observing the sterile field;

• ensuring, with the scrub practitioner, that all items passed to the sterile area have sterility assurance;

• assisting in the safe positioning of the patient on the operating table;

• maintaining the patient's rights and dignity;

• ensuring the patient's pressure areas are protected;

• ensuring that an electrosurgery pad is placed on the patient;

• connecting suction and electrosurgical and other relevant equipment;

• ensuring that suction bottles do not overfill;

• observing the scrub team and anticipating their needs, e.g. extra swabs;

• receiving and labelling specimens in accordance with local policy;

• preparing specimens for dispatch according to the surgeon's instructions;

• ensuring that a minimum noise level is maintained within the theatre;

• ensuring that the operating room doors are opened as infrequently as possible during surgery;

• passing messages for the surgeon and scrub team to the scrub practitioner, who will pass them on at a suitable moment;

• informing the scrub practitioner if they go off duty, and who has taken over this duty;

• assisting in swab, needle and instrument counts, as per department policy;

• ensuring that the theatre is never left without a circulating practitioner during an operation;

• sending for patients when requested to do so by the person in charge, in cooperation with the medical team;

• assisting the scrub practitioner with the clearing of trolleys and disposal of waste at the end of an operation and at the end of the list;

• assisting with the restocking of the theatre;

• ensuring that all relevant documentation is correctly filled in, including patient documents and theatre register.

Between each case on an operating list the theatre must be cleaned and prepared for the next case. This will include:

• disinfection after blood and body fluid spillage
• cleaning of operating table and horizontal surfaces with detergent
• cleaning of operating lights with detergent
• cleaning of all equipment used in the previous case, i.e. heel supports, table attachments, etc., with detergent
• removal of dirty instrument sets and any extra instruments
• disposal of suction bottle contents
• cleaning of the theatre floor with either a wet vacuum or a mop
• closure of rubbish bags and removal to an appropriate place for disposal.

The theatre practitioner should be aware of the potential risk of cross-infection of patients in the theatre. Each surgical wound should be treated as potentially contaminated to ensure complete isolation for each case. This procedure should be carried out as efficiently as possible to prevent delay between cases.

At the end of the theatre list terminal cleaning takes place. This will include:

- operating lights
- all wall-fixed and ceiling-mounted equipment
- all furniture, including wheels and castors
- horizontal surfaces and shelves
- operating room door handles and push plates
- floors
- scrub sink and taps
- kick buckets.

To work as a theatre practitioner the individual must provide patient care of the highest standard as well as gaining various technical skills and the underpinning knowledge. It becomes apparent that an individual has to have certain qualities to achieve this. These may include:

- a positive attitude, with consideration for others, which will ensure an efficient environment for patients
- honesty, integrity, stamina and dependability
- maintenance of patient confidentiality
- responsibility for updating personal knowledge and skills
- adaptability and flexibility in an area in which procedures and operating schedules may change frequently
- an ability to maintain a sense of humour, which can reduce stressful situations.

SUPPORT FOR STAFF

The theatre practitioner should recognize that the provision of total patient care in a highly technical area such as the operating theatre can lead to high levels of stress within the team. Therefore, an ability to cope with stressful situations is necessary. Each member of the team will have organizational pressures upon them, which can be manifested in their attitudes and behaviour. For example, surgeons are noted for their optimistic assessments of operating times,[17] which can lead to the list overrunning or to the cancellation of a case. Other critical incidents, such as the death of a patient on the operating table or the sudden arrival of a patient traumatically injured, can also cause high levels of stress in all members of the team.

Staff should be aware of the options available to them to deal with stress. Theatre managers should be able to undertake the role of professional advisers as and when the need arises. If a personal issue is causing the stress the occupational health departments of many hospitals offer a counselling service. Students and trainees may turn to their mentors or tutors.

To reduce stress in the working environment a good communication network is essential. Staff meetings can help to ensure that all staff are aware of future changes and allow them to voice their opinions.

Following the death of a patient in the theatre the hospital bereavement counsellor may be contacted to discuss the issue with the staff involved.

After any stressful incident the staff should be encouraged to discuss the event without apportioning blame. This should be a time to reflect whether the situation could have been dealt with differently, with perhaps a different outcome. This will allow staff to discuss their feelings and emotions within a supportive framework and prevent them harbouring thoughts that could lead to increased stress levels.

Educational support

There should be active educational support within each operating department, as these are considered specialist areas of care. For this to be achieved there should be a firm commitment from the managers and the necessary resources, which will depend on the size of the department, the number of learners and trainees and the levels of teaching required.

Many departments consider an educational coordinator to be an essential member of the team. This should ideally be a senior theatre practitioner who can advise on all aspects of theatre care. There should be close liaison with local colleges of health studies and education. Theatre practitioners should realize that it is not only students and trainees who require educational support, but all grades of qualified staff as well.

All new staff in an operating department should have an orientation programme tailored to their individual needs, which should include local policies and procedures. New staff should be allocated a mentor, to whom they can turn for support. Operating departments should have resources available with a quiet area for books, journals and teaching material for staff use.

Performance reviews should be carried out at regular intervals on all grades of staff, to encourage individual development and the undertaking of relevant courses. Staff should be encouraged to participate in the theatre policy committees and training programmes.

REFERENCES

1. NATN 1991 Operating department identifying non-medical staff skill mix. National Association of Theatre Nurses, London
2. Ayliffe GAJ, Lowbury EJL, Geddes AM, Williams JD (eds) 1993 Control of hospital infection. A practical handbook, 3rd edn. Chapman & Hall, London
3. Orr, N 1981 Is a mask necessary in the operating theatre? Annals of the Royal College of Surgeons of England 63: 390–392
4. Davis WT 1991 Filtration efficiency of surgical face masks: the need for meaningful standards. American Journal of Infection Control 19: 16–18
5. Berger SA, Kramer M, Nagar H et al 1993 Effect of surgical mask position on bacterial contamination of the operative field. Journal of Hospital Infection 23: 51–54
6. Babb JR, Davies JG, Ayliffe GAJ 1991 Test procedures for evaluating hand disinfection. Journal of Hospital Infection 18: Suppl B: 41–49
7. Ross C 1994 What cost ritual? British Journal of Theatre Nursing 4: 11–14
8. Whyte W 1988 The role of clothing and drapes in the operating room. Journal of Hospital Infection 11: Suppl C: 2–17
9. Medical Defence Union 1988 Theatre safeguards. Medical Defence Union, Medical Protection Society, Medical and Dental Defence Union of Scotland, National Association of Theatre Nurses, Royal College of Nursing, London
10. Seropian, R, Reynolds BM 1971 Wound infections after preoperative depilatory creams versus razor preparation. American Journal of Surgery 121: 251–254
11. Tunevall G 1988 Procedures and experiences with pre-operative skin preparation in Sweden. Journal of Hospital Infection 11: Suppl 13: 11–14
12. Kalideen D 1990 Preparing skin for surgery. Nursing 4: 28–29
13. AORN 1988 Recommended practices: preoperative skin preparation. AORN Journal 45: 950–958
14. Alexander JW, Fischer JE, Boyajian M, Palaiquist J, Morris MJ 1983 The influence of hair removal methods on wound infections. Archives of Surgery 118: 347–351
15. Kovach T 1990 Nip it in the bud. Today's OR Nurse 12: 23–26
16. NATN 1993 Principles of safe practice in the operating theatre. National Association of Theatre Nurses, London
17. Hindle A 1970 A simulation approach to surgical scheduling. Department of Operational Research, University of Lancaster

Care of the patient

During the 1980s and 1990s much literature has been published discussing the role of the nurse in theatre and focusing on the needs of the patient.[1-5] The issues of the nursing process, preoperative visiting, care planning, documentation of care, primary nursing and the named nurse within the operating theatre have been raised. This contrasts sharply with the theatre nurse of 1889, who was expected to have 'a level head, keen eyes, and a mind not easily irritated or confused, be able to keep out of the way whilst still being the greatest of help'.[6] The role of the theatre practitioner today is definitely not to 'keep out of the way', but to take an active part in all phases of patient care. It involves research-based practice to develop and maintain high standards in patient care.

The care of the patient in surgery covers five phases, each often based within a different geographical area and with different members of the team. Theatre practitioners and all involved in surgical nursing should strive to ensure that patient care is not fragmented because of this, and that continuity of care and communication regarding the patient (both verbal and written) is of a high standard. The importance of effective handover both pre- and postoperatively is discussed by Alin.[7,8] This identifies what information should be incorporated in a preoperative handover, in addition to a preoperative checklist (see Chapter 4). This includes:

- past medical and surgical history
- patient's perception of surgery
- patient's past experience
- patient's emotional state.

This will go some way towards minimizing the feelings the patient may have of being 'just another case on the list' or 'on a conveyor belt'. It is, however, helpful to consider the phases of care, in order to discuss and clarify the patient's needs and problems, and the theatre practitioner's role in relation to these:

- Preoperative phase – A and E/surgical ward
  Transfer of patient and reception to the operating department
- Care given in relation to anaesthesia – anaesthetic room
- Intraoperative phase – operating theatre
  Transfer of patient to the postoperative recovery room or recovery area
- Immediate postoperative recovery – recovery room
  Transfer of patient to the ward
- Postoperative phase – surgical ward, intensive therapy unit and high-dependency unit.

As can be seen above, these important areas of care are linked by transfers and receptions. These are important and often memorable times for the patient, and so will also be discussed here.

PREOPERATIVE PHASE
Preoperative visiting

The preoperative care given by theatre practitioners begins whenever possible with a preoperative visit to the patient on the ward. This aims to enhance the preparation and care the patient will have received from the ward nurses, and to consider specific areas of care to inform the patient about.

Offering patients information about pre- and postoperative procedures has frequently been shown to have a beneficial effect on their physical and psychological wellbeing postoperatively,[8-10] leading to fewer complications and a quicker recovery. Theatre practitioners have an important role to play in giving specific preoperative information. Nurses who work on surgical wards may have only a limited knowledge of what happens in the anaesthetic room, theatre and recovery room, and medical staff generally concentrate on giving medical information and obtaining consent. A preoperative visit by a theatre practitioner therefore has three advantages:[5]

- It enables the establishment of a supportive rapport with the patient.
- It enables the theatre nurse to obtain relevant information to assist in the planning of care, e.g. if the patient has arthritis this has implications for positioning.
- It allows the theatre nurse to offer information to reduce the patient's fear of the unknown and to minimize their stress, e.g. why they need to wear a gown, how theatre staff will be dressed, and briefly how they will be anaesthetized.

These advantages each have a direct effect on the quality of patient care, and so preoperative visiting would appear to be beneficial. It is important, however, that certain guidelines are followed in order to achieve these benefits.

Guidelines for preoperative visiting

- Allow adequate time – a hurried visit may do more harm than good, and 15 minutes is suggested as a minimum.
- Liaise with the ward nurses about any special concerns or needs the patient may have – these can then be concentrated on.
- Do not discuss any of the details of the surgery, prognosis or anaesthetic – these are the responsibilities of the medical staff.
- Try and arrange visits so that patients are received into the operating department by the theatre practitioner who visited them.
- Follow local policy with regard to dress for the visits. Wearing theatre clothing with protective outerwear is beneficial, as it allows the patient to see the normal clothes worn by theatre practitioners. It is important, however, that the clothes are changed when the theatre practitioner returns to theatre, for good infection control. Local policy and infection control advice must be followed. If theatre clothing is not able to be worn, some photographs of staff in theatre clothes may be helpful.
- Telephone the ward before your visit to check it is convenient to visit the patient.
- Liaise with ward nurses about what information the patient has already had. The

information given by the theatre practitioner should enhance this, not repeat it. The theatre practitioner's information should focus on what will happen to the patient when they arrive in the operating department; when they are being anaesthetized; when they are waking up; when they are in the recovery room. The theatre practitioner should not generally discuss postoperative care on the ward, or long-term recovery issues, which can more appropriately be discussed by other staff.

If such guidelines are followed the patient should enjoy and learn from the preoperative visit and the theatre practitioner should obtain information that will help in planning care for the patient. If a department is unable to facilitate preoperative visiting by theatre practitioners for all patients, an alternative process should be set up. This could involve:

- the use of information booklets for patients to read preoperatively.[2] These would need to be written by the theatre practitioners in order for them to be of greatest value
- an arrangement which allows ward staff to contact theatre practitioners when they feel a preoperative visit would benefit a specific patient – if the patient is very anxious or has specific questions, for example
- the use of a video, which patients could watch on the ward, to guide them through arrival in the operating department, clothing, and waking up, for example. Again, theatre practitioners would need to be involved in the making of such a video
- an arrangement which allows the theatre practitioner to see a group of maybe five or six patients together, in order to maximize the use of one 15-minute visit
- an arrangement which allows a group of patients to visit the operating department at an appropriate time. This can be especially useful for children, who could tour the areas concerned with their parents, on a Saturday morning or Sunday evening, for example.

Although each of these alternatives does allow the patient to receive relevant information from a theatre practitioner (either directly or indirectly), there are obvious disadvantages:

- They do not generally allow a supportive rapport to develop on a one-to-one basis.
- They do not allow the theatre practitioner to assess the individual patient's needs, and thus they focus entirely on information giving.

Theatre practitioners must therefore consider arrangements within their department and use imagination to consider how some, if not all, of the advantages of preoperative visiting can be realized.

Transfer of the patient to the operating department

Arrangements for the transfer of the patient to the operating department will vary from hospital to hospital, according to local policy and infection control advice. It will generally involve a ward nurse and a theatre porter or orderly. Their aim is to ensure as smooth a journey as possible for the patient, both physically and psychologically. Any special needs or concerns the patient has which may be relevant during the transfer should be communicated by the theatre practitioner (or ward nurse) to the collecting porter or orderly – for example if the patient is deaf and needs to lip read.

Reception of the patient in the operating department was fully discussed in Chapter 4 as checks and safety measures must be carried out before anaesthesia and are often undertaken by the theatre practitioner assisting the anaesthetist.

CARE GIVEN IN RELATION TO ANAESTHESIA

This is fully discussed in Chapter 4, as this care is generally given by the theatre practitioner assisting the anaesthetist in the anaesthetic room.

INTRAOPERATIVE PHASE

The intraoperative phase begins once the patient has been anaesthetized and transferred into the operating theatre itself. In order to consider the care a patient needs in the operating theatre, a structure and a format are helpful. The nursing process offers a structure for care, and a nursing model offers a format.

The nursing process

Although the term 'the nursing process' is now widely used in healthcare provision it is often used, and indeed perceived, incorrectly. Often, the nursing care plan and other documentation has a higher profile than the process itself. It is therefore necessary to define the term and relate it to surgical practice in the intraoperative phase, when most of the care is given by the theatre practitioner. An early and widely accepted definition of the nursing process is 'an orderly systematic manner of determining the patient's problems, making plans to solve them, initiating the plan or assigning others to implement it, and evaluating the extent to which the plan was effective in resolving the problems identified'.[11] The nursing process is therefore a problem-solving cycle and thus of relevance to all theatre practitioners. The terms used to identify the stages of the nursing process are assessment, planning, implementation and evaluation.

Assessment: 'determining the patient's problems'

Assessment of the patient's problems during the intraoperative phase requires information from four main sources:

- the preoperative visit by a theatre practitioner (or from ward staff)
- the operating list
- the surgeon
- practitioners' knowledge of the problems that face *every* patient who comes to theatre.

The theatre practitioner should make use of all such assessment information in order to effectively plan and implement care and prevent problems.

Preoperative visit As has been discussed, this allows the theatre practitioner to assess the patient fully. If it cannot be performed, the theatre practitioner must ensure that there is effective communication between the ward and the theatre when the patient arrives in the operating department. For example:

- if the patient has arthritis this will affect positioning

- if the patient is deaf this will affect care in the anaesthetic and recovery rooms
- the patient may speak only limited English.

Such assessment will ensure a high standard of patient care, and allow care to be properly planned, and if not performed will undoubtedly lead to delays.

The operating list In many circumstances, such as an emergency, the only information available to the theatre practitioner may be that on the operating list. Although this is obviously not ideal and will not be comprehensive, it can be helpful if studied and used thoughtfully. The basic information must include the patient's name, age and hospital number, the operation to be performed (and side if relevant), ward, surgeon and anaesthetist.

Name This may indicate the patient's nationality, a helpful piece of information for care in the anaesthetic and recovery rooms. A non-English name may alert the theatre practitioner to the fact that the patient may be of a different religion, and may need to keep various articles of clothing in place or various religious artefacts with them at all times. The name is obviously not foolproof, but is often a helpful indication and can prepare the theatre practitioner a little for the patient's needs.

Age A great deal of care can be planned once the theatre practitioner is aware of the patient's age. For example:

- Surgery on a baby or a child will need special paediatric instruments.
- Surgery on a baby or a child will necessitate a warm theatre and warm fluids to be used, owing to the problem of heat loss.
- Surgery on a very elderly person will mean aids for pressure area care are likely to be needed.
- Surgery on a very elderly person may mean a local or regional anaesthetic is more likely.

Finally, knowledge of the patient's age will assist the theatre practitioner receiving the patient to be prepared and to establish a rapport more readily.

Operation to be performed and side This is obviously essential for the theatre practitioner to know in order for the theatre furniture, instruments and equipment to be prepared. Assessment includes, for example, noting whether an operation is a repeat or a revision, which may require special instruments; the operation may also be likely to take longer, and a more experienced scrub person may therefore be needed.

Surgeon and anaesthetist Knowing who these are to be will enable the theatre practitioner to prepare correctly and efficiently according to their preferences.

An assessment based merely on the operating list, therefore, although not comprehensive, if considered thoughtfully is safe and allows the theatre practitioner to plan care.

The surgeon Again, if circumstances do not allow for a preoperative visit the surgeon can aid the theatre practitioner's assessment of the patient's needs, which can supplement the assessment based on the operating list. The surgeon will know the patient, their history, their medical problems and their needs for surgery. Asking the surgeon about the patient therefore may alert the theatre practitioner to information not available on the operating list. For example:

- the patient has had a previous limb amputation – relevant for positioning
- the patient has peripheral vascular disease and thus is at high risk of pressure area development
- the patient has terminal disease and thus may be depressed and withdrawn
- any planned preliminary procedures required, e.g. urinary catheterization.

This sort of information will assist the theatre practitioner in planning care and should minimize delays in theatre.

Knowledge of the problems that face every patient who comes to theatre An assessment based on the three areas above will mean the theatre practitioner can plan and implement care based on individual patients' needs and problems. This is vital, but is not sufficient alone. There are many potential problems and hazards that face every patient who undergoes surgery, and the assessment must include these in order to be comprehensive. Much of the care given in relation to these is the routine work of all theatre practitioners, but it is helpful to consider what problems all patients face:

- possibility of the wrong operation or on the wrong side
- foreign body possibly retained in the wound
- wound infection
- possibility of nerve/muscle damage
- possibility of corneal abrasion.

This list is not exhaustive: many other problems are more relevant in the anaesthetic and recovery rooms and thus are discussed in Chapters 4 and 7, as appropriate. The theatre practitioner should therefore be aware of these 'common' problems, and add them to their assessment of the patient's needs in order to plan care.

Planning: 'make plans to solve them'

Although the assessment stage of the process is undeniably the most important (care can only be as good as the assessment on which it is based), it is of little value unless the theatre practitioner uses the information to plan the patient's care during the intraoperative phase. Planning care therefore involves:

- preparing the theatre furniture, equipment and instruments appropriately
- arranging the theatre temperature
- ensuring that the scrub person has a good understanding of the surgery
- preparing equipment needed for any preliminary procedures
- preparing equipment needed to protect pressure areas
- ensuring that staff are all aware of any communication difficulties

and the preparation for any other care identified as necessary from the assessment.

Implementation: 'initiating the plan or assigning others to implement it'

Implementing the planned care is the next stage of the nursing process. This involves the theatre team putting the plan into action, the details of which will vary according to the patient's needs. In relation to the 'common' problems identified earlier, the care to be given is identified in the care plan later in this chapter, which illustrates the use of a nursing model. Obviously, details of how to implement care in relation to certain problems will vary from hospital to hospital, and local policies should always provide details.

The implementation stage therefore involves the theatre practitioner in caregiving, either directly or indirectly, to prevent problems, either actual or potential, affecting the patient. This will be discussed further later in the chapter.

Evaluation: 'evaluating the extent to which the plan was effective in resolving the problems identified'

The final stage in the nursing process is the evaluation of care given:

- Did it resolve or prevent problems occurring?
- Was it effective?

This involves the theatre practitioner observing the patient and asking these two questions about each aspect of care given. It does not mean that evaluation is carried out only at the end of the operation, or postoperatively. Evaluation is continuous: for example, the care that ensures the patient receives the correct operation is carried out while they are still in theatre. Care relating to the prevention of wound infection can be partially evaluated (was the aseptic technique breached in any way?) but consideration of whether wound infection has occurred can only be carried out when the patient is back on the ward. Further details as to when evaluation can take place can be seen in the care plan later in the chapter.

The theatre practitioner may be involved in both stages of the evaluation – this is helpful and necessary for individual patients, and for the theatre practitioner to improve care given to all patients.

Transfer of the patient to recovery

The postoperative phase is generally recognized as beginning when the patient is admitted to the postanaesthetic recovery room. This is an important journey, and one in which postoperative and postanaesthetic problems can arise. These are discussed in detail in Chapter 7. The theatre practitioner involved in the transfer, along with the anaesthetist, must ensure that:

- the patient is correctly positioned
- the patient is safe, i.e. cot sides are in place
- the patient is in a stable condition (i.e. not bleeding or having airway problems)
- the patient is adequately covered
- oxygen is administered if required
- other special equipment is available if needed, e.g. chest drain clamps, suction, airways, clip removers, wire cutters.

The theatre practitioner must also provide recovery room staff with a handover of relevant information, which must include:

- the patient's name and number
- the exact operation performed
- any special instructions, e.g. to sit up as soon as possible
- wound closure type, dressing and drains
- any specific problems (e.g. deafness, arthritis)
- any problems arisen in theatre (e.g. red area developed on sacrum).

The anaesthetist will hand over information regarding the patient's physiological condition, and information on drugs, anaesthesia and fluid balance.

IMMEDIATE POSTOPERATIVE RECOVERY

The role of the practitioner during this phase, and the transfer of the patient to the ward, is discussed in detail in Chapter 7.

POSTOPERATIVE PHASE

Following transfer of the patient to the postoperative ward (or unit), their care will be given by the nurses and other staff in that area. The role of the theatre practitioner during this phase is therefore simply to evaluate the care given in theatre and answer any queries the patient may have. This can be achieved by a postoperative visit. This can be of great value, especially if it is performed by the practitioner who visited the patient preoperatively and received them into the operating department.

The theatre practitioner must plan their visit at a suitable time, and ensure that they consider areas of care needing a late-stage evaluation. The theatre practitioner should not provide details of the surgery or the patient's prognosis, but leave this for the surgeon to discuss.

If theatre practitioners are unable to carry out postoperative visits routinely, there should be a system which allows the ward staff to request a visit for any patient who would particularly benefit. It is also necessary for the ward staff to communicate any relevant information to the theatre practitioners, for example if the patient had a red area on their elbow that was not previously identified, or they developed a wound infection 3 days postoperatively. These details are important for the theatre practitioner to evaluate care, and if possible to improve it for future patients.

The structure of the nursing process is therefore very relevant for the theatre practitioner, and using such a problem-solving approach should enhance the quality of care given.

NURSING MODELS

In all areas of healthcare professionals are striving to improve standards. Many are using a nursing model to help them achieve this. Nursing models are a fairly recent innovation, and therefore there is little evidence to confirm or deny that they make a significant contribution.[12] Nursing models identify the essential components of nursing practice, with the concepts and values required for the nurse to use them.[13] They therefore aim to provide a uniform approach to the patient, their needs and their care. This should mean that all nurses caring for a patient have the same aims, goals and care in mind, thus providing continuity of care even when continuity of the carers is not possible. This is relevant in surgical practice when, as identified earlier, care is given in different areas by different professionals.

Although a nursing model is reflected in the documentation of care, it is not merely the documentation, but includes the philosophy and values of those using it. Theatre nurses may therefore use a nursing model in one of two ways:

- The model used for the assessment, planning, implementation and evaluation of care given by theatre practitioners (in the five phases previously identified) differs from that used in the surgical ward.
- The theatre nurse uses the model that is used by ward staff pre- and postoperatively, to assess, plan, implement and evaluate the care given by them.

Theatre nurses must consider and identify the most appropriate model for them to use. A nursing model therefore provides a format for the structure of the nursing process, i.e. *what* to assess, plan, implement and evaluate. There are many nursing models which the theatre nurse must consider before choosing one. Three will now be briefly outlined.

Orem's model of nursing

Orem's model of nursing[14] is focused on the belief that a person is a functional, integrated whole, with the motivation to achieve self-care. Nursing care is therefore required when the individual is unable to achieve a balance between their self-care abilities and the demands made on these (Fig. 6.5). In relation to the nursing process, this model can be seen as follows:

- **Assessment** – the nurse must assess the demands made on an individual for self-care, and his ability to meet those demands. It also involves the nurse establishing reasons for the self-care deficit, and whether the individual's present state allows for safe involvement in care.
- **Planning** – goal-setting focuses on the restoration of self-care abilities and self-care needs.
- **Intervention** – involves facilitating each patient in the maintenance or re-establishment of full self-care, and can be wholly compensatory, partly compensatory or educative/developmental (see Fig. 6.5).
- **Evaluation** – this involves the nurse considering whether the patient is showing an increasing ability to undertake self-care.

Roy's model of nursing

Roy's model (Fig. 6.6) is known as an adaptation model for nursing.[15] It focuses on how a person – a whole system – responds or adapts to stimuli from within or from the surrounding environment.[16] The stimuli can be identified as either focal, contextual or residual:

- Focal stimuli – those that affect a person immediately and directly, such as surgery or infection.
- Contextual stimuli – the surrounding circumstances, which may influence a negative response to the focal stimuli, such as anaemia or a poor nutritional status.
- Residual stimuli – the beliefs and attitudes of an individual which will affect their current situation, generally developed from past experience – previous experience of hospital or surgery, for example.

Patients undergoing an elective operation, for example, need to adapt to the effect of the surgery and the anaesthetic (focal stimuli), their anaemia (contextual stimuli), and their bad memories of previous emergency surgery (residual stimuli).

A further component of the model are an individual's needs, which Roy divides into the following:

- Physiological – the structure and functioning of the body
- Self-concept – the way one perceives oneself
- Role function – concerned with fulfilling one's role in society
- Interdependence – the balance between dependence and independence.

In relation to the nursing process this model can be seen as follows:

- **Assessment** Roy identifies that assessment has two parts: first-level assessment aims to describe the patient's current behaviour, while second-level assessment describes the stimuli that caused that behaviour.
- **Planning** Goals focus on adjusting maladaptive behaviour to normal behaviour, and thus should be formulated with the patient and should be observable and measurable.

OREMS UNIVERSAL SELF-CARE NEEDS

1. Sufficient intake of air
2. Sufficient intake of water
3. Sufficient intake of food
4. Satisfactory eliminative function
5. Activity balanced with rest
6. Time spent alone balanced with time spent with others
7. Prevention of danger to self
8. Being 'normal'

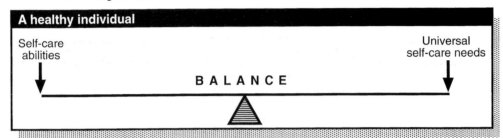

A healthy individual

Self-care abilities

Universal self-care needs

B A L A N C E

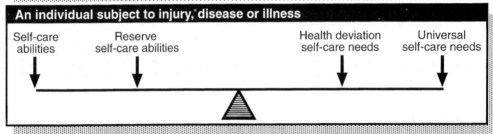

An individual subject to injury, disease or illness

Self-care abilities

Reserve self-care abilities

Health deviation self-care needs

Universal self-care needs

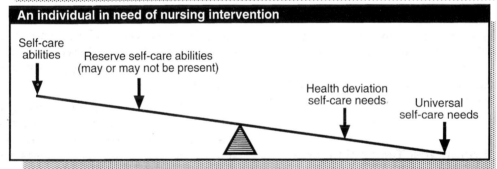

An individual in need of nursing intervention

Self-care abilities

Reserve self-care abilities (may or may not be present)

Health deviation self-care needs

Universal self-care needs

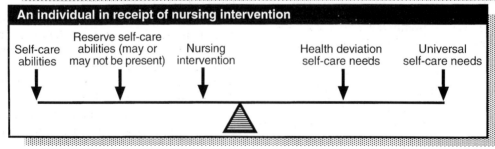

An individual in receipt of nursing intervention

Self-care abilities

Reserve self-care abilities (may or may not be present)

Nursing intervention

Health deviation self-care needs

Universal self-care needs

Figure 6.5 Orem's model of nursing.

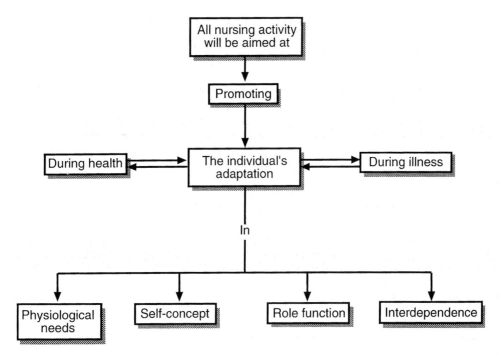

Figure 6.6 Roy's model of nursing.

• **Implementing** Nursing action is aimed at adjusting the stimuli which have led to maladaptive behaviour.

• **Evaluation** This considers the extent to which the individual has adapted to the stimuli with the assistance of nursing and medical care.

Roper, Logan and Tierney's model of nursing

This model was originally developed by Roper,[17] and has been developed into its most recent form by Roper, Logan and Tierney.[18] It is a systems model of nursing which tends to view human beings as a collection of interrelating biological, psychological and/or social systems.[19] These systems can be divided into a number of components, and human beings function best when all their systems are in a state of balance, both individually and collectively. Roper et al believe one of the best ways of understanding human beings is in terms of the activities they perform (Fig. 6.7). Further components of the model are the life-span, the dependence/independence continuum, and the factors that affect the activities of living.

In relation to the nursing process the model can be seen as follows:

• **Assessment** The activities of living are used as a basis upon which the assessment of individual needs takes place. Assessment is a continuous process, as patients' needs frequently need reassessing.

• **Planning** Goal-setting involves documenting all actual and potential problems.

• **Intervention** This involves selecting the most appropriate nursing action in an effort to meet goals which have been previously determined with the patient.

• **Evaluation** This involves re-examining each activity of living to establish whether the desired goals have been achieved.

This model has been chosen to illustrate the use of the nursing process and a nursing model in the operating theatre for the following reasons:

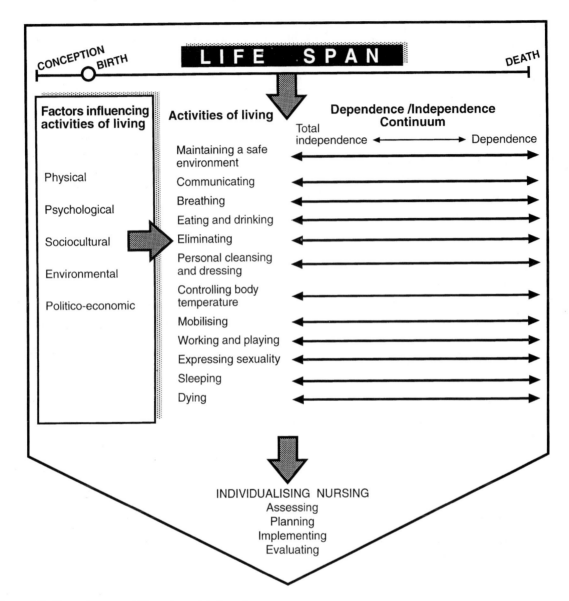

Figure 6.7 Roper, Logan and Tierney's model of nursing.

1. The concepts are easily understood and it is reasonably jargon free. This is important in the operating theatre, where models of care are relatively new.

2. The model is based on biological systems, and is therefore largely 'physical' in nature. This is relevant in the operating theatre when the patient is undergoing surgery, a major physical event in their lives.

3. The model allows for actual and potential problems. This is important, as preventing the many potential problems associated with surgery is an essential part of the theatre practitioner's role.

The care plan shown in Appendix 3 identifies the assessment, planning, implementation and evaluation of care given to a patient undergoing a major surgical operation. Although these problems may not all be relevant for a patient undergoing minor surgery, there are many problems faced by almost all patients. The care plan documents:

- Assessment – the patient's normal routine in each activity of living, and problems in relation to surgery
- Planning – the aim of care in relation to each problem
- Implementation – the care given
- Evaluation – how the care was evaluated.

It also includes a column for 'rationale', which gives the reasonings, or references as to why a

certain intervention is recommended. Many of these are discussed in the next section on major issues in care, or in the previous chapter on anaesthesia. Rationale and references would not normally be documented on a care plan.

Obviously this documentation is lengthy and needs adaptation for practical use. It is important, however, that all care provided by the theatre practitioner is documented in some way. Theatre practitioners must therefore strive to find a practical method of doing this (see Chapter 2 – Record keeping).

REFERENCES

1. Shaw H 1983 What aspects of the nursing process are applicable in theatre nursing and how can they be implemented? NATN News 20: 11–13
2. Leonard M, Kalideen D 1985 So you're going to have an operation. NATN News 22: 12–21
3. Nightingale K 1988 The ideal and the actual – preoperative visiting re-visited. British Journal of Theatre Nursing 25: 12–13
4. Copp G 1988 Intra-operative information and preoperative visiting. Surgical Nurse 1: 27–29
5. Wicker P 1987 The role of the nurse in theatre. Senior Nurse 7: 19–21
6. Francis M 1889 Asepsis for the nurse. Cited by Wicker P 1987[5]
7. Alin K 1991 Pre-operative handover. Surgical Nurse 4: 4–9
8. Alin K 1991 Post-operative handover. Surgical Nurse 4: 23–27
9. Boore J 1978 Prescription for recovery. Royal College of Nursing, London
10. Davis B 1984 Pre-operative information giving and patients' post-operative outcomes: An implementation

study. Nursing Studies Research Unit, University of Edinburgh
11. Yura H, Walsh M 1978 The nursing process, 3rd edn. Appleton Century Crofts, New York
12. Chalmers H 1988 Introduction. In: Choosing a model of nursing. Hodder and Stoughton, Bath
13. Riehl J, Roy C 1980 Conceptual models for nursing practice. Appleton Century Crofts, Norwalk
14. Orem D 1985 Concepts of practice, 3rd edn. McGraw Hill, New York
15. Roy C 1976 Introduction to nursing: an adaptation model. Prentice Hall, Old Tappan, New Jersey
16. Pearson A, Vaughan B 1986 Nursing models for practice. Heinemann, London
17. Roper N 1976 Clinical experience in nurse education. Churchill Livingstone, Edinburgh
18. Roper N, Logan W, Tierney A 1996 The elements of nursing, 4th edn. Churchill Livingstone, Edinburgh
19. Aggleton P, Chalmers H 1987 Models of nursing, nursing practice and nurse education. Journal of Advanced Nursing 1: 573–581

FURTHER READING

Wicker P 1990 A reassuring presence. Nursing Times 86: 59–61

Major issues in patient care

The previous section discussed the care of the patient in the five phases of surgical intervention and identified the role of the theatre practitioner. The use of a care plan based on a nursing model (with rationale) has highlighted that there are many problems common to all patients undergoing surgery. It is acknowledged that the problems encountered by patients undergoing 'minor' or day-case surgery have not been discussed; these are, however, outlined in Chapter 1, in the section on day-case surgery. This section will now discuss the major issues of patient care in the intraoperative phase and outline the role of the theatre practitioner in relation to these issues. Major issues of care not included are discussed in the more relevant chapters (Chapter 4, Anaesthetic practice or Chapter 7, Recovery practice).

Some issues of patient care as identified on the care plan are not expanded upon in this section, i.e. electrosurgical burns, eye damage and anxiety. These are discussed elsewhere in this book, or the rationale and further reading are provided on the care plan.

This section will therefore discuss the following issues:

- pressure area care
- positioning the patient
- ensuring that the patient has the correct operation
- ensuring there is no swab, needle or instrument retained in the wound
- prevention of infection.

PRESSURE AREA CARE

Pressure sores have a multitude of other names with which the theatre practitioner will become familiar:

- pressure ulcers
- bed sores
- decubitus ulcers
- pressure insults

- distortion ulcers
- trophic ulcers
- ischaemic ulcers.

This chapter uses the term pressure sores, as it is the most commonly used, is easily recognized and clearly identifies the importance of pressure – an important consideration for the theatre practitioner.

The prevention and treatment of pressure sores is a huge topic, with an immense amount of literature. This section will therefore focus on:

- the definition, incidence and effects of pressure sores
- the causes of pressure sores and the role of the theatre practitioner
- the identification of risk factors and the provision of care by theatre practitioners
- aids to prevent pressure sore development
- the role of the theatre practitioner in pressure sore prevention.

DEFINITION, INCIDENCE AND EFFECTS OF PRESSURE SORES

A pressure sore may be defined as an area of necrosis caused by excessive and prolonged pressure,[1] a useful definition as it denotes the key issues in relation to pressure, i.e. amount and duration, which will be discussed here. The incidence of pressure area problems is a major concern in many areas of healthcare provision – care of the elderly units, medical and surgical wards, accident and emergency departments, community care and elderly mental illness units, for example – and is often said to have reached epidemic proportions.

There is a wealth of literature in relation to care in these areas, in contrast to pressure area care in the operating department, which has only recently become a focus for clinical research – the relationship between pressure area damage and the operating department was first suggested by Hicks.[2] Indeed, Petersen[3] states that during a stay in hospital one of the most intensive pressure traumas a patient is subjected to is the operating table, and Moore et al[4] identify that 'during a stay in hospital, a surgical patient is nowhere more likely to develop pressure sores than on an operating table'.

The costs of pressure sores – economic, physical and emotional – are great, and affect both the patient and the hospital. Formation of a pressure sore will mean the patient inevitably has a prolonged hospital stay and treatment for the sores, both of which are expensive for the hospital to provide. For the patient, as well as the inconvenience of a prolonged hospital stay, the problems of pain, infection, debility and effect on body image are immense. A further cost to care providers has recently been identified as the cost of litigation in terms of damages awarded to patients who have developed pressure sores. All theatre practitioners should be aware of the increase in such litigation, and consider that lack of effective care provision is seen in law as negligence. This is especially important owing to the extent of the problem: Versluysen[5] suggests that surgical patients, especially the elderly, form the largest single group susceptible to pressure sores. A recent study by Bridel[6] shows a theatre-generated incidence of 12.5%, similar to those reported by Versluysen[7] and Kemp et al.[8]

The emphasis of modern care has therefore shifted the debate regarding the treatment of pressure sores (although this continues) to focus on their prevention. This involves the identification and detection of risk factors that predispose to pressure sore formation, and the provision of interventions necessary to reduce them. It is first necessary to understand the aetiology of pressure sores and how this relates to operating department practice.

CAUSES OF PRESSURE SORES

The causes of pressure sores can be identified as pressure, shearing and friction.

Pressure

Sustained pressure is seen as the principal cause of pressure sore formation. Although this does not generally directly harm living tissue it does compress blood vessels, causing ischaemia and resulting in a lack of nutrient and oxygen supply to the tissues and a build-up of metabolic waste. Tissue death therefore occurs from anoxia, rather than from mechanical disruption of the tissues.[9] Two factors are relevant in relation to pressure – amount and duration.

Amount of pressure

Blood normally flows through the capillaries at a pressure of 25–30 mmHg, oxygen and nutrients being absorbed by the tissue cells. If more pressure is on the capillaries than within them circulation will be impaired, leading to hypoxic tissue damage. Fernandez,[10] for example, identified that if pressures of more than 40 mmHg are exerted on an area, then capillary distortion occurs; at over 80 mmHg capillary collapse occurs and tissue necrosis follows.[10] Capillary pressures often exceed the level of 25–30 mmHg, especially over bony prominences during surgery, and hence tissue damage may occur. This is of great relevance to the theatre practitioner, as interface pressures of 260 mmHg have been found under the sacrum in a study by Redfern et al.[11] Gendron[12] takes this one step further and identifies pressures that are sufficient to cause tissue ischaemia in a supine patient:

- 20–40 mmHg at the occiput
- 30 mmHg at the spine
- 40–60 mmHg at the sacral area
- 30–45 mmHg at the heels
- 30–40 mmHg at the costal margins and knees (prone).

A safe pressure is therefore generally considered to be 32 mmHg – the same as capillary pressure, although Bridel[13] considers this to be in dispute and a baseline of 32 mmHg too simplistic to use as a minimum safe level. The theatre practitioner should be aware that although pressure injuries can occur anywhere, there are vulnerable sites which will need extra protection.

Although these are useful pieces of research, Bridel[13] suggests that the research results relating to intensity and duration of pressure vary considerably, and often use animal skin as a basis for experimentation. The theatre practitioner must therefore read such research thoroughly and critically, in order to evaluate its usefulness.

Duration of pressure

Duration of pressure rather than intensity is thought to be the more important factor. Petrie and Hummel[14] state that the patient can stand a great amount of pressure for a short time without sustaining tissue damage, or a low amount of pressure over a longer period. Healthy individuals can tolerate external pressures of up to 100 mmHg on bony prominences for short periods without incurring tissue ischaemia.[15] However, low constant pressures of 70 mmHg on bony prominences have been shown to cause microscopic changes in healthy individuals after 2 hours.[16] Indeed, prolonged surgical procedures have been identified as a very significant factor in pressure sore formation.[17]

This is relevant for the theatre practitioner as patients undergoing major surgery can be in position on the operating table for many hours – often more than 2 – and as such have been shown to record pressures of 91 mmHg on the occiput and 52.3 mmHg on the sacrum.[16] Furthermore, theatre trolleys and tables have long been cited as very significant factors in the aetiology of pressure sore formation,[18] and this is supported by more recent evidence.[4]

Shear

Shear occurs when a force is exerted on the body, the skin remains in a fixed position and the underlying tissues and skeletal system move. The outer layers of the skin therefore slide, resulting in damage to the underlying structures. This will cause constriction and distortion of the microcirculation (which is already compressed by pressure), and possible tearing of the underlying tissues. The theatre practitioner should therefore be aware that when moving an operating table bearing an anaesthetized patient, the weight of the patient is likely to move the tissues attached to bone, but that other structures such as skin and subcutaneous tissue will stay fixed to the support surface (operating table), thereby causing a shear force and possible tissue damage.

Friction

Friction occurs when shear exceeds the pressure on an area and the skin begins to move against its environment.[10] The forces of shearing and friction may occur if poor technique is used for transferring the patient to the table and adjusting their position. Whenever possible, therefore, conscious patients should be allowed to position themselves on the operating table. This is likely to achieve a more natural position, and alleviate as much pressure as possible. If this is not possible, a patient transfer system such as canvas and poles, rollers and air transfer devices should be used, as these minimize the risk of trauma due to shear or friction.

Adjusting an anaesthetized patient's position on the operating table by sliding creates a shear force that tends to fold and tear the tissues of the buttocks. The tissues may then be left in combined compressive and shear stress for the duration of the operation.[19] Whenever possible, therefore, changing the patient's position after anaesthesia has been given should be avoided. Any tissue damage that is not over a bony prominence is likely to have resulted from shear,[20] and could therefore possibly have been prevented. Plastic film dressings can be used to protect the patient's skin from friction, but it must be remembered that they do not reduce pressure. Pressure-relieving aids are still required.

IDENTIFICATION OF RISK FACTORS AND THE PROVISION OF CARE

Assessment of the individual patient will take place either during a preoperative visit or by using the alternative methods of assessment discussed earlier in the chapter. This must include an assessment of the risk of pressure sores, and should therefore involve liaison with the ward staff. A pressure sore risk calculator can be used, together with the nurse's own professional judgement. Hibbs[21] states that this is essential, as some patients with a no-risk score may develop pressure sores.

It is imperative that the most vulnerable patients are recognized at an early stage, therefore any assessment must be consistent and thorough; an agreed assessment tool should be used for this purpose. Flanagan[22] suggests the growing importance of such scales in today's climate of financial constraint and the fear of litigation. This is as important in the operating theatre as in other areas of healthcare. The advantage of using a recognized assessment tool is that consistency between staff is more likely, and that many possible contributing factors will be considered. There are several pressure sore risk calculators available, many based on the initial assessment scale devised by Norton et al.[23]

Norton pressure sore risk assessment scale

The Norton pressure sore risk assessment scoring system[23] was the first such rating scale developed, and originates from research in the 1950s in geriatric hospitals. It is based on five main risk factors:

- general physical condition
- mental state
- activity
- mobility
- continence.

A score is given for each risk factor, with a descending rating, 4 being a 'good' score and 1 being a 'bad' score. Scores can therefore vary

between 20 and 5. The research concluded that a score of 14 identified a patient at risk of a pressure sore, and a score of 12 as the level below which pressure sore development appeared to be inevitable (Fig. 6.8).

Recent research suggests that general physical condition and continence appear to be the most important factors, and that the Norton scale overpredicts pressure sores by 64%.[24] A further study, however, found that the Norton scale did not predict pressure sore development accurately, with 14% of patients identified as not at risk developing pressure sores.[25] Flanagan,[22] however, states that the majority of those patients had had recent surgery and hence their scores dropped postoperatively, and that the time spent on the operating table is not considered by the Norton scale.

Waterlow pressure sore prevention treatment policy

This policy was published in 1985[26] and includes a risk assessment tool, guidelines on the effective use of preventative equipment, and a first-stage wound classification management tool. It is now the most widely used method of risk assessment in the UK.[22] The risk assessment tool is based on risk factors identified as relevant by the literature at the time:

- build/weight for height
- continence
- skin type
- mobility

Physical condition		Mental condition		Activity		Mobility		Incontinent	
A		B		C		D		E	
Good	4	Alert	4	Ambulant	4	Full	4	Not	4
Fair	3	Apathetic	3	Walk/Help	3	Slightly	3	Occasionally limited	3
Poor	2	Confused	2	Chairbound	2	Very	2	Usually/urine	2
Very bad	1	Stuporous	1	Bedfast	1	Immobile	1	Usually/doubly	1

Figure 6.8 The Norton pressure sore risk assessment scale–scoring system key. A total score of 14 or below equals at risk.

- sex/age
- appetite
- special risks:
  — tissue malnutrition
  — neurological deficit
  — major surgery/trauma
  — medications.

The patient is given a score for each section, which are added together to obtain a cumulative risk status, with a score of 10 indicating a patient at risk, 15–20 high risk, and 20 or over very high risk (Fig. 6.9). This scale would seem appropriate for surgical patients, as it has more detail than the Norton scale and includes surgery as a risk factor.

Braden scale

The Braden scale was developed from research in nursing homes in the USA.[27] It is composed of six risk categories:

- sensory perception
- moisture
- activity
- mobility
- nutrition
- friction/shear.

It is therefore the only scale to assess the risk of friction/shear. Each risk category is scored from 1 (least favourable) to 3–4 (most favourable), with a minimum possible score of 6, showing a high-risk patient, and a maximum score of 23, showing a low-risk patient. Research identifies a score of 16 or below to be the point at which patients are at risk of developing pressure sores.[28,29] This scale is used widely in the USA, and studies suggest it is the most appropriate tool for research in relation to reliability and validity.[27,29] It is used by Bridel[6] in her study of pressure sore risk in the operating theatre, which concludes that it compares favourably with the

Build/weight for height		Risk areas Skin type	Visual	Sex/age		Special risks	
Average	0	Healthy	0	Male	1	Tissue malnutrition	
Above	1	Tissue paper	1	Female	2	e.g. terminal cachexia	8
average		Dry	1	14–49	1	cardiac failure	5
Obese	2	Oedematous	1	50–64	2	Peripheral vascular	5
Below	3	Clammy	1	65–74	3	disease	
average		Discoloured	2	75–80	4	Anaemia	2
		Broken/spot	3	81+	5	Smoking	1
Continence		**Mobility**		**Appetite**		**Neurological deficit** e.g. diabetes/CV	
Complete/	0	Fully	0	Average	0		
catheterized		Restless	1	Poor	1	Multiple sclerosis	4–6
Occasionally	1	Apathetic	2	N/G tube	2	Motor/sensory loss	
incontinent		Restricted	3	Fluids	2	Major surgery trauma	
Catheterized	2	Inert/traction	4	only		Orthopaedic spinal	5
incontinent		Chairbound	5	NBM	3	(below waist)	
of faeces				anorexic		On table over 2 hours	5
Doubly incont.	3					Medication	
						Steroids/Cytotoxic	
						Anti-inflammatory	
Score: 10+ at risk, 15+ high risk, 20+ very high risk							

Figure 6.9 The Waterlow pressure sore risk assessment scale. Several scores per category can be used.

Norton and Waterlow scales, and results support its use in future research.

The theatre practitioner should therefore discuss risk assessment tools with surgical ward staff, in order for the most appropriate to be used. Most are now available on pocket-sized cards for easy use. Flanagan[22] warns against an assessment tool being used only on admission, or as a substitute for sound clinical judgement. The patient's score must therefore be reviewed at regular intervals, and preoperative and postoperative scores are essential.

Whichever scale is chosen, it is essential that it is used consistently. The scales have different scoring systems, with the Norton and Braden scales using a lower score to identify a patient at high risk of pressure sore development, and the Waterlow a low score to indicate a low-risk patient; hence the potential for confusion exists. Pre-, intra- and postoperative documentation should allow the scale used and the patient's score at specific times to be recorded.

Whichever risk calculator the theatre practitioner uses, it must be used in conjunction with thorough observation of the patient's preoperative condition, the nurse's professional judgement, an understanding of the risk factors identified, and an awareness of other factors, such as those that directly relate to the surgery and anaesthesia.

What are the risk factors?

Clinical research provides us with accurate clues to the factors that identify a patient to be at high risk of developing a pressure sore due to surgical intervention. This is a fairly new area of research, and the findings are constantly necessitating developments in operating department practice, in order to reduce the risk for each patient. The following identifies and explains risk factors, using the research available to date. This should always be supplemented by a review of up-to-date research to ensure that all possible measures for the prevention of pressure sores are used.

Gendron[19] identifies three common factors in patients who developed unexplained 'burn-like' injuries (concluded to be pressure sores) after

lengthy surgical procedures. Other factors identified in the literature are the patient's age and weight, anxiety, nutrition, general anaesthesia, moisture, position used for surgery, and heat. These factors will now be discussed and the role of the theatre practitioner identified.

Length of procedure

The duration of surgery is a relevant factor in pressure sore prevention. The incidence of pressure sores is increased in patients whose surgery lasts longer than 2 hours.[30] The theatre practitioner must consider that the period of immobility is longer than the actual length of the operation. The patient is often given a premedication which has a sedative effect: movement and mobility are therefore likely to be decreased for some time preoperatively. In addition, transfer to the operating department, induction of anaesthesia and postoperative recovery, both in the recovery room and on the ward, all add to the length of the actual surgery, thus the period of immobility is even further extended. Any problems related to sustained pressure, shear or friction are therefore compounded by this extra time. This is an important factor and means that individuals not normally at risk from pressure sore development become at high risk, as identified by Stewart and Magnano.[31]

Vascular surgery resulting in lower blood pressure

Patients who require vascular surgery are at high risk of developing a pressure sore because their circulation is already compromised. This is of relevance to the theatre practitioner, as these patients are often operated on for this very reason, i.e. to improve their circulation and/or bypass any obstructions. These operations are difficult and require surgical dexterity and thoroughness. This, and the extent of the disease, therefore means the surgery generally lasts more than 2 hours, increasing the risk of pressure sore development.

Lowering of blood pressure, whether for the entire operation or intermittently (as in vascular surgery), creates a condition whereby a peripheral area – such as a heel – will have a reduced blood circulation. This is compounded by an increase in pressure if the patient is placed in the supine position for example, leading to a decreased local blood supply. The theatre practitioner should be aware of the effects of hypotension, and liaise with the anaesthetist to ensure that hypotensive periods are kept to a minimum.

Sustained pressure due to immobility

A healthy person continually shifts position to remove localized pressure in an area of their body which is generally perceived as discomfort. This occurs whether the person is awake or asleep, and is the body's natural defence against pressure sores. This ability is, however, lost when the patient is anaesthetized. An essential component of anaesthesia is muscle relaxation, with the result that the patient is literally unable to move a muscle for the duration of the surgical procedure. However, it is also important to acknowledge that even when the patient is no longer anaesthetized postoperative analgesia may have a similar effect by reducing pain, sedating the patient and decreasing their spontaneous movements. Many of the preventative methods and aids described in the literature to reduce immobility would not be applicable for use in the operating theatre, for example 2-hourly turning and the use of specialized moving-air mattresses. In practical terms it is impossible to change the position of the patient during surgery without compromising the sterile field and denying the surgeon full access to the operation site. Furthermore, moving a patient with an open body cavity can cause great trauma, especially if the patient is anatomically unstable, as in orthopaedic surgery for example.

Consideration should however, be given to what parts of the patient could be moved during surgery. For example, Lawson et al[32] studied occipital alopecia in patients following cardiac surgery. They, found that a 14% incidence was reduced to 1% by changing the position of the patient's head every 30 minutes. This was also confirmed by further research.[12,33,34] Although the patient may not be able to be completely moved to relieve pressure some parts of the body could be carefully adjusted if the surgery and the surgeon allow: careful movement of the legs during surgery on the head, for example, can relieve pressure and allow the cells to receive oxygen. **This must only be done with the permission and knowledge of the surgeon.**

A further source of pressure in the operating theatre can be the placement of surgical instruments on the anaesthetized patient during surgery, or weight from a member of the surgical team leaning on the patient, as identified by Gendron.[19] These will add to the patient's weight, and increase the risk of tissue damage in weightbearing areas, such as bony prominences. There are therefore only limited interventions the theatre practitioner can make to relieve the pressure due to immobility during surgery:

- Encourage the anaesthetist to move the patient's head every 30 minutes, if this does not interfere with surgery.
- Carefully move the patient's extremities, with the permission of the surgeon, if this does not interfere with surgery.
- Ensure that surgical instruments are not left on the patient.
- Ensure that members of the surgical team do not lean on the patient.

Age of the patient

A linear relationship between increasing age and increasing incidence of pressure sores has been documented by Manley[35] and Anderson and Kvorning.[36] The physiological effects of ageing include a decrease in skin elasticity and a loss of skin resilience. Furthermore, Krouskop[37] suggested that the decrease in skin elasticity that occurs in ageing allows for a greater degree of transfer of the mechanical load from the supporting structures to the underlying tissues, including the vascular structures. Ischaemia of the tissues may therefore occur at a lower pressure density in the elderly.

The ageing process is also associated with arteriosclerotic changes, leading to peripheral vascular changes which affect the skin's blood supply and increase its vulnerability to pressure effects.

A patient's age therefore affects their risk of pressure sore development in various ways. In a study of 885 patients reported to have pressure sores, 85% were over the age of 65.[38] Theatre practitioners must therefore be aware of a patient's age and take all preventative measures possible.

Weight

Any substantial deviation from the ideal body weight can increase the risk of pressure sores. Patients should be considered nutritionally at risk if they are less than 90% or more than 120% of their ideal body weight.[20] Thin patients have little protection from body tissue over their bony prominences, and thus have high peaks of pressure in these areas. If the patient has suffered sudden wasting of fat and/or muscle this will predispose to pressure sores, as the microvascular structure of the soft tissues will have had insufficient time to adapt. Conversely, although the obese patient has plenty of fatty padding to distribute pressure, it is possible that any additional protection gained by this is insufficient to offset the increase in pressure caused by the extra weight. The theatre practitioner must therefore assess the patient's weight before surgery, in order to plan effective care. Consideration must be given to the position required for surgery and the distribution of the patient's weight in that position. In the supine position, for example, a disproportionate amount of weight is borne on the occiput, spinous processes, scapulae, sacrum and calcaneum. Generally the sacrum is the first tissue to break down in this position.[19]

Anxiety

The effect of giving patients preoperative information to reduce their anxiety, reduce postoperative pain, improve the quality of sleep, reduce postoperative infection and minimize length of stay in hospital is well documented.[39–41] It is also possible that this particular intervention may benefit the patient in terms of pressure sore development, as Krouskop[37] has suggested a hypothetical relationship between emotional stress and an increase in pressure sore formation. This is likely to be an area for further research.

Nutrition

The nutritional status of the patient undergoing surgery is also an important factor in the development of pressure sores. The patient is more likely to develop a pressure sore if their nutritional status is poor. Preoperatively patients may become obese owing to decreased mobility, or undernourished owing to pain, debility, dislike of hospital food and prolonged periods of being 'nil by mouth', especially if surgery needs to be repeated or if they have had many investigations preoperatively. It is also necessary to consider that nutritional intake is often poor postoperatively, with patients often feeling nauseous, having a poor appetite or being unable to eat because of the surgery.

Poor nutritional status will affect the integrity of the skin and supporting structures, especially collagen and elastin.[21] Important factors include iron, vitamins A and C, and calcium. For example, in otherwise healthy people a vitamin C-deficient diet has been found to contribute to delayed wound healing and a decreased resistance to the skin being torn.[42] Age is again relevant here, as a study carried out by the Health and Nutrition Examination Survey[43] reported that dietary intake data revealed deficiencies in intake of iron, vitamins A and C and calcium in the elderly. Furthermore, Scott et al[20] identify that low albumin levels are associated with pressure sore development in the elderly. If the patient has suffered a loss of protein, or has had an inadequate intake of protein, they may develop oedema of the body's dependent parts which predisposes to pressure sores and delays healing.[9] Finally, research has shown that 40% of patients admitted to hospital are nutritionally below par.[44] The theatre practitioner should therefore be aware of the patient's nutritional status and take appropriate measures to prevent tissue damage.

General anaesthesia

As well as causing the required muscle relaxation to allow surgery to be performed, general anaesthesia may also cause hypotension. The pharmacological effects of anaesthetic agents, the inhibition of sympathetic nervous activity, and the loss of baroreceptor control of arterial pressure that results from loss of consciousness, may produce hypotensive episodes.[45] This is relevant in relation to peripheral blood supply, which may be further compromised if blood loss due to surgery is great. Indeed, a study in 1979[46] discovered that hypertensive subjects could withstand higher external pressures before vascular occlusion occurred. Although none of the subjects was hypotensive, it seems logical that the trend towards vascular occlusion at lower levels of external pressure would continue in a relatively linear fashion. A patient who has a general anaesthesia may also have suppression of their immune system for a period postoperatively,[47] which may mean they are more likely to develop pressure area problems.

Moisture

Perspiration and incontinence of urine may contribute to the development of pressure sores. Norton et al's original study[23] identified that 39% of incontinent patients developed pressure sores, compared to 7% of continent patients.

Frictional damage is also increased as a damp patient–support interface has an adhesive effect, resulting in a greater coefficiency of friction.[48] Moisture, especially when allowed to accumulate, increases the risk of pressure sore development because it decreases the resistance of the skin and can lead to a 'soggy' or macerated skin surface. This therefore weakens the natural barrier of the skin – the epidermis.[27] Theatre practitioners can guard against this by ensuring that the surface the patient is lying on is clean and dry, and by observing for and removing any pooling of fluids used in skin preparation. It is also helpful to ensure the patient has an empty bladder prior to the commencement of surgery.

Position

A further risk factor in relation to pressure sore development is the position required for surgery. The patient undergoing an operation is likely to spend a great deal of time in an abnormal position (some more abnormal than others – lithotomy, for example). This has a great effect on the body, which evolved for standing, with only the feet designed to be weightbearing. Surgical positions alter this and mean that other areas of the body become weightbearing.

The position used for surgery is determined by the operation to be performed, and must allow good access for the surgeon and the anaesthetist. Each position used in theatre has a profound effect on the patient's cardiovascular and respiratory systems, and on their nervous and muscular systems, and on the development of pressure sore formation. The theatre practitioner should therefore consider each position and the location of pressure through bony prominences, and where any shear forces may be present, and take preventative measures by providing necessary padding and support. Although all positions are hazardous to some extent (see section on positioning), one study has shown that the most frequent skin pressure injuries occur in the supine position.[2]

Heat

Heating blankets, which are commonly used in operating theatres to keep patients warm, may actually aggravate pressure sore development.[49] Heat causes the patient's metabolic rate to increase, meaning there is a greater need for oxygen and nutrients, and may result in tissue damage if other risk factors are present. Further research by Stewart and Magnano[31] suggests that the time required for pressure damage may be shortened by the presence of heat. The theatre practitioner should be aware of this and consider carefully, with the surgeon and the anaesthetist, when it is appropriate to use heating blankets.

AIDS TO PREVENT PRESSURE SORE DEVELOPMENT

This is likely to be an area of great development in the future as the problem of pressure sore formation in the operating theatre becomes more widely acknowledged, and the clinical research improves in quality and quantity. Aids to consider at the present time include:

- **Thickness of the mattress** This is an important factor as it affects the interface pressures and hence the likelihood of pressure sore formation. A minimum of 8 cm is now the normal thickness of operating department table mattresses.[30] (See Chapter 5 for further information.)
- **Vacuum bead mattresses** These have been found to be helpful in reducing pressure sore development, particularly in elderly orthopaedic patients.[50] These are now widely used, and have the benefit of maintaining the patient's position as well as reducing the effects of pressure by moulding to the patient's body, and providing a wide area to evenly distribute the patient's weight.[51]
- **Low-pressure air mattresses** These provide additional comfort and protection for the patient in the pre- and postoperative periods while they are on theatre trolleys.
- **Dry polymer gel pad** (from Central Medical Supplies).
- **Liquid displacement cell mattress** (made by Charnwood Surgical Ltd).

These last two items have been shown to demonstrate reduced interface pressure measurements in key sites of the body compared to conventional operating table mattresses.[17,52] Theatre practitioners must therefore consider up-to-date clinical research in order to establish the value of all items available to prevent pressure sore formation.

ROLE OF THE THEATRE PRACTITIONER

The role of the theatre practitioner has been referred to throughout in this section in order to aid understanding of why actions are needed. The interventions where the theatre practitioner has an especially active role in pressure sore formation are therefore summarized below.

- Have a good working knowledge of the aetiology of pressure sores and the risk factors leading to their formation.

- Move the anaesthetized patient very carefully to avoid trauma due to shearing forces.
- Use a plastic film dressing in areas at risk of shearing force or friction.
- Assess the patient's skin preoperatively and document skin condition, using a recognized risk assessment tool if possible.
- Limit the period of immobility by moving the patient in the early postoperative phase in the recovery room.
- Liaise with the anaesthetist to ensure that hypotensive episodes are kept to a minimum.
- Encourage the anaesthetist to move the patient's head every 30 minutes – with the permission of the surgeon.
- Move the patient's peripheries if possible – with the permission of the surgeon.
- Prevent the surgical team leaning or placing instruments or equipment on the patient.
- Ensure the patient is on a clean, dry, wrinkle-free surface, and that they pass urine pre-operatively if possible; avoid pooling of fluids.
- Provide appropriate aids to prevent pressure sores and position the patient carefully using pads and supports where possible to relieve pressure on bony prominences.
- Discuss the implications of a heating mattress or blanket with the surgeon and anaesthetist.
- Consider clinical research when purchasing equipment and aids to prevent pressure sore formation: ask to see reports of clinical trials.
- Evaluate the condition of the patient's skin postoperatively. This should also be performed when the patient is back on the ward, as pressure sores acquired in theatre may only appear hours or days later. Typically they develop 1–3 days after surgery.[20]
- Communicate with ward staff about patient's pressure area care, either in writing or verbally. Ensure all care given in relation to pressure area care is documented.
- Liaise with all members of the operating department team, and teach junior colleagues and learners about good pressure area care.

REFERENCES

1. Beland J, Passos J 1981 Clinical nursing: pathophysiological and psychosocial approaches, 4th edn. Collier Macmillan, London
2. Hicks D 1971 An incidence of pressure sores following surgery. ANA Clinical Sessions, Miami, pp 49-54
3. Peterson N 1976 The development of pressure sores during hospitalisation. In: Kenedi R, Cowden J, Scales J (eds) Bedsore biomechanics. Macmillan, London
4. Moore E, Green K, Rithalia S 1992a A survey of operating table pads and patient trolley mattresses. Journal of Tissue Viability 2: 67
5. Versluysen M 1985 Pressure sores in elderly patients. The epidemiology related to hip operations. Journal of Bone and Joint Surgery 67B: 10–13
6. Bridel J 1993 Pressure sore risk in operating theatres. Nursing Standard 7: 4–10
7. Versluysen M 1986 How elderly patients with femoral fracture develop pressure sores in hospital. British Medical Journal 292: 1311–1313
8. Kemp M et al 1990 Factors which contribute to pressure sores in surgical patients. Research in Nursing Health 13: 293–301
9. Torrance C 1981 Pressure sores: predisposing factors. The 'at risk' patient. Nursing Times 77: 5–8
10. Fernandez S 1988 Prevention and treatment of pressure sores. Care – Science and Practice 6: 17–21
11. Redfern S, Jeneid P, Gillingham M, Lunn H 1973 Local pressures with ten types of patient-support system. Lancet 2: 277–280
12. Gendron F 1988 Unexplained patient burns: investigating iatrogenic injuries. Brea, Cal, Quest, 170: 238
13. Bridel J 1992 Pressure sores and intra-operative risk. Nursing Standard 7: 28–30
14. Petrie L, Hummel R 1990 A study of interface pressure for pressure reduction and relief mattresses. Journal of Enterostomal Therapy 17: 212–216
15. Foster C, Mukai G, Breckenridge F, Smith C 1979 Effects of surgical positioning. AORN Journal 30: 219–232
16. Souther S, Carr S, Vietnes L 1973 Pressure tissue ischaemia and operating table pads. Archives of Surgery 107: 544–547
17. Neander K, Birkenfeld R 1991 Decubitus prophylaxis in the operating theatre? Journal of Tissue Viability 1: 71–73
18. Dyson R 1978 Bedsores – the injuries hospital staff inflict on patients. Nursing Mirror 146: 30–32
19. Gendron F 1980 Burns occurring during lengthy surgical procedures. Journal of Clinical Engineering 5: 19–26
20. Scott S, Mayhew P, Harris E 1992 Pressure ulcer development in the operating room: nursing implications. AORN Journal 56: 242–250
21. Hibbs P 1988 Pressure area care for the City and Hackney Health Authority: prevention plan for patients at risk from developing pressure sores – policy for the management of pressure sores. City and Hackney Health Authority, London
22. Flanagan M 1993 Pressure sore risk assessment scales. Journal of Wound Care 2: 162–167
23. Norton D, McLaren L, Exton Smith A 1962 An investigation of geriatric nursing problems in hospital. Churchill Livingstone, Edinburgh
24. Goldstone L, Goldstone J 1982 The Norton score: an early warning of pressure sores. Journal of Advanced Nursing 7: 419–426
25. Lincoln R, Maddox A, Patterson C 1986 Use of the Norton pressure sore risk assessment scoring system with elderly patients in acute care. Journal of Enterostomal Therapy 13: 132–138
26. Waterlow J 1985 A risk assessment card. Nursing Times 81: 49–55
27. Bergstrom N, Braden B, Laguzza A, Holman V 1987 The Braden scale for predicting pressure sore risk. Nursing Research 36: 207–210
28. Taylor K 1988 Assessment tools for the identification of patients at risk for the development of pressure sores. Journal of Enterostomal Therapy 15: 201–205
29. Bergstrom N, Demuth R, Braden B 1987 A clinical trial of the Braden scale for predicting pressure sore risk. Nursing Clinics of North America 22: 417–427
30. Pugh J, Millar B 1989 Mobility in the peri-operative phase. Surgical Nurse 2: 205–212
31. Stewart T, Magnano S 1988 Burns or pressure ulcers in the surgical patient? Decubitus 1: 36–40
32. Lawson N, Mills N, Oshsner J 1976 Occipital alopecia following cardiopulmonary bypass. Journal of Thoracic and Cardiovascular Surgery 71: 347
33. Elden W 1977 Occipital alopecia. Journal of Thoracic and Cardiovascular Surgery 73: 322
34. Poma P 1979 Pressure induced alopecia: report of a case after gynaecological surgery. Journal of Reproductive Medicine 22: 191
35. Manley M 1978 Incidence, contributory factors, and costs of pressure sores. South Africa Medical Journal 53: 217–222
36. Anderson K, Kvorning S 1982 Medical aspects of the decubitus ulcer. International Journal of Dermatology 21: 265–270
37. Krouskop T 1983 A synthesis of the factors that contribute to pressure sore formation. Medical Hypotheses 11: 255–267
38. David J, Chapman R, Chapman E, Lockett B 1983 An investigation of the current methods used in nursing for the care of patients with established pressure sores. Nursing Practice Research Unit, University of Surrey
39. Davis B 1984 Pre-operative information giving and patients' post-operative outcomes: an implementation study. Nursing Studies Research Unit, University of Edinburgh
40. Boore J 1987 Prescription for recovery. Royal College of Nursing, London
41. Hayward J 1975 Information: a prescription against pain. Royal College of Nursing, London
42. Irwin M, Hutchins B 1976 A conspectus of research on Vitamin C requirements of man. Journal of Nutrition 106: 823–879
43. Abraham S, Lowenstein F, Jonson C 1974 Preliminary findings of the first health and nutrition examination survey (1971–1972) Hanes, United States. In: Yurick A, Spier B, Robb S, Ebert N (eds) 1980 Age, person and the nursing process. Appleton-Century Crofts, Connecticut

44. Dickerson J 1986 Hospital induced malnutrition – a cause for concern. Professional Nurse August: 293–296
45. Yanick Harrington C 1987 Physiological monitoring. In: Kneedler J, Dodge G (eds) Peri-operative patient care, 2nd edn. Blackwell Scientific Publications, Boston, Chapter 19
46. Larson B, Holstein P, Lassen N 1979 On the pathogenesis of bedsores. Scandinavian Journal of Plastic and Reconstructive Surgery 13: 347–350
47. Stotts P, Pauls S 1988 Pressure ulcer development in surgical patients. Decubitus 1: 24–30
48. Lowthian P 1982 A review of pressure sore pathogenesis. Nursing Times 78: 117–121
49. Campbell K 1989 Pressure point measures in the operating room. Journal of Enterostomal Therapy 16: 119–124
50. O'Reilly M, Whyte J, Goldstone L 1981 A pressure sore survey. Nursing Times Theatre Nursing Supplement 77: 7–19
51. Dobbie A 1974 Accidental lesions in the operating theatre. NATN 11: 10–13
52. Moore E, Rithalia S, Gonsalkorale M 1992 Assessment of the Charnwood operating table and hospital trolley mattresses. Journal of Tissue Viability 2: 71–72

FURTHER READING

Bridel J 1993 The aetiology of pressure sores. Journal of Wound Care 2: 230–238
Bridel J 1993 Assessing trolley and table products. Nursing Standard 7: 11
Flanagan M 1993 Predicting pressure sore risk. Journal of Wound Care 2: 215–218
Foster C 1987 Positioning the patient. In: Kneedler J, Dodge G (eds) Peri-operative patient care. Blackwell Scientific Publications, Boston
Richardson B 1990 Pressure sores – a manager's perspective. Nursing Standard 5: 11–13
Wound Care Society 1995 Pressure sore development and prevention. Educational leaflet number 3. Wound Care Society, Northampton
Wound Care Society Pressure sore prevention – management and selection of equipment. Educational leaflet number 4. Wound Care Society, Northampton

---

Positioning the patient for surgery

Positioning the patient is an important aspect of surgical practice in all its phases. Care given in the preoperative, anaesthetic and postoperative phases must include safe positioning of the patient for both transport and transfer – to and from different departments, and between trolleys, beds and the operating table. Most patients undergoing surgery are sedated, some are unconscious, and all are dependent. The theatre practitioner must therefore have a good understanding of the following:

• requirements of the position used for surgery
• techniques and responsibilities in relation to patient positioning
• principles of patient handling and transfer
• principles of patient positioning
• commonly used positions for surgery
• effects of positioning on the patient
• hazards of positioning
• equipment used in positioning
• role of the theatre practitioner.

The transfer of the patient to the operating department occurs prior to the induction of anaesthesia. The various aids for patient transfer – canvases, 'patslides' and 'easyslides' are therefore discussed in Chapter 4, Anaesthesia.

REQUIREMENTS OF THE POSITION USED FOR SURGERY

The patient position used for surgery must allow good access for both anaesthesia and surgery, and ensure that the patient is safe and free from harm.

Surgical access

The prime determinants for patient positioning are safety and surgical access. In most cases this is straightforward, and the chosen position allows the surgeon to see, handle and operate on the required areas. In some instances, however, it is more complex and may necessitate moving the patient at specific points throughout the surgery. For example:

- Multiple access points may be needed, such as for an abdominoperineal resection.
- Multiple surgical teams may be needed, such as in major trauma surgery, when access to head, abdomen and limbs may be needed simultaneously.
- The patient may be unable to be positioned in the optimum position for access: a patient who has had a hip replacement may be unable to be placed in the lithotomy position for a gynaecological or urological procedure, for example.
- The surgical site may be shared with the anaesthetic requirements – in ENT surgery, for example.

In these circumstances the theatre practitioner, surgeon and anaesthetist must discuss and decide upon the optimum possible position, which maximizes surgical access when it is most required. In the event of multiple access sites being necessary a theatre practitioner must be available to assist with repositioning at all times.

Anaesthetic access

Good access for anaesthetic management is of equal importance when positioning the patient. However good surgical access may be in a certain position, it is of no value if the patient cannot be monitored adequately and their airway cannot be maintained. The anaesthetist must also therefore have good access, and this primarily involves:

- **Access to and support of the patient's airway** This will usually require easy access to the nose or mouth, and to the airway maintenance equipment used. In patients undergoing neurological or other head and neck surgery this is often not possible. Airway management in these instances needs careful planning, and a foolproof method of securing airway equipment is required.
- **Access to routes of drug, fluid and blood administration** This will usually require easy access to the patient's peripheral intravenous line in the hand, arm or foot. One technique is to place the patient's arm on an arm board, extended away from the body and the surgical field. In major surgery, where arterial and central lines are used, the upper chest and neck should also be accessible if possible. Adaptations are often required, depending on the surgical access needed, and should be planned by the anaesthetist, surgeon and theatre practitioner together.
- **Access to allow visual and tactile contact with the patient** This is necessary to assist in establishing the patient's physiological condition. Monitoring equipment is now standard for all patients, and offers a great deal of information, but an assessment by the anaesthetist and theatre practitioner of the patient's skin colour and condition, by colour and touch, remains essential. Positioning must therefore permit this. The patient's face should therefore be covered with towels only if it is absolutely necessary.
- **Access to monitoring equipment attached to the patient** Monitoring equipment is vital and must be accessible. An arm cuff used to monitor blood pressure throughout surgery, for example, should be accessible without disruption to the surgery in the event of a disconnection or a cardiovascular problem. Airway management, patient monitoring and the administration of anaesthesia all involve practices that continue throughout surgery. The anaesthetist must therefore be consulted before the patient is moved in any way, to ensure that anaesthetic practices are not disrupted. It is also necessary that the anaesthetist is aware of a change in position so that related physiological changes, such as a decrease in blood pressure, can be anticipated and expected and not cause alarm.

Patient safety

A final consideration in positioning, and one which is of prime importance, is that the patient should be safe and free from harm. This is vital, as the safety of an anaesthetized or unconscious patient is compromised in many ways:

• They cannot react to external stimuli, the reflexes are depressed and the muscles are paralysed. Positions used must therefore be safe and stable, and ensure that the patient does not fall.

• Their respiration may become obstructed by secretions or the tongue blocking the airway. Positions used must therefore be consistent with airway maintenance and access.

• They cannot move, and thus are at risk from pressure sore development. Positions used must therefore minimize potential pressure area damage.

• They have no joint mobility, and so ligaments, nerves and muscles are vulnerable. Positions used must avoid this.

• Their blood will pool in dependent areas, affecting both their circulation and their blood pressure. Positions used must minimize blood pooling, and patient movement must be slow enough to accommodate changes in circulating blood volume.

TECHNIQUES AND RESPONSIBILITIES IN POSITIONING

Self-transfer

A useful technique is for the patient to transfer themselves to the operating table whenever possible. This involves the theatre practitioner in the following:

• assessing whether the patient is able to self-transfer
• ensuring the self-transfer is safe, i.e. brakes are applied to both bed and trolley (or table), and the surfaces are at the same height
• instructing the patient how to transfer themselves
• observing the patient transferring, providing assistance if necessary.

Although this is obviously not suitable for the sedated or anaesthetized patient, it is helpful in many circumstances: when the patient is having a local anaesthetic, or has not received a premedication and is fully conscious, for example. This is common in day surgery units.

The advantages of self-transfer are that it allows the patient to find the most natural and comfortable position for themselves, and it minimizes patient handling and lifting for the staff.

Manual lifting

The majority of patient handling in the operating department will involve the manual lifting of the sedated, anaesthetized or unconscious patient.

Responsibilities

The responsibility for the safe handling and positioning of the patient lies with the theatre team. The responsibility for the correct final position lies with the surgeon, in conjunction with the anaesthetist.

There are many areas of care associated with correct and safe patient positioning which cannot be categorized as as either 'anaesthetic' or 'surgical' duties:

• preparation of equipment
• checking the operating table
• application of the indifferent or earthing electrosurgery electrode.

These always have been and will continue to be the theatre team's responsibility. It is therefore the responsibility of the team leader to identify and clarify who is to carry out these important aspects of patient care. This should avoid repetition while ensuring that vital tasks are performed.

The preparation of the operating table, attachments and any additional equipment, checking the operating table, application of the electrodes and assisting the anaesthetist and surgeon to position the patient should therefore be among the skills of all theatre practitioners.

PRINCIPLES OF PATIENT HANDLING AND TRANSFER

• The awake patient should be informed of any change necessary in their position.
• The patient should be allowed to transfer and position themselves whenever possible.

• The anaesthetist must be informed of any required movement of the patient.

• There must always be an adequate number of people to lift the patient.

• The anaesthetist should lift, or supervise the lifting of, the patient's head, in order to maintain the airway.

• The surgeon should lift any unstable or traumatized part of the patient, in order to observe and minimize damage.

• The patient should be lifted on an agreed signal or count from the team leader. This coordinates the lift and minimizes trauma to both patient and staff.

• The patient should be transferred gently to prevent physical injury.

• Patient monitoring and anaesthetic equipment should be reconnected with minimal delay.

PRINCIPLES OF PATIENT POSITIONING

The patient's position must be consistent with their vital functions of respiration and circulation. Bony prominences should be supported and cushioned whenever possible, in order to dissipate pressure and minimize pressure trauma. The patient should be covered as much as possible, for as long as possible. This serves to minimize heat loss and to provide them with as little loss of dignity as possible.

COMMONLY USED POSITIONS FOR SURGERY

The position used for surgery must allow good surgical and anaesthetic access, be consistent with vital functions, and mean the patient is safe and free from harm. There are many positions used for surgery, the most commonly used of which are supine, Trendelenburg, reverse Trendelenburg, lateral, prone and lithotomy. Each of these can be adapted to meet the specific needs of the patient, surgeon or anaesthetist.

Supine

This position is used for the transfer of all patients and for the administration for general anaesthesia in all patients, as well as being used for many operations. The patient lies flat on their back with the arms carefully positioned at their side, out on an arm board, or carefully folded and secured over the chest. The position is a fairly natural one for the patient and involves minimal disruption (Fig. 6.10). It is used for a wide variety of operations, including abdominal, breast and lower limb surgery.

Adaptations The supine position can be adapted easily to improve surgical access for many types of surgery, for example:

• the use of an arm board to allow access to the axilla for breast/axilla surgery
• the slight turn of the head to allow access to an eye, ear, side of the neck or head
• the abduction of a leg to allow access to the groin for varicose vein surgery.

Trendelenburg

This position involves a head-down tilt with the patient normally in the supine position. The extent of the tilt will vary between approximately 20° and a steeper tilt of 35–40° (Fig. 6.11).

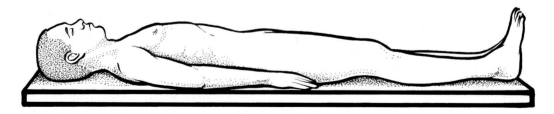

Figure 6.10 The supine position.

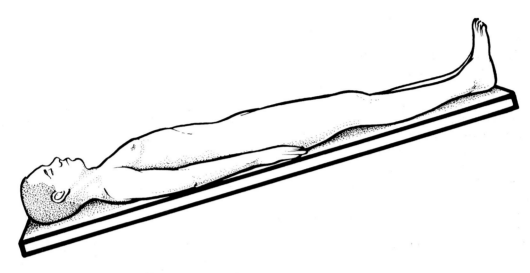

Figure 6.11 The Trendelenburg position.

The Trendelenburg position is commonly used for lower abdominal surgery, such as gynaecology. The benefit is that it allows the free contents of the abdominal cavity to fall under gravity towards the diaphragm and means that the area of surgery (the uterus, for example) is not obstructed in any way; surgical access is thus improved. It is also commonly used in surgery on the lower limb, such as varicose vein surgery, to reduce bleeding at the operative site.

Adaptations Varying degrees of tilt can be used as required. Also, the principle of the Trendelenburg position (allowing abdominal contents to fall away from the operative site) can be used in positions other than supine, for example the lithotomy position can be given a degree of Trendelenburg tilt, to assist in viewing the lower abdominal contents during a laparoscopy and dye procedures.

Reverse Trendelenburg

This involves tilting the operating table to place the patient (who is usually supine) in a head-up, foot-down position. It is used for head and neck surgery. The benefit of the position is that it allows good venous return from the operative area and creates a less vascular field. It is there-fore of benefit in neurological, thyroid and ear, nose and throat procedures, which involve surgery on very vascular structures.

Adaptations The degree of tilt can be adapted to the specific needs of the surgeon and anaesthetist, and the patient's particular physiology. If a large degree of tilt is required it is necessary to use a foot rest to prevent the patient slipping (Fig. 6.12).

Lateral

The lateral position involves carefully turning the anaesthetized patient on to their side, in order to allow good surgical access to the other side (Fig. 6.13). In order for the patient to be stable and safe, and to cause minimal physiological disturbance, the following features must be incorporated:

- The head must be supported.
- The dependent arm must be protected by a pad placed high in the underlying axilla.
- The upper arm must be supported on a special arm rest.
- The dependent iliac crest and bony prominence of the lower leg must be protected as much as possible to avoid pressure necrosis.

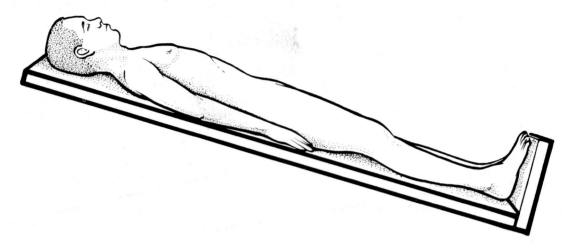

Figure 6.12 The reverse Trendelenburg position.

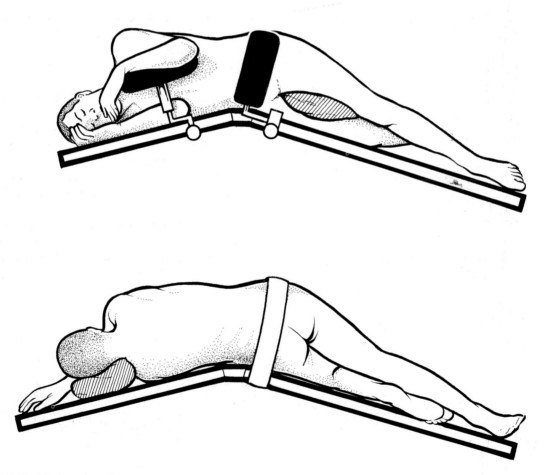

Figure 6.13 The lateral position.

- The legs should be protected with pillows in between them, and slightly bent to achieve stability.
- The pelvis and chest must be carefully stabilized with the use of special supports and table additions.

The lateral position is used for surgical access to the hip, kidney or thoracic cavity. More recently its use has increased in neurosurgery, for access to the cervical spine and posterior fossa, and to the lumbar spine for a microdiscectomy, an alternative to lumbar laminectomy. It is also used in a modified way for the administration of an epidural or spinal anaesthetic.

Adaptations These include variations in the flexion of the body – a large degree may be needed for renal surgery, for example, and a semilateral position may be used for hip surgery.

Great care is needed when using the lateral position in order to ensure that the patient is secure and safe from damage. The physiological effects of this position on the patient are dramatic, particularly within the cardiovascular and respiratory systems. The anaesthetic and airway management needs very careful planning and consideration, and at least three assistants are needed to help the anaesthetist position the patient. Further reading on this is recommended, and Anderton et al[1] provide excellent information on the physiology, hazards and care needed for the lateral position.

Prone

The prone position also needs great care to achieve, and has many physiological effects on the patient. Following the administration of general anaesthesia (and any other necessary procedures such as urinary catheterization) the patient is turned to lie on their front, with their back uppermost and the arms carefully positioned at their side, or raised upwards towards the head. The head is either carefully turned to one side, or positioned on a horseshoe ring (Fig. 6.14).

The prone position is used when surgical access is required to a posterior aspect of the body, such as a skin lesion on the back requiring plastic surgery. It is also used in neurosurgery as an approach to the spine, for the removal of a prolapsed intervertebral disc by a laminectomy, for example.

The position is achieved by a coordinated turn and must include the following:

- Head in as normal a position as possible.
- The face resting on the forehead only, and properly padded.
- The eyes must be completely free from pressure.
- The arms should be positioned above the head whenever possible.
- If surgical access to the head and neck is required, the arms should be positioned and secured at the patient's side
- Supports must be used to minimize pressure over bony prominences (such as knees and feet).
- The soft tissues such as the breasts and male genitalia must be carefully positioned to avoid pressure trauma; the breasts should be displaced laterally if large.

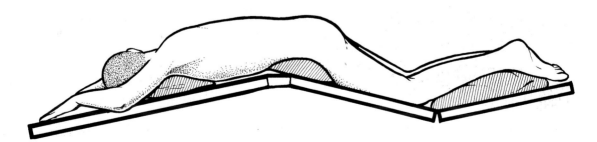

Figure 6.14 The prone position.

• A method of support must be used that will eliminate the possibility of mechanical pressure on the large blood vessels of the groin and abdomen. This is achieved by the use of a support which raises the patient above the table and exerts pressure only on bony prominences, or by a vacuum bead mattress.

Before turning the patient into the prone position the endotracheal tube must be totally secured to prevent accidental extubation, and the eyes must be carefully protected by protective shells and adhesive tape, or commercially available adhesive plasters.

Adaptations These can be made to improve surgical access by adjusting the operating table to flex the patient's legs or spine to the required degree. Other adaptations previously mentioned include the position of the head: either full face down on a horseshoe, or to the side; and the arms: above the head, or to the side. Anderton et al[1] provide excellent rationale for these adaptations and information on more extreme, but rare, adaptations. It is highly recommended further reading.

Lithotomy

The lithotomy position is achieved by lifting the patient's legs from the supine position upwards and outwards on to special supporting poles, which have canvas stirrups into which the patient's ankles are placed, thus providing good surgical access to the vagina, perineum, penis and rectum (Fig. 6.15). The knees and hips are flexed, and the hips abducted.

The lithotomy position is used for many surgical procedures, mainly gynaecological and urological: dilatation and curettage, laparoscopy, vaginal hysterectomy, cystoscopy, transurethral resection of the prostate and sigmoidoscopy, for example. It is also a common position in the UK for childbirth, despite the additional work against gravity it presents the mother with.

Moving the patient into the lithotomy position requires a minimum of the anaesthetist and two assistants, and is achieved as follows:

• The patient is placed on the operating table in the supine position.

• The arms are secured across the chest.
• The lithotomy poles are placed in position.
• The lumbar support may be placed in position.
• The patient is lifted on their canvas down the operating table, with their head and cervical spine supported by the anaesthetist.
• The legs are lifted together and the ankles placed in the canvas supports;
• The end of the table is removed or folded down.

Adaptations Adaptations of the lithotomy position may be necessary if the patient has arthritic or immobile joints and cannot achieve the position. It is essential that force is never used, but that the position is adapted by lowering the poles or using less abduction, for example.

The lithotomy position may also be adapted by adding a degree of Trendelenburg tilt (head down), thus allowing the abdominal contents to fall towards the diaphragm. This gives a good view of the reproductive organs and is thus very valuable for a laparoscopy and dye, for example, in which good vision is essential in order for the surgeon to diagnose any problems.

EFFECTS OF POSITIONING ON THE PATIENT

The more diverse a surgical position is the more extreme its effects on the patient will be. The more natural positions, such as supine, should be used whenever possible, to minimize the physiological disruption. The lateral, prone, lithotomy and more diverse positions (not discussed here) should be used with caution, and only when surgical access cannot be achieved in any other way. The more 'unnatural' positions present more challenges for anaesthetic and airway management, and have more dramatic physiological effects on the patient. The body systems most affected by the surgical position are the cardiovascular system, the respiratory system, nerves, muscles and joints, and the skin.

Cardiovascular system

Throughout the administration of anaesthesia and the surgical procedure there are many influ-

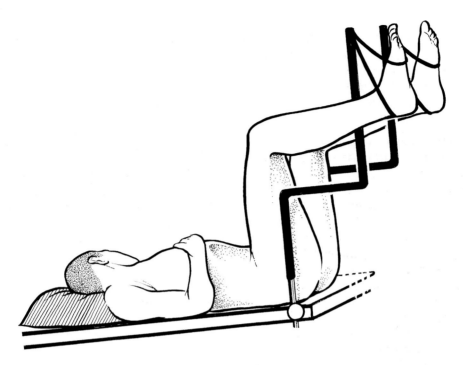

Figure 6.15 The lithotomy position.

ences on the patient's cardiovascular system. The specific effects of the surgical position include:

- Pooling of blood in dependent areas
- Impaired venous return from the lower half of the body due to atonal muscles and intermittent positive pressure ventilation
- Reduced cardiac workload in the supine position
- The physical effects of various positions on the major blood vessels of the body – the rotation of the neck may impede jugular drainage or vertebral artery supply if severe, for example, and the calf veins are compressed in the lithotomy position by the pressure of the pole on the leg
- Reduced circulating blood volume in the lithotomy position.

Respiratory system

The many effects of general anaesthesia and surgery on respiration include depression by drugs, and the mechanical disruption of the diaphragm by retraction, for example in liver surgery. The effects of the surgical position used include:

- Reduced blood flow to the uppermost lung in the lateral position
- The effect of the weight of the abdominal contents on the diaphragm in the supine, Trendelenburg and lateral positions, leading to impaired movement
- Reduced lung volume due to raised diaphragm in the supine, Trendelenburg and lateral positions
- Reduced lung volume in the dependent lung in the lateral position owing to the weight of the uppermost lung.

Nerves, muscles and joints

Positioning a patient so that the weight is borne through or stretches major nerves can have major postoperative effects, which may be either temporary or permanent. Nerve injuries may be caused by compression, traction, ischaemia or laceration.[2] Prevention of the first three is particularly important for theatre practitioners. Whichever position is used there is potential for nerve damage to occur, for example:

- Compression of the saphenous or lateral popliteal nerves caused by pressure from lithotomy poles
- Stretching of the brachial plexus of the upper arm if the head is not supported in the lateral position
- Pressure on the ulnar and radial nerves in the supine position if the arms are compressed on the mattress or screen support
- Pressure on the supraorbital nerve from the endotracheal tube connectors, as identified by Barrow,[3] or a badly fitting face mask
- Stretching of the brachial plexus of the upper arm caused by overextension of the arm on an arm board for breast or axilla surgery, in an adapted supine position (Fig. 6.16).

Muscles and joints are also greatly affected by the position used for surgery and the adjustments necessary to attain such positions. Strange aches, pains or sensations postoperatively may be worrying for the patient, and often the nurses on the surgical ward, who may not be aware of the position used for surgery and the effects of these positions on the muscles and joints, for example:

- Lack of support for the lumbosacral curve in the supine position may cause postoperative backache.
- Hyperextension injury to the knee can be caused when ankles are supported in the supine position.
- The cervical spine can be damaged when a patient is moved down the table to achieve the lithotomy position.
- Lack of support for the lumbosacral curve in the lithotomy position may cause postoperative backache.

Skin

The most traumatic effect of the surgical position on the patient's skin is that of necrosis due to pressure. The physiology of pressure sore devel-

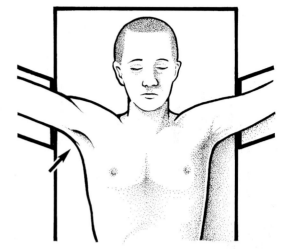

Arm extension should <u>not</u> exceed 90°

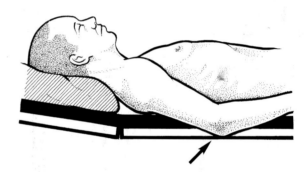

Figure 6.16 Incorrect positioning.

opment, the risk factors and the role of the theatre practitioner in the prevention of pressure sore development have already been discussed. It is, however, also necessary to consider pressure sore development in relation to the position used for surgery. Every position has potential pressure area problems; these can be illustrated by considering the supine, lateral and prone positions.

Supine position

The pressure areas at risk in this position are similar to those of concern to nurses in many hospital and community settings: the sacrum, coccyx and heels, owing to weight through these bony prominences. The patient in theatre has an additional problem, in that they cannot move at all, and thus further areas may be compromised, such as the head (occiput), scapulae, vertebrae and elbows (olecranon) (Fig. 6.17).

Lateral position

The pressure areas are at great risk in this position as the bony prominences are not used to weightbearing, and the position is often used for lengthy surgical procedures such as renal surgery and hip replacement. The areas of concern are therefore the shoulder (acromion), the hip (pelvic bones), knee (medial and lateral condyles) and ankle (malleolus) of the lowermost leg, and the knee and ankle of the uppermost leg. An area that must not be forgotten is the side of the head and the ear – a structure of cartilage and soft tissue not designed to be weightbearing. The results of prolonged pressure on the ear can include soreness and tingling postoperatively, to a necrotic pressure sore which may take many months to heal (Fig. 6.18).

Prone position

The exact areas of concern in the prone position will depend on the nature of the support used, and will essentially be those areas of weightbearing through bony prominences – the toes, knees (patella), pelvis, chest and shoulders (acromion process). Again the head is at risk, because of its own weight (approximately 10 lb), and the ear if the head is on its side. Soft tissues can also be at risk from pressure, and great care must therefore be taken with the positioning of the breasts and the external male genitalia to avoid pressure sore development in these vulnerable areas (Fig. 6.19).

HAZARDS OF PATIENT TRANSFER AND SURGICAL POSITION

Most hazards of surgical positioning relate to the cardiovascular and respiratory systems, the nerves, muscles, joints and skin, and have been identified and discussed above. Other hazards relate to incorrectly used equipment, faulty techniques and human error, and are thus preventable. The permutations of possible errors are numerous, but the following accidents are among those most likely to occur:

- 'whiplash' injury to the neck caused by incorrect patient position on the canvas
- injury to the lower limbs due to unstable lithotomy poles
- trauma from falling due to weak or faulty canvases or lifting aids
- trauma caused by unsupervised patient falling from the operating table
- trauma caused by the semiconscious patient falling from a theatre trolley, or from their bed in the postoperative recovery room
- trauma caused by part of the patient falling from the operating table – such as an arm or a leg
- injury from a canvas pole on the patient's elbow
- injury to the hip and/or lower back caused by not lifting the legs together into the lithotomy position

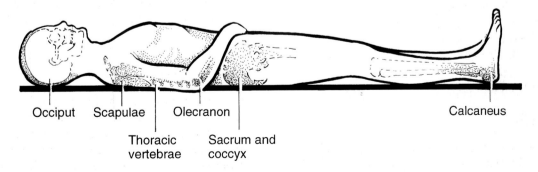

Occiput   Scapulae   Olecranon   Calcaneus

Thoracic   Sacrum and
vertebrae   coccyx

Figure 6.17 Pressure areas in the supine position.

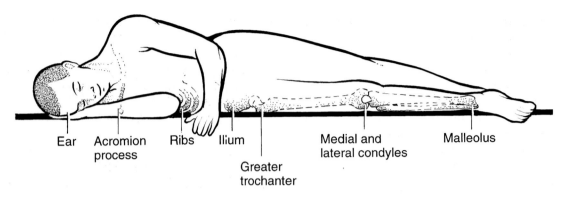

Figure 6.18 Pressure areas in the lateral position.

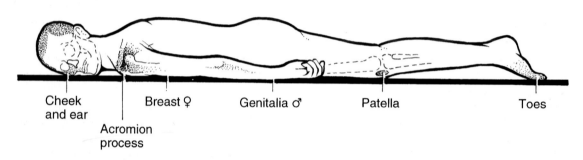

Figure 6.19 Pressure areas in the prone position.

- contact with metal causing electrosurgical burns
- trauma caused by stretching of drains, catheters and drips.

The following guidelines should therefore be used in conjunction with the principles for patient transfer and positioning discussed earlier, and should be an integral part of any operating department policy and practice:

- A designated person must be responsible for checking lifting aids, such as patient canvases.
- The patient must never be left unattended at any time.
- Guardrails or 'cot sides' must be used when transferring sedated, semiconscious and anaesthetized patients on trolleys or beds.
- All table attachments, such as lithotomy poles, must be checked once in position by a designated member of the theatre team.

- The patient must be checked for contact with metal before the surgical drapes are applied.
- One member of the lifting team must be responsible for the safe transfer of drips, drains and catheters, etc.
- The patient's legs must be lifted simultaneously into the lithotomy position.
- The patient's arms must be supported when poles are inserted into the canvas.

EQUIPMENT FOR POSITIONING AND TRANSFER

The basic equipment of bed, trolley and operating table must first be carefully checked by a designated theatre practitioner for the following:

- **Stability** – that it does not move when brakes are in the on position. A moving target can be detrimental when lifting, for both patient and staff. The operating table should also be stable, in that once a position is attained it is maintained. An operating table which loses height throughout surgery is a great inconvenience: it can mean the surgical team are operating at a lower than ideal height. It can also mean inaccurate physiological measurements are obtained – if the anaesthetist is measuring central venous pressure using manual apparatus, for example.

• **Provision of a tip-down position** – all beds, trolleys and the operating table must have a tip-down mechanism that is easily reached and quick to use. This may be necessary if the patient vomits, or has some other airway obstruction. It must therefore be in working order at all times, and all staff must be able to use it.

• **Facilities for emergency equipment** – the sedated, anaesthetized, unconscious or immediately postoperative patient is always dependent – on the anaesthetist, theatre practitioners and recovery room nurses. The trolleys and beds used for transfer to and from the operating department must therefore have the facility to accommodate emergency equipment in case there are airway problems: oxygen, tubing and mask, and airway adjuncts, such as a Guedel airway and Laerdel face mask. This equipment must also be present in both the operating theatre and anaesthetic room, and thus in close proximity to the operating table itself. Checking that these items are both present and in working order should be an integral part of every operating department's policy and working practices.

• **Cleanliness** – all surfaces used for patients must be clean before use, and provision made for their cleanliness to be maintained throughout the operating list. All theatre practitioners and those included in the transfer of the patient must be vigilant that any blood, vomit or fluids are cleaned away as soon as possible, to prevent cross-infection between patients.

Other equipment

There is a wide variety of equipment used in addition to the operating table to achieve the required position for surgery. All should be checked for cleanliness, stability, and that antistatic covers are intact before use. The range of equipment used will vary greatly according to the theatre specialty. Table 6.1 identifies items that are considered standard positioning equipment/table attachments, with their functions or common uses.

ROLE OF THE THEATRE PRACTITIONER

As identified earlier, the positioning of the patient for surgery is neither an 'anaesthetic' nor a 'surgical' duty, but an important area of care in which all theatre practitioners should be knowledgeable and competent. The following are essential skills:

• Checking the operating table and patient trolleys for safety, cleanliness and working order
• Lifting the patient using correct manual handling techniques, under the direction of the anaesthetist and the surgeon
• Preparation of the operating table and equipment for commonly used positions, such as those described in this chapter
• Alteration of the operating table position as required by the surgeon or anaesthetist. This must include
— brakes
— head tilt
— Trendelenburg and reverse Trendelenburg tilt height
which may all be needed in an emergency
• Providing the patient with as much dignity and warmth as possible
• Talking to the patient undergoing a local anaesthetic and explaining any positional changes to them
• Providing all aspects of pressure area care (see previous section)
• Checking the patient is correctly and safely positioned *before* the surgical drapes are applied, and this must include the following considerations:
— Is the canvas/sheet clean, smooth and dry?

— Is anaesthetic equipment such as ventilator tubing firmly attached and free from tension?
— Are all intravenous and other lines and catheters secure and free from tension?
— Is the return electrode (patient plate) correctly and securely applied?

Although these considerations and necessary actions must be within the skills of *all* theatre practitioners, it is good management sense for each operating department to identify *who* should routinely undertake these important aspects of patient care. The problem with something that is 'everyone's job' is that it is either done by everyone, thereby wasting time, or it is done by no-one, with far-reaching consequences. Operating department policy should therefore designate a particular person to undertake such duties.

Table 6.1 Standard equipment used for positioning the patient

Equipment/table attachment	Function/common use
Arm board	Extension of the arm for breast surgery or anaesthetic access
Leg board	Abduction of the legs during varicose vein surgery
Lithotomy poles	To support the legs for lithotomy position
Arm supports	To prevent patient's arms falling off the table in the supine position, for example
Vacuum bead (evacutable) mattress	To secure the patient in the exact position, and distribute weight evenly and widely
Horseshoe head ring	To attain head stability in the prone position and/or in neurosurgery
Ankle supports	To decrease pressure on the heel and enhance venous return in the calf
Foot board	To support patient's body weight and prevent slippage in the reverse Trendelenburg position
Pelvic, sacral and thoracic supports	To stabilize the patient in the lateral position
Pillows, pads and variously sized soft supports	To use as required to provide stability and distribute pressure

REFERENCES

1. Anderton J, Kean R, Neave R 1988 Positioning the surgical patient. Butterworths, London
2. Burge P 1990 Peripheral nerve injuries. Surgery 86: 2059–2063
3. Barrow D 1955 Supraorbital neuropraxia. Anaesthesia 10: 374

FURTHER READING

Groah D 1990 Positioning and draping. In: Operating room nursing perioperative practice. Appleton and Lange, Norwalk, Chapter 2
Miner D 1987 Patient positioning: applying the nursing process. AORN Journal 45: 1117–1127
Underwood M, Jameson J 1990 Preventing nerve injuries. Technic 83: 11–13

Ensuring that the patient has the correct operation

The responsibility for ensuring that the patient has the correct operation lies with the clinician, assisted by the theatre practitioner. Further reading on the issues relating to responsibility and accountability, and the ultimate responsibility of the surgeon, can be found in the section on medicolegal issues in Chapter 2. This is an area of great concern to all members of the team and also to the patient – incidents where the wrong operations have been performed invariably make headline news, and concern both healthcare professionals and public alike. Mistakes that lead to a patient undergoing the wrong operation include the following:

- operating list unclear or identifying the operation or side of operation incorrectly
- operating list unclear or incorrectly identifying exactly which digit or tooth (for example) to be operated on
- mistakes in the production of the operating list
- the patient's identity band being unclear, incorrect or missing
- the operation site being incorrectly marked
- abbreviations being used on the operating list
- patient being confused with a patient with the same or a similar name.

Errors can therefore occur at any stage of the hospital stay. Operating department managers, surgeons, anaesthetists and ward managers should consider every stage of the patient's admission, care before surgery and transfer to theatre in order to identify correct and fool-proof procedures at every stage. This should be clearly laid out in the form of a policy, procedure or clinical practice, and be available for all staff to read. Consideration should also be given to every stage of the production of the operating list, in order to ensure that errors do not occur here. Although it is not often possible to identify how and why human error occurs, it is possible to consider factors which may contribute to an incorrect operation being performed:

- late and frequent changes to the operating list after its original production
- staff at any stage working under pressure or with constant interruptions, e.g. admitting the patient, writing the list, typing the list, collecting the patient, etc
- no formal policy, clinical practice or procedure for sending patients to theatre and receiving them into theatre
- staff at any stage being unfamiliar with the patients and with correct policy.

Operating department managers and theatre practitioners must consider these and any other contributing factors that can be identified, and strive to remove or reduce them. For details of how to guard against the patient having the wrong operation see Box 6.1.

The general procedure for checking the patient must include the following:

- The patient is correctly labelled on admission with an identity band.
- The patient should be sent for by the nurse in charge of the theatre, by name and hospital number, and collected by a porter with these details in writing.
- The patient's identity, consent and necessary documentation must be checked by the ward nurse when the patient leaves the ward. Consent and all details must correspond exactly with those on the operating list.
- The patient's identity, consent and necessary documentation must be checked by a theatre practitioner, the operating surgeon and the patient's anaesthetist when the patient is received into the operating department. Consent and all details must correspond exactly with those on the operating list.
- The operating list, once produced, should not be altered except in exceptional circumstances and any alterations should be subject to strict procedural rules.

Box 6.1 Theatre safeguards.[1] Reproduced with permission.

The correct patient and the correct operation

Safeguards

1. The patient should be identified in the anaesthetic room by the full name and hospital number on the identity bracelet. Questioning the premedicated patient is undesirable and unreliable, particularly with children. An additional check should be made against the theatre list.

    The consent form is a valuable additional documentary check on the identity of the patient, the type of operation proposed and the site and side of the body. Always check it in the anaesthetic room.

2. The person sending for the patient has the responsibility for ensuring that the correct patient has been brought into the anaesthetic room or the operating theatre. The anaesthetist should check the consent form and examine the other records accompanying the patient before giving any anaesthetic to make sure that they relate to that patient.

3. In cases where a patient is to have a spinal or epidural anaesthetic rather than a general anaesthetic, and if no anaesthetist is present, the practitioner who is to perform the operation or to carry out the examination should be responsible for ensuring that the correct patient has been brought for operation and that the correct side, limb or digit is identified.

4. It is the surgeon's duty to see the patient before he is anaesthetized and to make sure that the accompanying documents relate to that patient. If the surgeon cannot personally examine the patient's clinical records before the start of the anaesthetic he should delegate this responsibility to the surgical assistant.

5. Before beginning the operation, the surgeon or the assistant should check that the patient's full name, hospital number, and date of birth and the nature of the operation, as set out on the operation list, correspond with the entries in the clinical notes and on the identity bracelet.

6. The operation list should be drawn up by a member of the surgical team and should indicate the nature and site of the proposed operation. Operation lists should be altered as little as possible and never by telephone. Authorization must be by the responsible clinician in conjunction with the nurse in charge of the theatre. Any alteration of the operation list should be made on every relevant copy by a person to whom the task is specifically delegated and notified to the anaesthetist.

7. In each case, all the forenames and the hospital number should be recorded legibly and used for identification purposes. Underline the surname to avoid doubt.

8. Write references to the procedure or site in full. Avoid abbreviations – especially 'l' and 'r'.

9. Use the word 'right' only to indicate the side of operation.

10. The site of the operation should be marked by a member of the surgical team before the patient arrives in the theatre if possible. An indelible skin pencil should be used.

11. To avoid ambiguity about the digit on which the operation is to be performed, fingers should be described as: thumb, index, middle, ring and little, and not as: thumb, first, second, third and fourth.

    Toes should be described as: hallux for big, second third, fourth and fifth or little.

    To avoid confusion arising from the palm facing up or down, the surgeon and nurse should check on the positioning of the hand before the operation.

Admission, labelling and ward procedure

Safeguards

1. Label all patients admitted for operative procedures immediately on admission.

2. It is the responsibility of the nurse in charge of the accident and emergency department to label each unconscious patient admitted through the department. Identity bracelets are the most reliable means of labelling unconscious patients.

    The identity bracelet should be of a reliable design and should bear the patient's full name, hospital number and date of birth. Identity bracelets for children should be child-proof.

    If the identity bracelet is removed from a patient for any reason, take special care to ensure that no mistake is made about his identification. His name can be written in indelible ink on his skin.

3. Deal with day patients who are to undergo operative procedures in the same way as in-patients and label them properly.

4. The nurse in charge of the theatre or a specifically designated person should be responsible for sending for the patient with the agreement of the anaesthetist. Send for patients by name and number only, and never, for example, as the 'next patient'. Where it is the practice for a porter from the theatre to collect the patient from the ward, he should take with him a legible note of the full name and hospital number of the patient.

5. The senior ward nurse should be responsible for checking that all patients who are to undergo operations have been properly labelled and are dispatched correctly, accompanied by the correct documents.

6. Using a skin marker, label the side and site of operation where appropriate.

ROLE OF THE THEATRE PRACTITIONER

1. The theatre practitioner must be familiar with and understand the recommended practice for ensuring that the patient has the correct operation, as identified in the *Theatre Safeguards*.[1]*

2. The theatre practitioner should ensure that operating department policy is based on the recommended practice in *Theatre Safeguards*.[1]

3. The theatre practitioner must ensure that all patients are checked in accordance with *Theatre Safeguards* (see Box 6.1),[1] and that the correct patient is brought into the anaesthetic room.

4. The theatre practitioner must ensure that the person who checks the patient into the department, or takes any other steps to ensure the patient has the correct operation, documents this and signs any necessary documentation.

5. The theatre practitioner must ensure that the surgeon and anaesthetist both check the patient and the necessary documents before the patient is anaesthetized.

6. The theatre practitioner must ensure that adequate time is allowed for all checking procedures, and that checks are conducted in a calm and professional manner, with no interruptions. No theatre practitioner, anaesthetist or surgeon should ever become blasé about the possibility of the wrong operation being performed.

7. The theatre practitioner should teach junior colleagues and learners the correct checking procedures, and assist in teaching medical staff, and insist that all learners understand the correct procedures.

8. Local operating department policy should identify the following:

- Who exactly may undertake reception of the patient?
- What exactly is to be asked directly of the patient, and what can be established from the ward nurse? This is important, as the premedicated patient should not be questioned repeatedly. It may be acceptable for the patient's 'nil by mouth' time,

false/loose teeth and any allergies, for example, to be established from the documents or from the ward nurse. *This must be clearly identified in local policy.*

- The procedure to follow when a discrepancy is found when checking the patient into the operating department. This should identify the following actions:
  — ensure ward nurse remains with the patient to provide comfort and reassurance
  — communicate directly with the theatre practitioner in charge, surgeon or anaesthetist regarding the discrepancy
  — reassure the patient and provide explanation once the necessary action has been decided on
  — inform the person in charge of the department, the ward nurse and the theatre receptionist if any subsequent changes to the operating list are necessary, and ensure that lists in theatre and anaesthetic rooms are changed
  — liaise with ward staff and medical staff in order to reduce problems occurring in future if possible.

The theatre practitioner should be aware that the premedicated patient should not sign a consent form, as they are under the influence of drugs – the value of their written consent is therefore questionable (see section on consent in Chapter 2).

9. The theatre practitioner must ensure that all staff are aware of *Theatre Safeguards*[1] and local operating department policy, and exactly what they are checking and why, i.e. that they have established the patient's identity, and that consent and other documents correspond exactly with the operating list.

10. If any member of the team is unsure of any patient or list details at any time they must voice this concern, and establish that the correct procedure is being undertaken. If a wrong operation is performed the theatre practitioner must document this according to hospital policy, including an incident form. Staff should have the support of their manager, and a trade union or professional body representative to assist them with the necessary documentation and subsequent inquiries.

Theatre Safeguards is due to be updated in 1998

11. The theatre practitioner should ensure that a clearly legible operating list is present in theatre at all times during the session. One must also be available in the anaesthetic room, with the theatre receptionist and on all the relevant wards. If a written list is not available, surgery should wait until medical staff supply one.

REFERENCES

1. Medical Defence Union 1988 Theatre safeguards. Medical Defence Union, Medical Protection Society, Medical Defence Union of Scotland, National Association of Theatre Nurses, Royal College of Nursing, London

Swabs, needles or instruments being retained in the wound after surgery

This is a very real problem and an area of great concern to all members of the surgical team. It is also of great concern to patients, that something might be 'left inside', and thus is a major issue in patient care. The effects of a foreign body retained in a surgical wound will vary according to what the item is, where it is retained, and the general condition of the patient. It may cause any of the following, for example:

- slow or delayed wound healing
- irritation, discomfort or pain at the wound site
- referred pain in another area of the body
- infection of the wound
- infection of a body cavity, e.g. peritonitis.

This last may have a detrimental effect on the patient, especially if they are unwell for other reasons, and can be a contributing factor if the patient should die.

Almost any item used in a surgical procedure can be retained in a wound, although the most common are:

- swabs
- scalpel blades or fragments of blades
- needles from non-traumatic sutures, or loose needles
- screws, or detachable parts of instruments.

For information on the responsibility and accountability of members of the surgical team the theatre practitioner must read the section on medicolegal issues relating to the operating department, in Chapter 2.

This section will outline the recommended practice for swab, needle and instrument counts, produced by all professional bodies concerned with operating theatres,[1] on which all department policies should be based, and identify the role of the theatre practitioner in relation to counts.

PERFORMING COUNTS

The theatre practitioner will quickly become familiar with the term 'swab count', and when these are carried out. It must be understood, however, that every item used in an operation must be counted, as any of them can be retained. This therefore includes:

- swabs
- blades
- instruments
- atraumatic and loose needles
- hypodermic needles
- bulldogs
- tapes
- slings
- screws/nuts/any detachable instrument parts
- items used to hold instruments together, e.g. rubber bands.

For details of how to perform counts see *Theatre Safeguards*[1] and the following section for how to put these safeguards into practice.

- Use of appropriate cleaning fluids
- Disposal of linen and clinical waste in the correct way, using appropriate bags as identified by local policy and national guidelines.

Preoperative patient care

- Bath/shower
- Gown/shave/hair removal
- Specific preparation, e.g. bowel preparation
- Skin preparation.

Staff/management

- Occupational health guidelines and support relating to staff presence in the operating theatre – with colds or infective lesions, for example
- Provision of clothing for use in the operating theatre only: hats, theatre suit and footwear
- Correct use and disposal of face masks
- Correct use of protective clothing. Aprons, gloves (sterile and non-sterile), gowns and eye protection must be available and worn according to the risk of the clinical situation, with regard to universal precautions and staff safety
- Hand washing – correct hand washing is essential in the prevention of infection in all areas of the hospital, including the operating department. Theatre practitioners must be aware of correct hand-washing techniques, and when hand washing is required. This is separate from scrubbing up, and includes hand washing by anaesthetic, circulating and recovery personnel
- Safe handling and disposal of sharps in the anaesthetic room, operating theatre and recovery room
- Written operating department policies should be available in every theatre, which include infection control practices as outlined above. They should be written by a multidisciplinary team in liaison with other experts within the hospital, such as pharmacy (cleaning fluids), infection control and microbiology (use of masks/clothing/waste disposal), and engineering (maintenance programmes).

Aseptic technique

- Correct scrubbing-up procedure
- Correct gowning procedure
- Correct gloving procedure
- Maintenance of aseptic technique by the scrub practitioner
- Close observation for any breaks in sterility by both scrub and circulating theatre practitioners
- Correct draping procedure
- Safe handling and disposal of sharps into an approved sharps container
- Single-use items to be used once only, and not resterilized.

OTHER DEPARTMENTS

Housekeeping/hotel services Domestic/cleaning staff are employed by the housekeeping departments of most hospitals. The theatre practitioner must liaise with this department to ensure that operating theatre cleaning is performed as and when required, and is of an adequate standard.

Ward staff Ward staff are responsible for the preoperative care of the patient, and the theatre practitioner must liaise with them in relation to any problems or difficulties – patients being inadequately prepared for theatre, for example.

Engineering The engineering department is a vital link in the prevention of infection, by providing, monitoring and maintaining adequate ventilation systems within the theatre suite. The theatre practitioner should be aware of the monitoring procedures, and who to contact with any problems.

Infection control nurse The infection control nurse is an excellent resource and the theatre practitioner should contact him or her for advice on any patient problem or disease with which they are not familiar. They are also involved with monitoring the spread of infection in the hospital, and may be involved in investigating infections which appear to originate from the operating department. The infection control nurse would be an essential member of the policy team of the operating department in relation to infection control policies.

Microbiology/bacteriology The microbiologist will be able to advise on the treatments and precautions necessary for patients with rare conditions. They will also be able to help with policy/practice decisions by assisting the theatre practitioner to evaluate the clinical research available on controversial topics such as the use of face masks and length of scrubbing-up time.

Sterilizing and disinfecting services The theatre practitioner should be aware of the working of this department, especially relating to the turnaround time of instruments, the method of checking the expiry date of instruments, and quality control mechanisms to check that autoclaves are working correctly.

Occupational health This department can advise on particular staff problems in relation to infection control and needlestick injuries. They should be involved in policy making in the operating department as appropriate.

FURTHER READING

Ayliffe G, Collins B, Taylor L 1990 Hospital acquired infection. Butterworth-Heinemann, Oxford, Chapters 5 and 16
Gould D 1994 Infection control in high risk environments. Nursing Standard 8: 57–61
Royal College of Nursing 1994 Guidance on infection control in hospitals. Royal College of Nursing, London
Ross C 1994 What cost ritual? British Journal of Theatre Nursing 4: 11–14

Taylor M 1993 Universal precautions in the operating department. British Journal of Theatre Nursing 2: 4–7
Taylor M, Quick A 1994 MRSA in the operating department. British Journal of Theatre Nursing 3: 4–7
Walker A, Donaldson B 1993 Dressing for protection. Nursing Times 89: 60–62
Walsh M, Ford P 1989 Nursing rituals – research and rational actions. Butterworth-Heinemann, Oxford

7

Recovery practice

J. Sharp

As part of the operating department the recovery room provides facilities for the care of the highly dependent postoperative patient. Operational policies will determine the extent of this service, including at what stage patients are transferred to the ward or other high-dependency units. These times vary according to clinical need and practice: in some situations patients remain in the recovery room for several hours and will be maintained on life support, including respiratory ventilation.

The area should be light to allow observation of the patient's pallor and well ventilated to reduce the concentration of exhaled anaesthetic gases. If children and those with special needs, including the very old or people with learning disabilities, are to be nursed there should an area where the parent, guardian or carer may be with the patient during the recovery process. Further design considerations for recovery rooms are discussed in Chapter 8.

This section will outline basic principles of recovery room practice, including aspects of patient care planning and implementation.

Equipment

As part of daily routine all essential equipment is checked, clean and ready for use. Equipment required for each bed space is as follows:

- oxygen outlet, flowmeters, tubing
- fixed and variable-performance oxygen masks, nasal catheters and prongs
- t-piece attachment for use with laryngeal mask or endotracheal tubes
- syringe to deflate cuffs of laryngeal mask or endotracheal tube
- suction unit with a supply of suitable catheters and Yankauer ends
- a range of oropharyngeal and nasopharyngeal airways
- selection of swabs, adhesive tape, dental rolls, mouthcare pack, syringes, needles and cannulae
- vomit bowl, tissues
- gloves
- waste bin
- sharps disposal bin
- bin for reusable contaminated equipment
- Mapleson C breathing system or self-inflating bag with face mask
- ECG monitor, electrodes and recording paper;
- pulse oximeter
- sphygmomanometer and stethoscope or automatic blood pressure measuring equipment. A full range of cuff sizes should be available.

The following equipment should be easily accessible:

- intubation equipment, laryngoscope, various blade sizes, fibreoptic laryngoscope, tracheal tubes and introducers
- anaesthetic machine with ventilator and disconnection alarm
- intravenous infusion sets and cannulae, including central venous lines and manometers
- transducer equipment for invasive monitoring

- blood warmer
- pressure infusion bag
- Wright's respirometer
- bronchoscope
- cricothyroid puncture set
- tracheostomy set
- chest drain
- infusion pumps for administering drugs
- glucometer
- thermometer suitable for recording subnormal temperatures
- blood gas syringe (preheparinized)
- tubes for haematology
- peripheral nerve stimulator
- insulation blanket
- electric fan
- defibrillator.

Drugs for use in emergency situations:

- cardiac arrest
  — adrenaline
  — atropine
  — bretylium tosylate
  — calcium
  — lignocaine
  — sodium bicarbonate
- reintubation
  — Suxamethonuim;
- anaphylaxis
  — antihistamine, i.e. diphenylhydramine
  — adrenaline
  — hydrocortisone
- Malignant hyperpyrexia
  — Dantrolene
- full range of crystalloids and colloid solutions.

Miscellaneous equipment:

- clock with sweep hand clearly visible
- cupboard for controlled drugs and other drugs
- refrigerator for drugs
- screen to offer privacy when carrying out nursing care
- torch.

Additional equipment required is a paediatric trolley with a full range of equipment appropriate for the clinical management and resuscitation of children of all ages.

CARE OF EQUIPMENT AND FABRIC OF ROOM

The equipment will need to be serviced regularly by engineers in order to ensure safety. Planned preventative maintenance policies should be agreed and documented according to manufacturers' recommendations and strictly adhered to.

All practitioners should know how the equipment functions and is maintained, how to report a fault and who is responsible for repairing it.

- Know your equipment.
- Know your hospital policy.

All surfaces and equipment should be checked and damp dusted on a daily basis.

Patients should be transported to the recovery room on a bed. Beds brought to the recovery room from the wards or theatre should be:

- clean, with clean linen
- adjustable height
- with facilities for attachment, such as infusion pole, back rest, cot sides, traction
- with head-down tilt/foot elevation
- with locking wheels
- with a comfortable, easily cleanable mattress
- with a fire blanket, for possible evacuation of patient on mattress.

General considerations

All staff who work in recovery rooms must be educated and trained to the highest professional standard so that they can provide optimum care for patients and respond to the potentially life-threatening circumstances that may arise at any moment.

A basic understanding of anatomy, physiology and pharmacology relevant to anaesthetic and surgical procedures must be supplemented by practical training in airway management and resuscitation. A full understanding of monitoring requirements and equipment, as well as nursing of patients in a range of specialties, is mandatory.

Formal assessment to agreed standards should be made during and at the completion of training. Progress should be documented and deficiencies identified and promptly rectified. Assessment should cover knowledge and understanding as well as practical competence.

All staff should participate in regular in-service training and education to keep them proficient in skills which are used infrequently where appropriate and with agreed policies.

Specialized skills should be made available to staff:

- defibrillation
- intravenous drugs administration
- topping up of established epidurals
- assessment of the extent of the areas of anaesthesia following regional anaesthetic techniques
- preparation and use of patient-controlled analgesia equipment.

Post-basic courses in anaesthetic (ENB182) and operating department (ENB183) nursing provide training.

Training can be reinforced by rotating staff through areas such as intensive care, respiratory and coronary care units.

PATIENT CARE IN THE RECOVERY ROOM

Care planning is part of the process which assures individualized patient care. It also provides a means of documenting care throughout the patient's stay in hospital. A nursing care plan has four main elements:

- assessment
- planning
- implementation
- evaluation.

Assessment/planning

As part of care planning recovery nurses should visit patients preoperatively, using this time to talk and give information and to listen in order to identify individual needs. The practitioner should encourage patients to talk through their problems and fears. The visit will initiate assessment and planning as the nurse is able to establish orientation, emotional state, mobility, vision, hearing and any communication problems.

Following the arrival of the patient in the recovery room it is necessary to make an initial assessment to plan the care needed. Below is a format that is very easy to remember and which encompasses most of the activities relevant to the acute stage of recovery:

- A = Airway
- B = Breathing
- C = Conscious state, Circulation, Comfort and Cold
- D = Drips, Drains, Drugs
- E = Environment
- F = Feel the patient.

Although a framework is provided for care plans there is room to be flexible so that the care plan becomes relevant to the area and is individualized for the patient. An example care plan is shown in Appendix 4.

Implementing

The practitioner should be competent to carry out the care that has been planned. Assistance may be required to give the patient complete care.

Evaluating

The care is then evaluated and it should be evident whether it is adequate or whether a further course of action is needed.

TRANSFER OF THE PATIENT TO THE RECOVERY ROOM

Recovery staff should be given the following information:

- patient's name and age (check this against notes and identity bracelet)
- surgical procedure and name of surgeon
- brief summary of the patient's condition, including pre-existing disease
- any potential airway or circulatory problems and state of dentition
- type of anaesthetic given
- details of vital signs
- details of analgesia/antiemetics and anticipated needs
- antibiotics given and when next dose is due
- blood loss
- fluids given and future requirements
- urine output
- significant preoperative factors, such as problems with communications or emotional state
- monitoring required
- postoperative orders, including oxygen therapy investigation required.

The recovery practitioner is handed the anaesthetic record, prescription sheet and fluid chart along with the theatre care plan notes and X-rays.

Before the practitioner takes responsibility for the patient they should check the whereabouts of the anaesthetist in case they need to make contact urgently. If the documentation is in order and the practitioner is competent to take over the responsibility of care, the anaesthetist may leave the recovery room.

The handover to recovery staff will include:

- the operation performed
- skin closure and dressings
- care and placement of drains/catheters
- special nursing requirements, such as patient positioning
- documentation signed.

THE IMMEDIATE RECOVERY PERIOD

Continuous individual observation is required on a one-to-one basis until the patient is able to maintain his or her own airway. Remember to follow the format A, B, C, D, E, F when making an initial assessment.

Airway/breathing

On accepting the care of the patient the practitioner should assess the patient's airway and breathing. This should include how the patient is breathing, the depth and rate, the use of artificial airways, the patient's colour, whether the breathing is noisy, denoting partial obstruction or spasm, and the oxygen saturation. From this the practitioner can plan and implement the necessary care. The patient should be nursed on their side or supine, depending on the anaesthetist's or surgeon's instructions or whether there is a laryngeal mask in place. Occasionally a patient may be brought to the recovery room in a sitting position. Stability must be ensured and access to the patient's head maintained.

• On observation the patient should look well perfused, although those who have undergone major surgery may look pale, but should not look cyanosed.

• The patient's head should be at the correct end of the bed or trolley to facilitate head-down tilt should this become necessary.

• The breathing should be regular, with no signs of labouring, and respirations will be approximately 10–24 per minute, unless there is any underlying cause to depart from this.

• The chest should rise and fall with both sides expanding evenly; there should not be a rocking motion.

• The breathing should be quiet; this may be confirmed by feeling expired breath on the back of the hand.

• If the patient is shivering oxygen consumption will increase.

• Suctioning of the airways may be required: take care during this procedure to be gentle, to prevent mucosal damage and laryngeal spasm.

• If the unconscious patient vomits postoperatively they should be turned immediately into a lateral position, the head tilted down and suction applied if necessary. If the patient is awake, sit them up and offer a vomit bowl and tissues. Stay with the patient.

• Some patients may require jaw support in order to prevent airway obstruction by the tongue. Pull the jaw forward with the fingers at the angle of the jaws just under the ears to prevent obstruction. It is important that this is done cautiously in patients who may have arthritic necks. Sometimes the use of a cervical collar will prevent injury (Fig. 7.1).

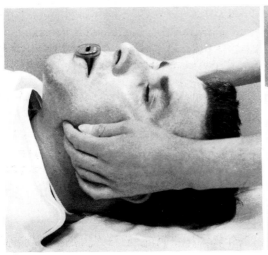 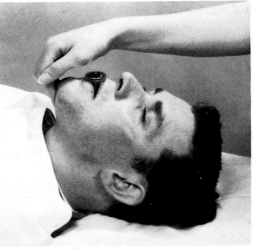

A   B

Figure 7.1 Maintaining the airway in an unconscious patient. A. The fingers are placed behind the angle on each side of the jaw, and are lifted slightly forwards. B. Alternatively, the chin can be lifted forward.

The recovery practitioner must always stay at the patient's head until they are conscious and can maintain their own airway.

Communication will be important as the patient is waking: it should be remembered that hearing is the first sense to return in the recovering patient.

OXYGEN THERAPY

Various methods of delivering oxygen are described below.

The Hudson mask This is a clear plastic mask shaped to fit the face. The flow of oxygen determines the percentage given, as follows:

- 2 litres/minute = 28%
- 4 litres/minute = 40%
- 6 litres/minute = 60%.

The mask may be used with Venturi valves, which allow the delivery of specified concentrations of oxygen. Postoperatively oxygen concentrations of 40% are usually prescribed, but these may be higher or lower according to the patient's need.

MC mask This is a clear plastic mask with a sponge protection around the area that contacts the face, designed to be comfortable for the patient.

Nasal catheters and prongs Small catheters with sponge protection which are placed in one nostril, or prongs which consist of two nasal tubes fixed in place around the patient's ear. These methods of delivering oxygen may be better tolerated than masks, but should not be used if a Guedel airway is in place as flows will be inadequate, or if high concentrations of oxygen are required as humidification will not be achieved.

Endotracheal tubes, Guedel airways and laryngeal masks The functions and uses of these artificial airways have been described in Chapter 4. Practical aspects of their management are described below.

- *Guedel airways* Used postoperatively to maintain a clear airway in the recovering patient; may be left *in situ* until the patient rejects the device. The airway should be monitored: if there are signs of laryngeal spasm it may be necessary to withdraw the airway slightly to prevent irritation of the larynx or cords. The airway may be used in combination with a mask or endotracheal tube, and suctioning of bronchial secretions may be carried out through the tube or airway with a fine catheter (Fig. 7.2).

- *Laryngeal masks* The patient may be returned to the recovery room with a laryngeal mask; when they regain consciousness they will normally gag on the mask, at which time the cuff should be deflated prior to removal.

- *Endotracheal tubes* The patient may be returned to recovery with an endotracheal tube in place. Prior to removal the cuff must be deflated and the patient be breathing spontaneously.

Following the removal of any artificial airways oxygen may be administered by mask until saturation levels are within normal limits. When breathing and saturation levels are satisfactory oxygen therapy may be discontinued. The patient should be observed for at least 15 minutes to ensure that oxygen saturation levels remain at 94% or above (see Pulse oximetry below). If this is not achieved the anaesthetist may prescribe the continuation of oxygen therapy during transfer and until the patient improves in the ward.

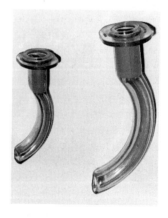

Figure 7.2 Guedal airways (7 and 12 mm, pvc).

Some basic nursing points:

- Sit the patient up if possible.
- Encourage the patient to cough and to take deep breaths.

Postoperative hypoventilation or airway obstruction may be caused by:

- central nervous system depression caused by anaesthetic agents
- depression of respiratory muscles caused by muscle relaxants used in anaesthesia
- airway obstruction caused by mucous secretions, laryngeal oedema or obstruction by the tongue.

These are recognized by:

- slow or shallow respirations
- audible gurgling respirations
- wheezing respirations
- auscultation
- cyanosis, restlessness, rapid pulse rate.

Pulse oximetry

This electronic monitor provides continuous non-invasive measurement of the patient's blood oxygen saturation levels (SaO_2) by measuring the absorption of selected wavelengths of light through living tissue. The monitor usually includes a photoelectric plethysmograph which measures peripheral blood flow and displays this as a pulse rate. Pulse oximetry will provide early warnings of hypoxia and may be used to ensure adequate oxygenation during procedures such as intubation.

Saturations are measured through a light probe which clips gently to a finger, earlobe or, in some cases, adheres to the nose. The probes will not record satisfactorily if nail polish is worn or if there is excessive movement.

Oxygen saturation measurements should be above 96% when the patient is receiving oxygen and not less than 94% when not.

Cardiovascular monitoring

Pulse

The pulse should be monitored regularly to check the rate, depth and regularity. Variations may be caused by shock, medication, or raised intracranial pressure. The depth of the pulse will indicate whether or not the patient has a good cardiac output; an irregular pulse may be a sign of cardiovascular disease. Checks on peripheral pulses will be necessary following vascular surgery, for example the dorsalis pedis pulse after femoral popliteal surgery.

Blood pressure

The recording of blood pressure is an important aspect in monitoring the progress of the recovering patient. There are two main methods of recording blood pressure: invasive or direct, or non-invasive.

Invasive methods Cannulae are placed in a peripheral artery and vein – usually the radial, although in some cases the femoral artery may be selected. The cannulae are attached to transducers which convert the internal vessel pressure into a waveform or digital display on a monitor.

Central venous pressure monitoring Central venous cannulation involves catheterizing the superior or inferior vena cava via a large peripheral vein to record pressure within the vena cava or right atrium. The catheter may be inserted directly or, if intended to remain *in situ* for long periods, may be tunnelled beneath the skin. Tunnelling is a precaution against infection entering from the skin site. Triple-lumen catheters are used if the patient requires continuous monitoring and therapy. Central venous catheterization is performed for the following reasons:

- central venous pressure (CVP) monitoring
- intravenous fluids, blood or blood products administration
- to provide long-term venous access
- administration of drugs, including cytotoxics
- parenteral feeding.

CVP may be measured by a manometer, which is a calibrated column of fluid for measuring pressure; the set-up is described in Chapter 4. The catheter may also be attached to a transducer and readings displayed on a monitor.

The normal pressure range is 3–10 cmH$_2$O; high CVP readings indicate fluid overload or cardiac dysfunction, low readings suggest a reduction in blood volume.

Non-invasive methods A sphygmomanometer is used for recording blood pressure. This consists of a hand-pumped inflating cuff attached to a calibrated column of mercury. The cuff is placed on the arm and secured above the antecubital fossa or on the leg above the popliteal fossa. Care must be taken to ensure correct positioning, both for access and to prevent peripheral nerve damage. The cuff should be 20% wider than the diameter of the limb used, and the patient should be advised to straighten the limb during inflation. The cuff should not be positioned on a limb that is used for intravenous infusion as this can cause reflux of the fluid into the giving set.

Electrical devices which automatically read the blood pressure and record this on a display are recommended. This equipment uses a cuff in the same way as a sphygmomanometer and similar precautions should be taken as outlined above.

Electrocardiograph

The electrocardiogram (ECG) records the electrical currents associated with cardiac contraction. These are conducted via electrodes fixed to the patient's skin and are then amplified electronically and displayed as a trace on a monitor. The use and functions of ECG are further described in Chapter 4.

The wound

Wound dressings should be observed for signs of postoperative bleeding: if there is seepage then a pressure dressing should be applied over the original dressing. Swelling may occur and is an indication of haematoma; any concerns must be reported to the surgeon.

The location and type of wound drain should be noted; accurate observations of fluid or blood loss, in both volume and rate, should be recorded.

COMMUNICATION

When the patient regains consciousness they should be reassured and told that the operation is complete, where they are and what time it is. The patient may find communication difficult but the sound of the practitioner's voice will be reassuring. Some patients may become confused or aggressive: the practitioner must react in a non-confrontational manner, offering continued support and reassurance.

The most important causes of confusion are cerebral hypoxia, hypoglycaemia, electrolyte imbalance and medications, especially benzodiazepines.

SLEEP AND REST

The patient should be allowed to sleep after consciousness has been regained. Noise levels in the recovery area should be minimized to encourage this.

ORAL FLUIDS

Many recovering patients will complain of a dry mouth. If the swallowing reflex is present and there are no contraindications resulting from the surgery, sips of water or moist sponge sticks may be offered. If drinks are not allowed it will be necessary to assess the condition of the mouth and carry out mouthcare if required. Dentures will have been removed preoperatively: unless there are clinical reasons these may be given to the patient as soon as their condition is stable.

Patients may vomit or feel nauseated; this could be caused by pain, or by the opiates used in pain relief. Antiemetics should be used to alleviate nausea and vomiting.

Nasogastric tubes are usually used following gastrointestinal and other major surgery. They should be secured to the patient's nose, taking care to avoid undue pressure on the nares. If nausea is felt by the patient relief may be achieved by aspiration. All aspirate should be recorded on the fluid balance chart.

INTRAVENOUS THERAPY

Intravenous therapy will depend on several clinical factors, including the patient's general condition, the nature of the operation and blood loss during surgery. Fluid replacement regimens will have been prescribed but these may need adjusting if the patient shows symptoms of hypovolaemia or circulatory overload. In hypovolaemia these are:

- pallor
- weak thready pulse, increased rate
- cold extremities
- collapsed veins
- falling blood pressure
- oliguria
- thirst.

In circulatory overload they are:

- distended veins
- a full, bounding pulse
- increasing blood pressure
- tachycardia
- breathlessness.

The intravenous cannula site should be checked to ensure there is no regress and that it is secured to the skin. Flushing should be carried out antiseptically; air should not be allowed to enter the line.

Commonly prescribed fluids are:

- Ringer lactate (Hartmann's solution)
- dextrose 4% with saline 0.18%
- 0.9% saline
- dextrose 5% in water
- plasma expanders
- blood and blood products.

To calculate the infusion rate use the number of drops per millilitre for the giving set used and apply the following formula:

$$\frac{\text{Total volume of fluid} \times \text{drop factor}}{\text{Total time of infusion per minute}}$$

$$= \text{number of drops per minute}$$

URINARY CATHETERS

Self-retaining urethral catheters are inserted into the bladder as part of the routine in major pelvic surgery and urology, where it is important to monitor the output of urine accurately. The minimum should be no less than 30 ml per hour; less than this should be reported to the clinician and signs of hypovolaemia should be noted.

Following certain urology procedures, particularly transurethral resection of the prostate, continuous bladder irrigation will be in progress via a three-way catheter. Monitoring of the output, including the irrigation fluid, is important as retention may be caused by blood clots obstructing the outflow. Explanations will have been given to the patient preoperatively and this should be reinforced by the practitioner.

STOMAS

Stomas are created surgically to act as a diversion because the intestinal or urinary tract is damaged by disease or trauma. They may be temporary or permanent. In most cases because of the altered body image and psychological stress the patient's preparation for surgery will have included education and counselling in order to reduce anxiety. The recovery practitioner should be aware of this and reassure the patient by reinforcing advice and sympathetically helping to allay their concerns.

Part of the preparation will include the siting of the stoma and selection of the appliance. The size of the appliance will be sufficient for the output and will fit closely around the stoma to prevent skin irritation. It should not be changed unless there are obvious problems.

BODY TEMPERATURE

Body temperature is measured in degrees celsius using either a clinical thermometer or an electronic device. Reasons for recording temperature include:

- to obtain a baseline
- as an indication of infection or deep vein thrombosis
- to check for incompatibility during blood transfusion
- to monitor in cases of hypothermia.

Electronic probes react rapidly and may be used orally, or in the axilla or ear. In pyrexia tepid sponging or fans may be used to reduce the temperature and to make the patient feel more comfortable. If the patient is cold or hypothermic, with recordings of 35°C or below, they should be warmed. A space blanket may be used but should not be placed directly next to the skin: a single sheet must be placed between the patient and blanket. Other warming devices may also be used.

MOBILIZING

Depending on surgical constraints patients should be encouraged to sit up supported by the use of head rests and pillows. In the immobile patient pressure sites should be protected, positions changed and regular passive movements encouraged.

ASSESSMENT OF CONSCIOUS STATE

- Awake: the patient is alert, conscious with eyes open.
- Drowsy: the patient's eyes are shut except when spoken to, but the patient will cooperate on request.
- Rousable: the patient opens their eyes and responds to a stimulus, such as calling them or stroking the earlobe.
- Coma: the patient does not respond to stimuli.

The Glasgow Coma Scale was developed by the Institute of Neurological Sciences, at the Southern General Hospital in Glasgow to assess head-injured patients but may be used in the recovery room to assess the conscious state of patients (Box 7.1). The REACT score (Box 7.2) is another method of assessment in the postanaesthetic recovery phase, as is the Salim score.

CIRCULATION

Circulation can be assessed by observing the perfusion status. Observe skin colour, temperature, moistness, pulse rate, blood pressure and conscious state during recovery from anaesthesia.

Adequate to good perfusion:

- warm pink dry skin
- conscious, alert and orientated in time and place
- pulse 60–100 per minute
- blood pressure greater than 100 mmHg systolic.

Box 7.1 Glasgow Coma Scale (GCS)

		Score
Eye opening	Nil	1
	To pain	2
	To commands	3
	Spontaneously	4
Motor response	Nil	1
	Extends	2
	Abnormal flexion	3
	Withdraws	4
	Localizes	5
	Obeys commands	6
Verbal	Nil	1
	Incomprehensible	2
	Inappropriate	3
	Confused	4
	Orientated	5

Patients in coma have a GCS of 7 or less. They fail to obey commands, express no sounds and do not open their eyes. The lower the score the more deeply unconscious the patient is.

Box 7.2 REACT score

Score assessment

R = Respiration
    0 Needs ventilation
    1 Spontaneous breathing with rate
       < 10 per min
    2 Spontaneous breathing with rate > 10 per min

E = Energy
    0 Does not move legs
    1 Moves legs but cannot sustain head lift
    2 Sustains head lift and moves legs

A = Alertness
    0 Awakens only with vigorous stimulation
    1 Awakens when gently stimulated
    2 Awake and seldom dozes

C = Circulation
    0 Systolic blood pressure < 80 mmHg or weak pulse at the wrist
    1 Systolic blood pressure 80 mmHg preoperative Vesting level
    2 Systolic blood pressure greater than preoperatively

T = Temperature
    0 Axillary temperature < 35°C
    1 Axillary temperature 35.0–35.5°C
    2 Axillary temperature > 35°C

Score of 10 Patient is fully recovered from anaesthesia
Score of 9 Patient still has residual anaesthetic effects
Score of 8 Not ready for discharge

(From Franlin KE and Murphy P. Nursing, April 1984. REACT – A new postanaesthetic recovery score)

This score assessment alone is not enough to decide if patient is ready for discharge. Criteria for discharge from recovery room is dealt with later in this chapter.

Inadequate or poor perfusion:
Two of the following:

- altered conscious state
- cool pale clammy skin
- pulse less than 60 per minute or greater than 100 per minute
- blood pressure less than 100 mmHg systolic.

No perfusion:

- unconscious
- cool pale skin
- absence of palpable pulse
- unrecordable blood pressure.

Complications and resuscitation

UPPER AIRWAY OBSTRUCTION

Indications of partial upper airway obstruction:

- noisy breathing
- snoring
- inspiratory stridor (crowing noise)
- laboured breathing.

Indications of total respiratory obstruction:

- silence
- no movement of air at airway
- signs of hypoxia develop rapidly
- dysrhythmia and bradycardia
- rocking movement of chest and abdomen.

Causes

- Obstruction of airway by tongue
- Foreign bodies in the pharynx
- Laryngospasm
- Vomit
- Mucosal oedema
- Secretions, blood or mucus.

Management

- Extend the neck, lift and pull the jaw forward.
- Insert airway.

If the obstruction is not cleared:

- Turn the patient on to left side.
- Tilt head of bed down.

- Suction aspirate from pharynx.

If obstruction persists:

- Suction aspirate under direct vision by use of laryngoscope.
- If vocal cords in spasm give oxygen via mask (Mapleson C).

If still unsuccessful intubation using muscle relaxant (suxamethonium) and ventilation may be required.

Less common causes of total respiratory obstruction

- Laryngeal oedema
- External pressure on trachea
- Paralysis of vocal cords owing to surgical trauma to recurrent laryngeal nerve
- Tracheal collapse.

Management

Laryngeal oedema:

- head-up position
- humidification
- steroids, diuretics, nebulized adrenaline
- endotracheal intubation.

External pressure on the trachea:

- if due to haematoma following neck surgery it is necessary to remove skin clips or sutures and evacuate the clot

- endotracheal intubation or tracheotomy may be necessary.

Damaged vocal cords or tracheal collapse:

- endotracheal intubation.

SHOCK

The signs of shock are as follows:

- pallor
- cold, clammy
- thin thready pulse
- tachycardia
- anaphylaxis
- low blood pressure
- diminished state of consciousness.

Types of shock

- Hypovolaemic/haemorrhagic
- Cardiogenic
- Anaphylactic
- Neurogenic
- Septicaemic.

Causes

Hypovolaemic/haemorrhagic:

- haemorrhage
- excessive urinary output.

Anaphylactic:

- allergic reaction, frequently to medication.

Management

Haemorrhagic:

- stop bleeding
- replace blood loss.

Hypovolaemic:

- replace lost fluid.

Anaphylactic:

- treat with antiallergic drugs; have full rescuscitation equipment standing by.

PNEUMOTHORAX

Causes

Pneumothorax is caused by a collapse of the lung due to air in the thoracic cavity caused by trauma, including stab wounds and following the insertion of CVP lines. It may also be caused by spontaneous rupture of lung cysts.

Treatment

- Insertion of thoracic drain attached to underwater drainage system to prevent ingress of air to chest
- Keep drainage system below chest level at all times to prevent back flow
- Observe patient's breathing.

DIABETIC PATIENTS

These patients will require dextrose and insulin to be given both interoperatively and postoperatively until they are back on to their usual regimen. The dextrose infusion should be established and then a pump for insulin attached. At first it may be necessary to do hourly blood glucose estimations, but this may be reduced as time goes on. Patients are prescribed a sliding dose of insulin, which is given according to the result of the estimation. Glucometers provide an accurate measurement of blood sugar levels.

The signs of hypoglycaemia (low blood sugar) are:

- hunger
- sweating
- mood changes
- tachycardia
- eventual loss of consciousness.

The causes of hypoglycaemia are:

- too much insulin
- insufficient carbohydrate
- strenuous exercise.

KETOACIDOSIS OR DIABETIC COMA

The signs of hyperglycaemia are:

- an acetone smell on the breath
- ketosis in veins

- acidosis leading to hyperventilation (blood pH below 7.4)
- glycosuria due to high blood sugar (over 10 mmol/l)
- skin hot and salty
- patient may drift into a coma.

Hyperglycaemia is caused by increased energy demands and inadequate treatment. Further investigations will be required if it is suspected.

Treatment

- Insulin to increase glucose metabolism
- Intravenous sodium bicarbonate to correct acidosis
- Intravenous saline and dextrose to correct dehydration
- Intravenous potassium with insulin therapy; potassium may be lost from blood into cells (previous cardiac arrhythmias).

BLOOD TRANSFUSION

Patients who have undergone major surgery often require blood transfusions according to the postoperative instructions. The following observations should be made:

- temperature
- pulse
- respiration
- urine output
- observe skin for rashes
- look for pain in back, headache.

If any adverse reaction is noted the infusion must be stopped and the clinician informed immediately.
 Most important causes are of confusion

- cerebral hypoxia
- hypoglycaemia
- electrolyte imbalance
- occasionally benzodiazepines.

CARDIAC ARREST

All staff should be familiar with cardiopulmonary resuscitation procedures, and receive regular training and updates. Recovery nurses need to have theory and practice skills to correctly manage cardiopulmonary arrest in patients with ventricular fibrillation (VF)/pulseless ventricular tachycardia (VT), asystole and electromechanical dissociation (EMD). The guidelines laid down by the Resuscitation Council (UK) should be followed and the algorithms used as a learning tool (Fig 7.3).

TRANSFER OF PATIENT TO THE WARD

Before any patient is discharged from the recovery area the staff should satisfy themselves on the following points:

- The patient is conscious, can maintain a clear airway and protective reflexes are present.
- Breathing and oxygenation are satisfactory.
- The cardiovascular system is stable. Consecutive readings of pulse rate and blood pressure should approximate the normal preoperative values or be at an acceptable level, commensurate with the planned postoperative care. Peripheral perfusion should be adequate.
- Temperature should be within normal limits.
  - Check postoperative orders:
    — oxygen therapy
    — monitoring requirements
    — fluid balance, i.v. regimen, urinary output
    — adequate provisions for analgesia and antiemetics
    — check wound, dressing, drains and document
    — ensure nursing records are in order.

Only when these criteria have been met should the ward staff be contacted to take over responsibility for care. If oxygen therapy is part of the postoperative plan notify staff at this time.

 Transfer of care takes place in recovery. The recovery nurse gives face-to-face handover to a competent nurse who will take responsibility for continuing care on the ward. Handover is a vital component of patient transfer, and details include:

- The patient's name, type of anaesthetic and surgery performed

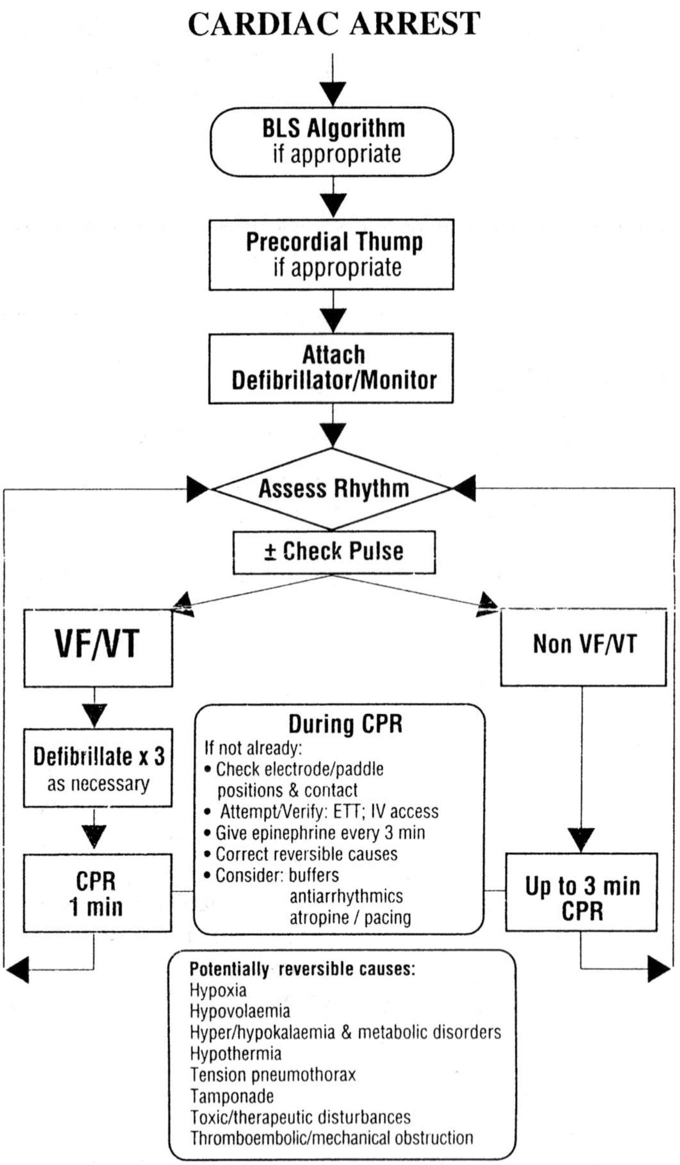

CARDIAC ARREST

Figure 7.3 The ALS algorithim for the management of cardiac arrest in adults. Note that each successive step is based on the assumption that the one before has been unsucessful. Reproduced with permission from the Resuscitation Council UK.

- Time of arrival in recovery room
- Brief explanation of airway management
- The time the patient regained consciousness
- Clinical observations, any special concerns or instructions
- General condition of patient
- Positioning, including pressure areas
- Wound site, skin closure, type of dressing; whether or not there is any oozing, or if pressure dressing has been necessary
- Fluid balance, infusion lines, drains, catheters, nasogastric tubes, etc.
- Drugs given in recovery: analgesia, antiemetics, antibiotics and any further instructions

- Nausea and vomiting: have oral fluids been tolerated? should the patient be nil by mouth?
- If a patient has a controlled device for analgesia or an infusion pump in place, the dose, administration and record of how much has been given should be checked
- All actions should be recorded in the care plan.

Medicines

Prior to the administration of any pharmaceutical the practitioner must be aware of local and national rules and procedures for the safe administration of medicines. The *British National Formulary* and manufacturers' literature will provide advice on dose, cautions, contraindications and side effects.

ADENOSINE

Indications for use

Paroxysmal supraventricular tachycardia.

Dose

The initial dose is 3 mg given rapidly into a central or peripheral vein, followed by a saline flush. Repeat injections after 1–2 minutes of 6 and 12 mg may be given if the initial dose is ineffective. The injection must be give rapidly to achieve adequate and effective blood levels, as the half-life of adenosine is only 10–15 seconds. Patients must be monitored cardiovascularly when this medication is used.

The major advantage of adenosine is that it may be used for a broad complex tachycardia of uncertain aetiology. However, its use may cause the patient to experience strange feelings and may result in severe chest pain. Bronchospasm may be induced or worsened in patients who have asthma.

The effects of adenosine are enhanced by dipyridamole and antagonized by theophylline.

Contraindications

Second- or third-degree atrioventricular block and sick sinus syndrome.

ADRENALINE

Indications for use

Emergency treatment of acute anaphylaxis, asystole, pulseless ventricular tachycardia, ventricular fibrillation and electromechanical dissociation. Adrenaline is used as the first medication in cardiac arrest protocols.

Dose

In cardiac arrest the initial intravenous dose is 1 mg. Where intravenous access is delayed 2 mg may be given via the tracheal tube; 5 mg may be given intravenously if a fourth dose is required in EMD or asystole.

For anaphylaxis first-line treatment is adrenaline intramuscularly 0.5–1 mg (0.5–1 ml adrenaline 1–1000) repeated every 10 minutes according to blood pressure and pulse.

Use

Adrenaline is a directly acting sympathomimetic amine that possesses both α- and β-adrenergic activity. In the doses used for resuscitation adrenaline stimulates both α_1 and α_2 receptors to produce arterial and arteriolar vasoconstriction. The resulting use in systemic vascular resistance maintains a higher blood pressure during cardiopulmonary resuscitation. The net effect of this is to produce an increase in cerebral and coronary perfusion.

The effects of adrenaline on β_1 receptors are both an increase in heart rate and the force of contraction, which are potentially harmful as they increase myocardial oxygen requirements and may increase ischaemia.

In cardiac arrest a dilution of 1 in 10 000 (1 mg in 1000 ml) is used, the dose being 10 ml of the solution every 2–3 minutes.

AMINOPHYLLINE

Indications for use

Relief of bronchospasm. A bronchodilator used in asthmatics, the therapeutic ratio of aminophylline is very narrow, which means that the difference between the therapeutic dose and toxic dose is small. It is important to check before giving an initial loading dose whether the patient has been taking aminophylline or theophylline.

Dose

The loading dose of 250–500 mg (5 mg/kg body weight) is given by slow intravenous injection over a period of 20 minutes. Maintenance if required in patients not previously treated with theophylline is 500 µg/kg/hour by slow intravenous injection.

AMIODARONE

Indications for use

Resistant tachyarrhythmias, Wolf–Parkinson–Wright syndrome.

Dose

A loading dose of 5 mg/kg in 100 ml of 5% dextrose is given over 1–4 hours via a central or large peripheral vein. The maximum dose is 1.2 mg in 24 hours.

Amiodarone increases the duration of the potential in atrial and ventricular myocardium, hence the QT interval is prolonged.

Most of the side effects of amiodarone are not relevant in the emergency situation, although nausea is common.

ATROPINE

Indications for use

Asystole, sinus atrial or nodal bradycardias with hypotension. With neostigmine for reversal of neuromuscular block.

Dose

The recommended adult dose for asystole is 3 mg intravenously. For the treatment of symptomatic bradycardia an initial dose of 0.5–1 mg intravenously is required; repeated doses may be necessary.

Atropine antagonizes the action of the parasympathetic neuromuscular acetylcholine at muscarinic receptors. It therefore antagonizes the effect of the vagus nerve on both the sinoatrial node and the atroventricular node (AVN), increasing sinus automaticity and facilitating AVN conduction respectively.

Following intravenous administration in particular, blurred vision, dry mouth, urinary retention and acute confusional states may occur.

BRETYLIUM TOSYLATE

Indications for use

Refractory ventricular tachycardia (VT), refractory ventricular fibrillation (VF).

Dose

Given intravenously the initial dose is 5 mg/kg body weight. A 500 mg preparation is available for emergency use.

Bretylium is an adrenergic neuron-blocking agent. Its initial action is to cause an increase of noradrenaline. The antiarrhythmic action of the agent may take some time to become established and basic life support must be continued for at least 20 minutes after administration.

CALCIUM

Indications for use

Electromechanical dissociation caused by severe hyperkalaemia, severe hypercalcaemia or overdose of calcium channel blocking agents.

Dose

The initial dose of 10 ml of 10% calcium chloride (6–8 mmol calcium) may be repeated if necessary. Calcium is given during cardiac arrest only when there is a specific indication, as high concentrations have detrimental effects on the ischaemic myocardium and may impair cerebral recovery. Calcium chloride should not be given immediately before or after sodium bicarbonate without first flushing the intravenous line. It must not be injected into small veins as this causes tissue necrosis.

CYCLOSINE

Indications for use

Nausea and vomiting.

Dose

By intravenous or intramuscular injection 50 mg three times daily. Side effects include blurred vision, dry mouth and drowsiness.

DANTROLENE, DANTRIUM INTRAVENOUS

Indications for use

Treatment of malignant hyperthermia.

Dose

By rapid intravenous injection 1 mg/kg body weight, repeated as required to a cumulative maximum of 10 mg/kg.

DEXAMETHASONE

Indications for use

Dexamethasone is a steroid used for the treatment of anaphylaxis, acute allergic conditions and cerebral oedema.

Dose

0.5–20 mg initially by intravenous injection.

DEXTROSE 50%

Indications for use

Treatment of hypoglycaemia causing unconsciousness.

Dose

Up to 50 ml of 50% given intravenously.

DIAMORPHINE

Indications for use

An opiate analgesic used to control moderate and severe pain.

Dose

By subcutaneous or intramuscular injection, 5 mg repeated every 4 hours if necessary. By slow intravenous injection one-quarter to half intramuscular dose.

Most common side effects include nausea, vomiting and drowsiness. In larger doses may produce respiratory depression and hypotension.

DIAZEPAM

Indications for use

Status epilepticus and febrile convulsions, as a sedative.

Dose

By slow intravenous injection 2–10 mg; not more than 5 mg/min into a large vein.

DICLOFENAC SODIUM

Indications for use

A non-steroid anti-inflammatory agent (NSAID) used in postoperative pain relief.

Dose

Initially after surgery 25–50 mg over 15–60 minutes.

The medication is contraindicated in patients with hypersensitivity to aspirin or any other NSAID; it results in a worsening of asthma, and should not be used for patients with a history of peptic ulceration or in the elderly.

DIGOXIN

Indications for use

Supraventricular arrhythmias, particularly atrial fibrillation.

Dose

Emergency loading dose by intravenous infusion 250–500 µg over 10–20 minutes. This may need to be reduced if any other cardiac glycosides have been taken in the last 24 hours.

Digoxin is a cardiac glycoside that slows the conduction of impulses through the conducting systems of the heart, increases myocardial contraction and may cause arrhythmias.

It is advisable to check that the sodium potassium concentration is greater than 40 mmol/l: monitor with an ECG. Dose may need to be reduced when treating elderly patients.

DIHYDROCODEINE TARTRATE

Indications for use

Moderate to severe pain.

Dose

Intramuscular injection up to 50 mg every 4–6 hours. For side effects see Morphine/diamorphine.

DOPAMINE

Indications for use

Cardiogenic shock in infarction or cardiac surgery.

Dose

By intravenous infusion 2–5 µg/kg per minute initially.

Dopamine offers inotropic support as a cardiac stimulant, acts on β receptors in the cardiac muscle and increases contractility with little effect on heart rate.

Dosage is critical: low doses induce vasoconstriction and increase renal perfusion; higher doses lead to vasodilation and may exacerbate heart failure.

DOXAPRAM

Indications for use

As a respiratory stimulant.

Dose

For postoperative respiratory depression. Intravenous injection over at least 30 seconds, 1–1.5 mg/kg repeated if necessary after 1 hour. Alternatively by intravenous infusion 2–3 mg/min adjusted according to response.

EPHEDRINE

Indications for use

Reversal of hypotension caused by epidural anaesthesia.

Dose

3–6 mg repeated every 3–4 minutes up to a maximum 30 mg. Monitor with ECG when administering intravenously.

FLUXAZENAL

Indications for use

To reverse the effects of benzodiazepines.

Dose

By intravenous injection 200 µg over 15 seconds, 100 µg at 60-second intervals as required, to a maximum dose of 1 mg. Side effects include nausea, vomiting and flushing.

FRUSEMIDE

Indications for use

Pulmonary oedema, oliguria in renal failure.

Dose

Slow intravenous injection of 20–50 mg. May be infused at a rate of no more than 4 mg/min.

Precautions should be taken as frusemide is a nephrotoxic and otoxic agent. Potentiates damage to kidneys and ears caused by gentamicin and other aminoglycoside antibiotics. Hypokalaemia and hypotension may also develop.

GLYCERYL TRINITRATE

Indications for use

A short-acting vasodilator especially of the coronary arteries, used for prophylaxis and treatment of angina.

Dose

Sublingually 0.3–1 mg repeated as required. By intravenous infusion 10–100 µg/min. Transdermal as a self-adhesive patch, variable dose between 2.5 and 10 mg/24 hours.

NB: As a special precaution self-adhesive patches must be removed prior to defibrillation.

Monitor ECG when infusing agent as the patient may rapidly become hypotensive if there is postoperative bleeding.

GLYCOPYRRONIUM BROMIDE

Indications for use

An alternative to atropine in combination with neostigmine for the reversal of non-depolarizing muscle relaxants. When given intravenously it produces less tachycardia than atropine.

Dose

By intravenous injection for the reversal of competitive neuromuscular block, 10–15 µg/kg with 50 µg/kg neostigmine.

HALOPERIDOL

Indications for use

In the short term to quieten disturbed patients and to alleviate anxiety.

Dose

Intravenous injection of 5–10 mg will last for approximately 8 hours.

HYDRALAZINE

Indications for use

Moderate to severe hypertension; a vasodilator which may produce a rapid fall in blood pressure and tachycardia.

Dose

By intravenous injection 5–10 mg over 20 minutes; may be repeated after 20–30 minutes. Intravenous infusion initially 200–300 µg/min.

ISOPRENALINE

Indications for use

Symptomatic bradycardia unresponsive to atropine. Heart block. Its main use is in the emergency treatment of complete heart block and unstable bradycardia to maintain cardiac output until transvenous pace-making is established.

Dose

By intravenous infusion 0.5–10 µg/min. Monitor with ECG.

KETOROLAC

Indications for use

This NSAID may be used for the short-term management of moderate to severe pain.

Dose

By intramuscular injection; by intravenous injection over not less than 15 seconds.

Patients over 16 years initially 10 mg then 10–30 mg every 4–6 hours. In the initial post operative period the dose may be repeated 2-hourly. The daily dose must not exceed 90 mg; in the elderly and patients weighing less than 50 kg the daily dose should not exceed 60 mg. The drug is not recommended for children under the age of 16 years.

For contraindications see Diclofenac.

LIGNOCAINE

Indications for use

Ventricular premature beats, haemodynamically stable ventricular tachycardia, refractory ventricular fibrillation, laryngospasm.

Lignocaine is a local anaesthetic that possesses antiarrhythmic activity. It decreases ventricular automaticity by reducing the rate of diastolic depolarization. Its local anaesthetic action suppresses ventricular ectopic activity.

Dose

By intravenous injection, bolus dose of 100 mg given rapidly for ventricular fibrillation or 1 mg/kg for haemodynamically stable ventricular tachycardia. This may be repeated if necessary by an infusion of 2–4 mg/min. For laryngospasm 1 mg/kg bolus dose.

Features of lignocaine toxicity are largely manifested through the nervous system, with paraesthesiae, drowsiness, confusion and muscular twitching progressing to convulsions. Treatment is by stopping administration and management of the seizures.

METARAMINOL

Indications for use

Acute hypertension. A vasoconstrictor sympathomimetic raising bood pressure transiently by acting on the α-adrenoreceptors to constrict peripheral vessels.

Dose

By intravenous infusion 15–100 mg in 500 ml adjusted according to response.

METOCLOPRAMIDE

Indications for use

Nausea and vomiting.

Dose

Intramuscular or intravenous injection 10 mg. Daily dose should not normally exceed 500 μg/kg.

Side effects

Oculogynic crisis, where the eyes oscillate uncontrollably with alarming giddiness. Opisthotonus, with extensor spasm: the patient is 'as stiff as a board'. Drowsiness, dry mouth, muscle tremor.

METOPROLOL

Indications for use

Supraventricular tachycardia. This cardioselective β-blocking agent is used to slow the heart. It is less likely to precipitate asthma than propranolol. Use with caution in patients with obstructive airway disease.

Dose

Intravenous injection up to 5 mg at a rate of 1–2 mg/min, repeated after 5 minutes if necessary to a total dose of 10–15 mg. Monitor with ECG.

MIDAZOLAM

Indications for use

Occasionally useful in postoperative recovery for restless patients. Short-acting benzodiazepine used as a sedative.

Dose

Slow intravenous injection; usual range 2.5–7.5 mg given in 2 mg increments. Use lower doses in the elderly.

MORPHINE

Indications for use

Opioid analgesic for severe pain. Used intraoperatively as well as postoperatively. Doses of intraoperative analgesia may delay the need for an initial dose of morphine postoperatively. Widely used in conjunction with devices for patient-controlled analgesia.

Dose

10–15 mg 4-hourly subcutaneous or intramuscular injection.

By slow intravenous injection one-quarter to half the corresponding intramuscular dose. By weight 0.15–0.25 mg/kg adult.

The side effects of morphine include nausea, vomiting and drowsiness; larger doses may cause hypotension and respiratory depression.

Antiemetic agents should be given concurrently to suppress induced nausea and vomiting. Respiratory depression or hypotension can be reversed by naloxone.

Another effect of opiates to take into consideration is amnesia: patients will often appear to understand information given to them and participate in discussion, but later they have no recall of this. It is important to be aware of giving important information, especially to day patients, if this involves details of postoperative instructions. Opiates may also reduce the desire to pass urine.

NALOXONE

Indications for use

In opioid overdose.

Dose

By intravenous injection 100–200 μg every 2 minutes; further doses by intramuscular injection after 1–2 hours if required. Initially the dose should be titrated to each patient in order to obtain optimum respiratory response while maintaining adequate analgesia. Alternatively an infusion can be used, with adjustment of the rate to achieve the desired effect.

NEOSTIGMINE

Indications for use

Reversal of non-depolarizing muscle relaxant drugs.

Dose

50–70 μg/kg (maximum 5 mg). Atropine or glycopyrronium should be given at the same time to prevent the effects of bradycardia, excessive salivation and other muscarinic actions of neostigmine.

NITROPRUSSIDE

Indications for use

Hypertensive crises; also used in surgery for controlled hypotension. It is a short-acting vasodilator used intravenously. The infusion needs to be covered with black plastic or tinfoil to prevent decomposition caused by light.

Use cautiously if any evidence of hepatic failure as the cyanide ions may not be reduced in patients already receiving antihypertensive therapy. Monitor with ECG.

Side effects may include headache, dizziness, nausea and sweating.

NIFEDIPINE

Indications for use

Hypertension and angina.

Dose

Straight from the capsule directly under the patient's tongue; may be swallowed.

ONDANSETRON

Indications for use

Preventative treatment for nausea and vomiting.

Dose

8 mg orally 1 hour prior to induction of anaesthesia, followed by further doses of 8 mg at 8-hour intervals. Alternatively, at induction of anaesthesia a 4 mg dose either intravenously or intramuscularly.

Side effects are headaches, a sensation of flushing and warmth in the head.

PROCHLORPERAZINE

Indications for use

Nausea and vomiting.

Dose

Intramuscular injection 12.5 mg. Side effects include prolonged sedation in the elderly; dystonic reactions sometimes occur, particularly in young adults and children.

PROPRANOLOL

Indications for use

Supraventricular tachycardias, phaeochromocytoma, thyrotoxic crisis.

Dose

Intravenous injection 1 mg over 1 minute. Side effects are bradycardia, conductive disorders and bronchospasm.

When using β-blockers in patients with asthma or obstructive airways diseases, consider the risk of inducing bronchospasm.

PROTAMINE SULPHATE

Indications for use

Reversal of the anticoagulant effects of heparin.

Dose

Slow intravenous injection of 1 mg/100 mg of heparin. Side effects are bradycardia and hypotension. Excessive use will have an anticoagulant effect.

SALBUTAMOL

Indications for use

Bronchodilator used for the treatment of asthma.

Dose

Slow intravenous injection 250 µg. By inhalation of nebulized solution 2.5 mg. Metered aerosol 100 µg per puff.

SODIUM BICARBONATE

Indications for use

Metabolic acidosis, hyperkalaemia.

Dose

Should be titrated after regular blood gas analysis; small doses of 8.4% sodium bicarbonate given intravenously. In cardiac arrest where the arterial pressure is less than 7.0–7.1 calculate the appropriate dose using the formula below:

$$\frac{\text{Base excess} \times \text{weight (kg)}}{3}$$

SUXAMETHONIUM CHLORIDE

Indications for use

Short-acting depolarizing muscle relaxant, particularly for rapid-sequence intratracheal intubation.

Dose

By intravenous injection 60 µg/kg. Side effects are known as scoline apnoea. Where the patient has low or atypical plasma pseudocholinesterase enzymes, results in prolonged muscle paralysis. These patients require sedation and ventilation until the effects of the drug wear off, as is the case with dual block where repeated doses of suxamethonium have resulted in the development of non-depolarizing block following the initial depolarizing block.

VERAPAMIL

Indications for use

Supraventricular tachycardia.

Dose

The intravenous dose is 5–10 mg given over 2 minutes. A further dose of 5 mg may be given after 5 minutes if necessary. Patients need to be monitored with ECG.

Side effects are in common with other vasodilators, including flushing, headaches and hypotension. Verapamil must not be given to patients with broad complex tachycardia of ventricular origin.

Refractory hypotension may occur if used in combination with other antiarrhythmic agents. Interaction with β-blockers may be particularly severe, therefore this combination should be avoided. Verapamil also induces an increase in the plasma concentration of digoxin and may precipitate digitalis toxicity.

Patient-controlled analgesia

Patient-controlled analgesia (PCA) allows the patient to control the delivery of a drug to achieve effective pain relief with minimum side effects. The basic concept is that the patient is connected to a device containing a supply of opioid, e.g. morphine or diamorphine. When pain relief is required the patient activates the device by pressing a hand-held button. The demand for analgesia is met by a small predetermined dose of intravenous opiate which gives a plasma concentration that achieves analgesia while avoiding profound sedation and respiratory depression.

The PCA device is computerized and is programmed for the size of bolus dose (the amount of analgesic delivered in one dose) and the minimum time interval between doses (the lockout time or off-cycle). More sophisticated devices can be programmed to deliver a background infusion as well.

Dosage and frequency

The size of the bolus dose, the lockout time and any required background infusion rate may all differ according to hospital, surgical procedure or personnel involved, but should form part of a PCA protocol (see Appendix 5). For example, some users suggest a bolus dose of 1 mg morphine with a lockout time of 5 minutes, whereas others advocate a larger dose and a lockout time of 10 minutes.[1]

The Joint College Report[2] suggests that 'in order to improve the efficacy of analgesic administration, the dose and frequency should be adjusted in response to the needs of each patient, who should have an individualized regimen'.

Implementation and limitations

The initial use of PCA by the patient is normally supervised by a pain nurse as part of the acute pain service, or by a recovery nurse. He or she normally reinforces the instructions that were given prior to the operation. PCA has been shown to be of most value in the control of postoperative pain, and is ideally suited to the treatment of acute localized pain. PCA is not recommended for the treatment of generalized pain, such as in osteoarthritis, and the prolonged use of opioids is not advised.

It is essential that patients who have been selected as suitable for PCA therapy receive thorough preoperative counselling (see below).

Safety

Sophisticated PCA devices give the medical team control of the medication delivery. To eliminate the risk of overdosage, once a demand has been made the lockout period or off-cycle is activated, which prevents the patient receiving another dose for a specified time. Once this predetermined period has elapsed, further demands will be met. Demands made during the lockout period are usually recorded by the system. Regular monitoring should enable the dose and lockout period to be adjusted according to the patient's needs.

Benefits

Patient acceptance of PCA is very high. Because patients are reassured that analgesic is readily available and there will be no delay in administration, they suffer less anxiety and discomfort. Experience has shown that patients are satisfied with their pain relief, are comforted by the system's presence and feel happy that they are not taking up the nurses' valuable time. In one study, examining over 8000 pain assessments, patients were reported as having little or no pain on 92.6% of occasions.[3]

PCA has consistently been shown to improve the quality of pain relief while reducing the impact on nursing time.[4] In addition, several informal studies have shown improved efficacy, reduced opioid dosage, fewer postoperative complications and earlier discharge from hospital compared to routine intramuscular therapy.[4–6]

Unlike intramuscular bolus opioids, PCA allows the quantity of pain relief to be tailored to each individual and there is minimal delay between pain perception and pain relief.[6]

Selection of suitable patients

In general, patients undergoing all types of surgical procedure should be suitable for PCA. According to market research conducted in early 1993, the following types were highlighted as benefiting from PCA.[7]

- those undergoing general surgery
- orthopaedic patients, especially those thought likely to experience a great deal of pain
- those undergoing thoracic and abdominal surgery
- those undergoing gynaecological and obstetric procedures
- paediatric patients.

Although it is difficult to give specific guidelines on which patients to select, there are a number of situations where PCA should *not* be provided.
These are:

- physical inability to operate the PCA demand button (alternatives to the patient pendant are available on request from Abbott Laboratories)
- a history of chronic obstructive airways disease
- head injury
- previous severe side effects or allergy to morphine and related drugs
- impaired mental status, judged preoperatively by the anaesthetist and ward sister
- marked metabolic disorder, i.e. electrolyte and fluid imbalance, sepsis, etc.
- history of previous narcotic drug abuse.

REFERENCES

1 Gould TH et al 1992 Policy for controlling pain after surgery: effect of sequential changes in management. British Medical Journal 305: 1187–1193
2 The Royal College of Surgeons of England – The College of Anaesthetists 1990 Commission of the provision of surgical services: Report of the Working Party on Pain after Surgery, September 1990
3 Norcutt WG et al 1990 Introducing patient-controlled analgesia for postoperative pain control into a district general hospital. Anaesthesia 45: 401–506
4 Schug SA et al 1991 Treatment principles for the use of opioids in pain of a non-malignant origin. Drugs, 42(2) 228–239
5 Ready LB 1990 Patient-controlled analgesia – does it provide more than comfort? Canadian Journal of Anesthesia 37(7) 719–721
6 Mackie AM et al 1991 Adolescents use patient-controlled analgesia effectively for relief from prolonged oropharyngeal mucositis pain. Pain 46: 265–269
7 Spectrum Research 1993 Report into Acute Pain Services in Hospitals; June

FURTHER READING

British Medical Association/Royal Pharmaceutical Society of Great Britain 1996 British National Formulary No. 31 (March 1996) London

Pritchard AP, Walker VA 1984 The Royal Marsden Hospital manual of clinical nursing procedures. Harper and Row, London

Kaczmarowski N 1982 Patient care in the operating room. Churchill Livingstone, Edinburgh

Hatfield A, Tronson M 1992 The complete recovery room book,

Association of Anaesthetists of Great Britain and Ireland, 1993, Immediate post anaesthetic recovery.

8

Design considerations

S. A. Webster

This chapter is intended as a guide for those briefing the design team. It assumes that those commissioning a new operating department or day surgery unit, or refurbishing or extending an existing one, will appoint a professional design team to develop their brief. You should require the lead consultant of the design team to produce a project quality plan to define the roles and responsibilities of all those involved, including the briefing group, and to define what information needs to flow between the various parties.

The chapter briefly describes and illustrates matters of concern in designing operating departments and day surgery units. It is not an exhaustive briefing document, as you should expect your design team to have the necessary knowledge of ergonomics and technology to make their own contribution to the design process. Your briefing as client should therefore concentrate on **briefing by exception**. Concentrate on any special techniques that may be involved in the services to be provided, or any other social or cultural issues which may have to be addressed, as well as management preferences. For example, at the Chelsea and Westminster Hospital in London children are accompanied by their parents into the anaesthetic room and their parents are with them while they receive anaesthesia. The parents are also at the child's side when he or she recovers. This has an implication for the working space required around the trolley when the anaesthesia is being given, and for the space in the recovery area to accommodate such visitors.

CURRENT TRENDS AND THEIR IMPACT

Alvin Toffler, in his book *The Third Wave* (1981) speculated on the rise of the 'prosumer' society, in which a great proportion of a person's work will involve the production of goods and services for personal or family use. As individuals become more involved in satisfying their own needs he saw them gaining skills and knowledge in areas which previously were mystifying. As they gained new skills they would become more competent and demand greater participation in other areas too.

In the healthcare field he pointed to the use of pregnancy test kits, self-examinations, coin-operated blood pressure machines and the home use of instruments such as otoscopes, as indicators for the rise of a prosumer society. Linked to this is the increased importance of health as an indicator of the overall quality of life. As people become more knowledgeable and take more responsibility for themselves their expectation of becoming full partners in their healthcare will grow.

There are also demographic changes. Changes in age distribution, fertility rate, urbanization, work status and education will all profoundly influence the future of the facilities we are contemplating. For example, as we are living longer and our fertility rate is slowing down the proportion of older people in our population continues to grow. We already distinguish between the 'young old' in their 60s and the 'old old' in their 80s. Our longer lifespan is due primarily to an improved standard of living and advances in healthcare. Our older population will demand greater services from the healthcare system: they tend to have a greater number of chronic health problems, require more visits to the doctor, require a longer period of recovery after treatment and need more hospital-based care than the younger population. What does this say for the design of our day surgery units? What does it say about the reducing number of acute beds in hospitals?

Or, for example, choices are being made by couples on how many children to have and whether to have them at all. Because childbirth is now more a matter of choice it is reasonable to anticipate that parents to be will want to make more decisions about the healthcare their children receive. Closer attention will have to be paid to the needs of the child undergoing surgery and recovering in postanaesthesia recovery rooms, and to children attending day surgery units.

Or, again, both parents already have become more involved in looking after infants. This means that baby feeding and changing places need to be included which both men and women can use.

It seems to be sensible to keep an eye on lifestyle shifts and demographic trends because some of the decisions we make now in designing operating theatres and day surgery units must be based on speculation about the way we will live in the year 2000 or 2020.

When it comes to building, where capital improvements and construction costs are significant, planning for the long term is essential. Whether planning for long- or short-term goals, however, the result is not static. There has to be enough elasticity in the strategic plan to allow the plan to be altered as the need arises.

The planning process itself must be a learning experience because there are opportunities to learn from the process as well as its results.

TRENDS IN THE PROVISION OF SURGICAL SERVICES

Over the last 20 years the organization and provision of surgical services have been greatly influenced by a general drive for improved efficiency and economy, as well as by the continued rapid rate of technological innovation and by demographic change. The impact of day care has yet to be determined. It is worth noting that UCLA have opened an ambulatory cardiac centre, and the Central Middlesex in North London is contemplating extending elective surgery into an Ambulant Care and Diagnostic Centre. The need for major invasive techniques may be disappearing.

INTERIOR DESIGN

Undergoing surgery is by definition a traumatic experience, and the interior design of an operating department or day surgery unit should not add to the trauma. Good interior design can put patients at ease and help staff morale. A contented staff will produce good health outcomes. The interior design should create a cheerful and pleasant environment throughout the building while taking account of the restraints imposed by clinical requirements, e.g. access zoning, location of fixed equipment and services outlets. Users will take it for granted that the functional planning has been properly worked out. What they *will* remember is the quality of care and the environment in which they were treated.

CONTROL OF INFECTION

Until now microbiological considerations have predominated in the management of the operating department. For a long time the design of operating departments was largely determined by the idea of a 'clean' and a 'dirty' corridor. This was based on beliefs and theories which have not been vindicated by experience, and separate 'clean' and 'dirty' corridors are no longer a requirement. (see Chapter 3).

Access zones

The essence of the planning of an operating department or day surgery unit is the control of movement. It is not desirable to have unrestricted general access. Most spaces will be in one of the four following zones:

- a general access zone to which anyone entering the department is admitted
- a limited access zone to which those who need to enter parts of the department adjacent to the restricted access zone or the operative zone are admitted
- the restricted access zone to which are admitted those whose presence is associated with activities in the operating zone
- the operating zone: the area surrounding the operation site and the preparation room.

Security policy for these departments must be compatible with that for the whole hospital. Access to the departments and to staff changing rooms should be controlled.

Planning an operating theatre department

WORKFLOW AND MOVEMENT PATTERNS

Repetitive movement patterns are major risk sources. When there is no separation between 'clean' and 'dirty', movement patterns must be identified. These are related to patients, escorts and visitors, staff, supplies and disposal. The various spaces within the department should be linked by a corridor which introduces a simple and economic workflow. A single corridor system is the simplest topologically and can produce the most economic plans.

PREPARATION PROCEDURES

The main source of microorganisms is people, particularly when they are moving about. The bacterial load can be reduced by keeping to a minimum the number and the movement of people in the operating zone and ensuring that a sufficient flow of air is moved away from the operating zone.

The number of movements required by the team to move the patient into the operating zone means that the risk of bacterial contamination is high at the times when the patient enters and leaves the operating room. Therefore sterile instrument trays should not be opened until the preceding operation has been completed.

Sterile trolleys should be laid up preferably in a separate preparation room with direct access to the theatre. The doors to the preparation room should remain closed until the next patient is in the theatre.

The major source of cross-infection is the patient's own body. It could be questioned whether some of the more exotic laminar flow regimens that have been promoted in the recent past are valid, as they only deal with exogenous microorganisms (see Chapter 3).

ACCESS ZONES IN THE OPERATING THEATRE DEPARTMENT

Figure 8.1 illustrates suggested layouts for the various access zones described earlier.

CLEANING

Cleaning is a major task in the working of the operating room. Sufficient space has to be provided for cleaning equipment and materials to be stored locally.

MOVING THE PATIENT

Moving the patient should disturb the patient as little as possible and reduce interference with the conduct of clinical procedures to a minimum. The health and safety of the staff indicate that this should not require extraordinary physical effort from them.

There are several ways of moving the patient from a ward to the operating table and back again, characterized by the points in the journey at which the patient is transferred from one means of transport to another. Figures 8.2 and 8.3 illustrate possible access zones and service rooms related to these possible segregations.

GENERAL RELATIONSHIPS

Figure 8.4 shows the relationships of the principal spaces within an operating department. Although a single corridor system is the simplest, fire escape considerations may modify the eventual plan.

SPECIAL CONSIDERATIONS

• **Fire Safety** Fire safety principles apply to alterations and upgrading of existing buildings as well as to new projects.

Fire safety has two components, design and management. The Secretary of State has put responsibility for management on units. Ultimately safety will depend on how people behave in an emergency. The design should help orderly, safe evacuation, but only staff training can ensure that such measures succeed.

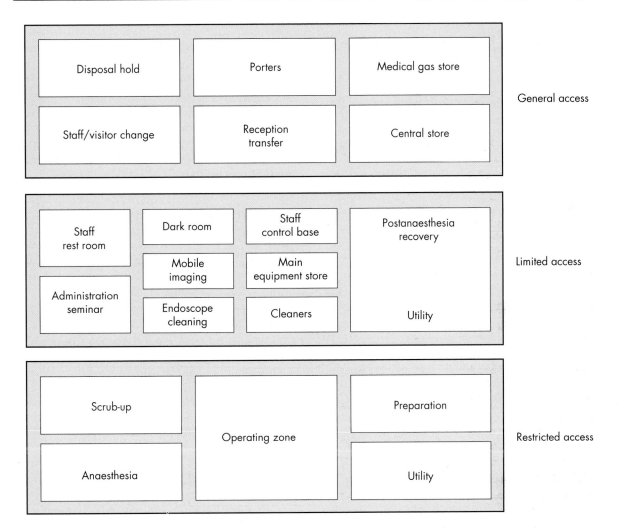

Figure 8.1 Access zones in the operating theatre department. (Reproduced with permission from NHS Estates 1991 Health Building Note 26.)

At the appropriate stages of the design process the architect and engineer will discuss and verify the proposals with the relevant fire authority. The briefing group should ensure that the project team and all other planning staff are acquainted with the structural provisions for fire safety and the design strategy for escape routes, fire barriers, etc., so that these become integrated into the way the department is run.

• **Views** If at all possible ask for windows to be provided to give a long view out of the department. If this is not possible, courtyards allow more rooms to enjoy natural daylight and ventilation.

• **Decoration and maintenance** Heavy mobile equipment is used throughout the department. Finishes have to be robust enough to withstand accidental impact and additional protection should be provided at likely points of impact. The designers will need to be advised of existing or proposed cleaning regimens when selecting materials and finishes.

Brief the designers to minimize areas needing frequent redecoration or which are difficult to

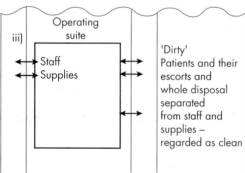

Figure 8.2 Operating suites – possible segregation policies. Clearly a twin corridor system requires more space. Achieving a single corridor system requires operational discipline. Consider whether the assumptions underlying segregation are justified in options i) – iii). (Reproduced with permission from NHS Estates 1991 Health Building Note 26.)

service or clean. Special consideration must be given to items such as doors, external corners, partitions and counter tops, which can be subject to heavy use. Point out good and bad features from the briefing group's experience.

There is a trend towards dispensing with flammable anaesthetic agents, which means that no antistatic provision is necessary in the floor. The design team will need to be advised on anaesthetics policy.

TECHNICAL SUPPORT FACILITIES

Communications and information technology

Information and management technology (IT) now has a central role in health management and health education.

Good communications are of great importance. IT systems selected should be consistent with local and national health service IT strategies.

Give detailed consideration to:

- the choice of system
- functions to be included in the system
- location of terminals
- access levels for information.

Functions may include:

- maintaining an appointment system:
  — confirming appointments with patients
  — checking that patients intend to attend
  — making appointments with other hospital departments
- running a patient management system:
  — communicating with health record services
- managing theatre lists and sessions
- transmitting urgent test results from pathology
- transmitting digital imagery to or from radiography
- managing materials and supplies
- providing clinical audit
- providing management and statistical information
- monitoring building security:
  — unauthorized access
  — tampering with secure storage locations

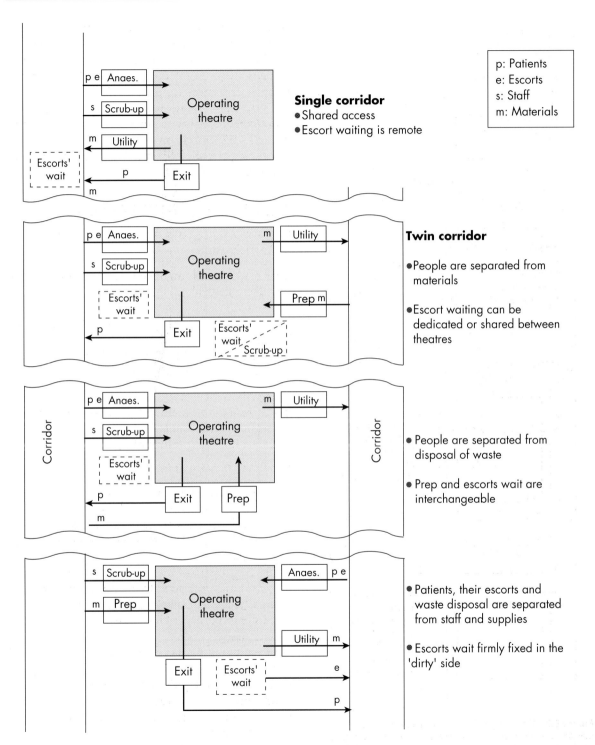

Figure 8.3   Operating suites – service rooms related to possible segregation policies. (Reproduced with permission from NHS Estates 1991 Health Building Note 26.)

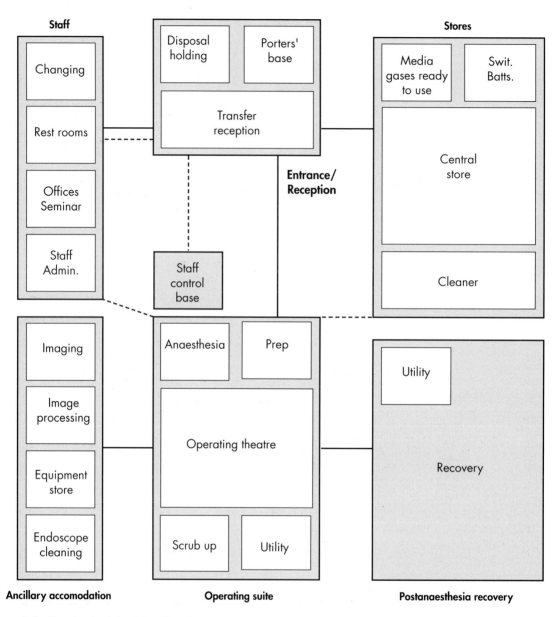

Figure 8.4 Functional relationships. The relationships of the principal spaces within an operating department. Although a single corridor system is the simplest, fire escape considerations may modify the eventual plan, ——— must be adjacent, ----- must be nearby. (Reproduced with permission from NHS Estates 1991 Health Building Note 26.)

— fire
• monitoring environmental conditions – line to hospital building management system (BMS)

A typical network for an operating department is shown in Figure 8.5.

Computer needs

Brief the design team to:

• provide sufficient space for working at VDUs
• ensure that lighting levels are compatible with the use of VDUs

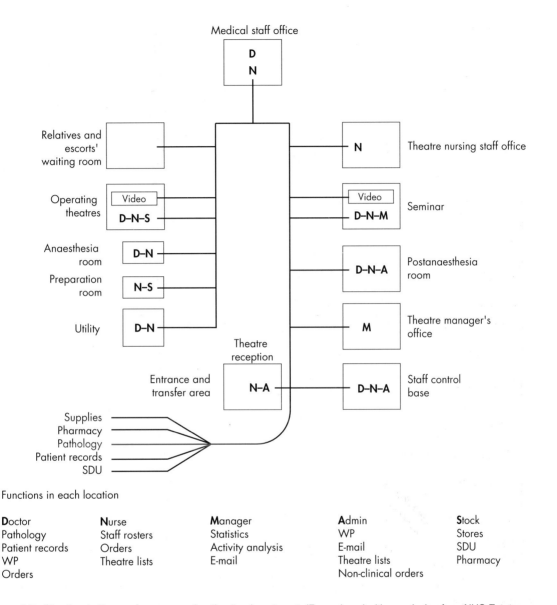

Figure 8.5 IT network diagram for an operating theatre department. (Reproduced with permission from NHS Estates 1991 Health Building Note 26.)

- provide means of controlling the noise of computer-related equipment
- provide means of dealing with the heat emitted by computer-related equipment
- anticipate the wireways associated with computer-related equipment
- provide sufficient power and uninterruptible power supplies

- consider the space required for periodic upgrades and routine maintenance.

Radiography

It is likely that film-based imaging will continue to be used for some time, and exposed film may be processed in the operating department.

Imaging techniques have, however, evolved considerably and rapidly, and provision for digital technology may be made. Ensure that the policy advocated is consistent with policies elsewhere in the hospital.

Medical gas pendants

Articulated motorized pendants which are adjustable both horizontally and vertically are generally recommended because they increase the number of ways in which the table and the operating team can be arranged. If ultraclean ventilation is envisaged it is possible to incorporate the services within the canopy framework.

Medical compressed air

In addition to the 4-bar supply of respirable air, each theatre should be provided with a 7-bar supply for surgical tools (see further below).

Ventilation

Conventional air conditioning systems provide filtered air at controlled temperature and humidity to the operating theatre. Patient well being cannot be maintained by ventilation only, and may have to be supplemented by other means, such as thermal blankets and heating pads.

The reduction of bacterial count is proportional to the volume of air supplied, which both dilutes the air in the theatre and prevents the entry of contaminated air from the periphery. Bacterial counts taken shortly after walls have been cleaned down and for areas such as the underside of operating tables would seem to question how beneficial ventilation systems are in counteracting the effects of convection, the movement of people and of turbulence caused by the opening and closing of doors (see Chapter 3).

Ultraclean ventilation (UCV) systems are alleged to provide operating sites within the theatre zone virtually free from contamination (see Chapter 3). As the flow of filtered air is discharged vertically downwards over the operating site, the possibility of staff introducing bacteria into the airstream is reduced.

Nevertheless, most cross-infection of patients is endogenous. The provision of UCV is costly.

The use of UCV means that theatre lighting will have to be shaped and positioned so as to minimize disruption to the air flow. Systems are available which incorporate lighting and service outlets fully integrated with the ventilation system. Cruciform arrangements are common.

For staff health and safety considerations pollution by spent anaesthetic gases should be minimized by active scavenging in the operating zone and by high rates of air change in postanaesthetic recovery areas.

Comfort remains a consideration. To some extent this will depend on the activity of the various staff in the theatre. Some members of the operating team are more active than others. An inactive, thinly covered patient may require a higher ambient temperature than the staff.

Supply, storage and disposal

The quantity and distribution of storage space required in an operating department can only be specified in terms of a known policy. Within the concept of 'briefing by exception' it is a major area where the operational policy must be carefully defined. Supply and disposal must be thought of integrally, supplies entering to be either consumed or deployed and then disposed of or recycled.

The briefing group should consider:

- whole-hospital supplies and disposal policies
- the different kinds of items supplied
- the delivery points
- the volume and location of storage spaces
- specialized storage requirements, particularly for controlled drugs.

Figure 8.6 shows preferred locations for storage and holding.

Efficient stock control increases working efficiency and leads to substantial savings in operating costs. Departmental stores management should be linked to the hospital supplies management system. It is essential to understand the materials handling policy for the whole hospital.

Room activity space	Medical and surgical sterile sup's	Pharmacy supplies	Controlled drugs	Pathology	Blood bank	Clean linen	Catering	Stationery	Housekeeping	Mobile equipment*
Entrance						○				○
Transfer						○				○
Reception office				△				●		
Porter's base										
Staff change/WC/SH						●				
Staff control base		●	●		●			●		
Anaesthesia	●	●	●			●				●
Operating theatre										●
Scrub-up	●									
Preparation	●	●								
Utility				△					●	○
Exit bay										△
Local equipment cupboard										●
Recovery	●	●	○					●		●
Utility (recovery)									●	
Mobile X-ray equip bay										●
Staff rest rooms										
Beverage bay						●	●			
Office/Seminar								●		●
Cleaners' room									●	●
Disposal hold										
Battery switchroom										
Central stores	●	●								
Equipment store										
Medical glass store										
Endoscope cleansing		●								

Key
* excluding trolleys and beds
● storage
△ holding
○ policy option

Figure 8.6 Location of storage and holding. (Reproduced with permission from NHS Estates 1991 Health Building Note 26.)

The lower the frequency of delivery, the greater the amount of money is tied up in a working stock of instruments and equipment.

Management systems and timetables for ordering, delivery and disposal should be devised and agreed with the managers of the hospital stores, sterilizing and disinfecting unit (SDU), the pharmacy, laundry, catering and portering services. Conventionally, stock levels are checked and replenished daily. If possible, supplies should be ordered on a whole-hospital basis; however, operating suites and postanaesthetic recovery staff may obtain items directly from the SDU or pharmacy.

Good working relationships between departments are essential. Good and safe handling procedures by staff are also essential.

Disposal

Special procedures are required for disposal or recycling instrument trays and clinical waste generated by surgery. Disposal and recycling procedures for infected material must be in accordance with hospital and departmental infection control policies.

Infected medical equipment must be sent to the SDU for decontamination. Used instrument trays, soiled linen bags and general rubbish bags should be labelled in accordance with hospital policy.

Materials for disposal associated with a particular patient must be held until after the used instrument tray has been checked in the SDU, and only then released.

Disposal of pressurized containers requires special attention (see SAB (88) 79 'LPG Aerosol Containers: Risks arising from storage, use and disposal').

Specially constructed containers should be used for sharps, particularly needles, to minimize the risk of injury to staff, particularly portering staff handling goods for incineration.

The briefing group should decide whether a disposal hold should be incorporated in the department, and if so, what its capacity should be. There are no hard and fast guidelines on this

and it must be determined by departmental disposal policy and experience.

Any department which generates a considerable quantity of material for disposal has a need for a disposal hold, as well as management procedures agreed with other relevant departments to remove it.

Figure 8.7 illustrates the major sources, routeing and destination of items for disposal or recycling.

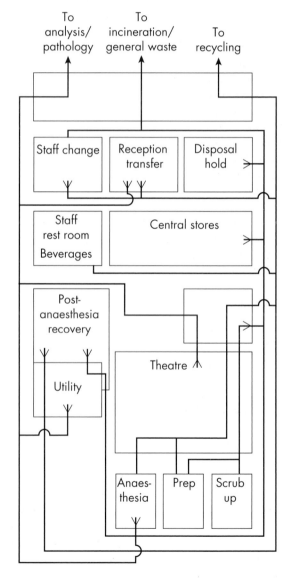

Figure 8.7 Routing of items for disposal, recycling or analysis. (Reproduced with permission from NHS Estates 1993 Health Building Note 52.)

PARTICULAR SPACES TO CONSIDER

Entrance and transfer areas

'Briefing by exception' calls for the briefing group to prioritize several factors in the management of the department, principally patient transport, control of infection, security, supplies and disposal.

A single point of access ensures security. It follows that the reception point should overlook the access to staff changing rooms, main storage area, disposal hold and the patient transfer area. The siting and design of the reception office should make it self-evident as a point of reception for visitors to the department. This office is the control centre for the department and provision must be made for IT. Space must be made for holding specimens and samples for despatch to the pathology department. Information essential to the control function, e.g. operating lists and departmental notices, needs to be displayed prominently.

Sizing the transfer area will be determined primarily by policies on moving the patient. A supervised waiting space for hospital porters should be provided near the entrance to the department.

Staff control base

A staff control base is the control point for coordinating staff activities, the movement of patients and the routeing of pathology specimens to reception for onward despatch. It must be easily accessible from the reception, administrative offices and operating suites.

Operating suite

The anaesthetic room

The need for an anaesthetic room depends on patient throughput. If flows are low anaesthesia may be induced in the operating theatre itself. If required, the anaesthetic room is reached from the limited access zones and leads to the operating zone.

The anaesthetic room is a quiet place in which a general or local anaesthetic is given to the patient. Consideration should be given to reassuring and relaxing the patient, for example by providing space for escorts to accompany the patient to this point, or by the incorporation of artwork in the ceiling.

Clinical procedures such as setting up intravenous infusions may be instituted here, and diathermy pads and monitoring equipment attached to the patient.

Patients may arrive on a trolley or a bed. Children may be accompanied by a member of the paediatric nursing team and a relative. The patient is then transferred to the operating table or top and positioned for surgery before or after anaesthesia is induced.

The patient is moved feet first into the anaesthetic room and then into the theatre. Privacy and an undisturbed environment are of great importance.

All anaesthetic rooms in a suite should be laid out identically. Workflow considerations predominate. *Any team should be able to lay their hands on whatever they need in any anaesthetic room in a suite without consciously looking for it.* Layouts should not be handed, to make services distribution easier, for example:

- A worktop and storage units should be located to the left-hand side of the patient.
- Services such as piped medical gases and vacuum outlets for associated equipment and anaesthetic gas scavenging should be on the right.

Ceiling-mounted services are not recommended. A separate surface is required for writing.

A lockable cupboard must be included for the temporary storage of controlled drugs issued to an anaesthetist for an operating session. Some drugs may require refrigerated storage. The briefing group must consider whether a controlled drugs cupboard is to be located in each anaesthetic room.

Some procedures may require a mobile examination lamp. It is essential that maximum illumination can be brought to bear on any part of the patient required. The worktop should be lit by a concealed source, and it should be possible to vary the level of the general lighting to reduce the glare for patients.

Double doors from the corridor into the anaesthetic room and from there to the operating room are required to pass the patient and the team through. These doors should have obscurable glass panels to allow inspection while maintaining privacy. Each such set of doors must be capable of standing open, should be wide enough to admit any associated equipment, and should close quietly.

There should be a clock with sweep second hand above the entrance to the operating theatre.

There should be a sink for clinical hand washing and rinsing anaesthetic instruments, sited at the end of the room opposite the position of the patient's head.

The operating room

This is the operating zone. During an operation the surgical team and assisting staff occupy distinct areas of the room, centred on the patient. The patient, scrub team, anaesthetist and assistant occupy the central area, together with the equipment being used in the procedure.

Most of the equipment and most members of the surgical team are positioned either side of the patient on the table, with the exception of the anaesthetist, the assistant and the anaesthetic equipment at the head of the table. The remaining space is used by staff indirectly involved in the procedure who are responsible for provision, management and removal of equipment and supplies. Special surgery may require the team to cluster at the head or the foot of the table.

Notionally the operating team will occupy a circle centred on the patient. With the supporting team occupying the remainder of the space the resultant room tends to be square. In practice, a room of 7.5×7.5 metres provides sufficient space for most procedures.

A minimum clear height of 3 metres from finished floor level to ceiling is usually recommended for unrestricted adjustment of the operating lamps and other ceiling-mounted equipment. Doors through which beds or trolleys pass must be wide enough to allow them through with attachments, including sterile drapes, and should be capable of standing open.

A high level of general lighting should be provided, together with a special ceiling-mounted light to illuminate the operating area.

The electrical outlets, medical gases and vacuum points and anaesthetic scavenging points must all be conveniently sited.

Additional facilities such as lighting controls, diagnostic imaging screens, clock, and writing surface and swab count record are usually arranged on a theatre control panel which can easily be seen by the operating staff.

Natural daylight is appreciated by staff. A view out is much preferred, but this requires a window in an outside wall. A second-best option is to allow for 'borrowed light', but this may need obscured glass to maintain privacy.

Operating microscopes The briefing group should give particular attention to the size and weight of any operating microscopes which may be required. Guidance should be given to the design team in order to position it exactly where it will be required.

Ceiling mounted or mobile? A mobile microscope is preferable if it is to be used by several different surgical specialties, each for a limited period in a working session. Consideration then must be given to moving and storing a bulky but delicate instrument. An operating microscope requires a rigid supporting structure to avoid vibration.

Dedication of theatres Reserving an operating room for a single specialty which may be a surgeon's preference, is not always possible. The briefing group should consider with such surgeons as may use the equipment the extent to which such a reservation can be justified.

Scrubbing and gowning area

This space, reached from the limited access zone, leads directly into the operating zone. The number of staff scrubbing simultaneously will vary but usually does not exceed three. The scrub team should be able to see a clock, and if possible be able to see into the theatre. It may be useful to have a view through to an adjoining scrubbing and gowning area in case someone needs assistance from a circulating nurse.

There should be sufficient space to store sterile packs of gowns and gloves for at least one session. Such supplies should not be placed over a trolley on which an open gown pack is presented or exposed to accidental splashing. There should be provision to collect used towels and pack wrappers.

Preparation room

This space, reached from the limited access zone, leads directly into the operating zone. There should be sufficient space to allow a scrub nurse and assistant to prepare a sterile trolley and also to provide parking for sterile trolleys for the next case.

The nurse preparing a sterile trolley will scrub up in the scrubbing and gowning room, but don gloves in the preparation room.

Staff must be able to readily locate items required. As in the case of the anaesthetic room, the layout should be common to all preparation rooms, but if the theatre it serves is dedicated to a particular type of procedure there must be an area set aside for items particular to that procedure.

The door into the operating room must be wide enough to allow laid trolleys to pass through without compromising their sterility.

Utility

This space is reached from the operating zone and leads to the limited access zone. Here equipment used in the operating room is cleaned, fluids are emptied, and mops and buckets needed for cleaning the operating room floor between cases are stored.

Commonly surgeons wishing to examine a specimen do so in this space, and so facilities for clinical hand washing should be provided.

For disposal of fluids a slophopper sink and drainer may be provided. The sink can also be used for filling buckets and for examining specimens. *For health and safety reasons the slophopper should be set at a height convenient for lifting and emptying of buckets.*

Sealed and labelled disposal bags, bagged linen, bagged waste and other miscellaneous items generated during an operation are collected for removal.

There must be space for storing disposal bags and specimen containers, and hook clips for storage of mop handles and heads.

Patient exit bay

This space leads from the operating zone back to the limited access zone. Exit bays are commonly shared between two operating rooms. They should be large enough to park two beds or trolleys awaiting the return of patients from the operating room.

Postanaesthetic recovery

Patients are brought from operating rooms to this space while they recover and await transfer to the wards. While here they still require the attention of anaesthetists and other trained staff. As they recover consciousness patients are disorientated and probably in some pain, and so the decor should be as pleasant as possible. Austere colour schemes should be avoided.

Lights in the ceiling should be positioned to avoid causing glare to patients' eyes. Background lighting should not be harsh, but local lighting must be available to help in clinical examination. Any windows should preferably have a pleasant outlook.

Space should be provided for escorts to be at the patient's side when they recover.

Two beds per operating room should be provided as a minimum. The briefing group should consider the average time that will be spent in the recovery room and the number of cases to be operated on during a session.

The briefing group will need to take account of hospital transportation policy when working out arrangements for the delivery, despatch and parking of beds and trolleys.

Because anaesthetists are still responsible for the patient while they are recovering, the recovery room should not be remote from the operating rooms.

There should be piped oxygen, 4-bar medical compressed air and medical vacuum outlets and other services available to each bed space. Wall-mounted delivery points are common, but mobile equipment suspended from racking increases the possible uses of the space. A further option is to use delivery points suspended from the ceiling. This gives the greatest flexibility, but at some cost.

The postanaesthestic recovery room must be mechanically ventilated because the air is polluted by anaesthetic gases exhaled by patients.

A nurses' base should be placed to provide an overview of all the recovery beds and with direct access to both clean and dirty utility spaces:

- Clean utility should provide storage for consumables and equipment and, subject to policy, drugs.
- The dirty utility should be equipped for the storage, preparation for use and disposal after use of vomit bowls, bedpans, urine bottles and for urine testing. A small amount of storage is required for items for processing.

A local equipment store may be provided.

Endoscope cleaning room and store

This space is reached directly from the operating theatre or endoscopy room where these procedures take place. The acoustic and visual privacy of the theatre for the patient undergoing the procedure is paramount. There should be separate clean and dirty zones. The dirty area is for reprocessing used equipment. The clean area is to store reprocessed equipment. Endoscopes and accessories which cannot be autoclaved may be cleaned and disinfected in the dirty area. Accessories may be sterilized and suction bottles automatically emptied, washed and disinfected. Alternatively, these items may be returned to the sterile services department. The briefing group must advise the design team which approach is to be followed.

For the dirty area, advise whether there is to be:

- an automated endoscope washer/disinfector
- an automated suction bottle washer/disinfector
- twin sinks with double drainers

- working space (with worktop autoclave)
- storage for consumables
- suction to irrigate tubes and cannulae
- ultrasonic cleaner for flexible accessories.

Toxic and hazardous substances are used. Brief the designers that the toxic vapours should be immediately removed by extraction ventilation to prevent inhalation.

Protective clothing is worn when mixing/dispensing toxic solutions of glutaraldehyde. Storage is required for goggles, gloves, impermeable aprons and respiratory protection.

For the clean area advise on the extent of provision of:

- storage for flexible endoscopes
- storage for flexible accessories for endoscopes
- storage for other accessories for endoscopes.

Provide clinical hand-washing facilities and pedal-operated sack stands for associated waste disposal.

Image processing

If film is to be used in the operating department provide a space equipped with power and water supplies, a sink and drainer and a benchtop automatic processor. There should be storage space for a small quantity of chemicals.

The design team should be referred to the COSHH Regulations 1988 and subsequent amendments.

Imaging equipment bay

The bay provides parking for mobile image intensifiers and storage for lead aprons and gloves worn by staff. The design team will need to be told that the use of X-ray or laser equipment will require the approval of the local radiation/laser protection adviser.

Facilities for staff and visitors

Garment changing

Changing rooms are needed in operating departments so that staff and visitors can change from everyday outdoor clothes or working hospital uniform into theatre clothing, including footwear. They should be able to place their outdoor clothes in secure storage racks or lockers, select theatre clothing of the appropriate size from the range presented, change, put on theatre footwear and move through the access zones to places of work. The process is reversed when leaving the department.

The arrangements for storing outdoor clothes and uniforms and for receiving soiled theatre clothing and footwear must be convenient and orderly. Recent developments in the layout of swimming pool changing rooms merit study. Greater throughput for both sexes can be achieved in a limited space by using unisex cubicles rather than single-sex communal changing rooms.

Storage and washing of theatre boots or clogs requires special consideration. Facilities in the cleaners' room may be used to wash them. Boots and clogs, whether clean or dirty, should be stored tidily on a designated and easily accessible boot rack in a space that is well ventilated. Clean and dirty boots should be separated.

WCs should be located adjacent to the changing area and not within it.

Rest rooms

Rest rooms are by definition places where staff can escape for a brief period from the stress of the work in the department, and so the interior decor should be both cheerful and relaxing. A pleasant outlook is usually appreciated.

The briefing group will have to take account of the hospital policy on catering and ensure that the department catering policy is consistent with it. This will determine the extent to which any pantry needs to be provided, or whether simpler facilities for making beverages and perhaps preparing snacks with a microwave is more appropriate. Any catering provision will imply the supply and disposal of consumables, and may also include a requirement for washing up.

The briefing group must decide on a policy for the provision of spaces for medical, nursing staff,

assistants and orderlies, which may be varied according to local custom and practice or for cultural reasons.

There should be telephone links to outside the department, provision for writing notes and for reading.

Offices

The changing nature of administrative work means that all offices should be provided with IT outlets and telecommunications as well as conventional facilities for writing case notes.

Consider 'hot desking'. In many organizations it is no longer considered necessary to provide a dedicated workstation for each member of staff. For example, consider whether it is necessary to provide a separate office for clinical nurse teachers in addition to the office for theatre nursing staff.

The brief may need to include:

- **Manager's office** The theatre manager's office need not be sited within the access zones of the theatre itself. Visitors to this office are not expected to change. It should be adjacent to the theatre reception office. It is the base for administrative work and for carrying on confidential discussions with staff and relatives or escorts.
- **Medical staff office** The medical staff office should be next to the rest room(s). As well as being a possible location for confidential discussions, it is likely to be used for dictating case notes.
- **Theatre nursing staff office** This may also be used for confidential discussions and will be used for storing records.

Seminar room

Hygiene considerations and garment changing regimens mean that it is not easy for staff to leave the department for training. A seminar room may therefore be provided. This space may also serve as the base for the clinical nurse teacher. There should be lockable storage for dedicated equipment.

Consider whether training can take place in the rest rooms. It may be possible to double up on the use of space by skilful timetabling.

Ancillary spaces

Relatives' and escorts' waiting room Relatives and escorts of patients undergoing surgery are likely to be feeling anxious. A room in which they can wait after escorting their relative or friend into the anaesthetic room and before meeting them again in the postanaesthesia recovery room should be provided. The decor should be pleasant and calming. A pleasant outlook should be provided if possible.

This room should be near the recovery room and out of the main traffic flows of the department. It needs facilities for making drinks and telephone calls.

Storage

Within the stores area there should be a place for administrative work, with local filing, information and telephone outlets.

A number of discrete stores should be provided:

• **A central departmental store**, subdivided into separate areas for general consumables, disposables and stationery; a sterile supply section for preset trays and other sterile packs from the SDU and commercial sterile disposables (e.g. sutures, implants). Controlled drugs should not be held here. Liaison with the SDU manager is needed to ensure that the shelving and racking provided is similar to that in the SDU itself. Space should be allowed for loading and unloading sterile preset instrument trolleys without compromising the trolleys.

• **Main equipment store**, for bulky items not in daily use. Most of these are floorstanding, so designated parking bays should be identified for each item of equipment known at the time of briefing, together with the provision of additional space for unknown items, which will have to be based on a best guess. Because of the value of this equipment the store should be secure.

• **Local equipment storage**, immediately adjacent to the operating suites for items in daily use.

• **Disposal hold**: the floor should be clearly marked into zones for various types of waste, to allow rapid collection and to reduce the staff cost associated with collection and disposal. Part-height dividers provide greater integrity.

• **Mobile imaging equipment** needs a designated space to park with access to mains power for recharging.

• **Medical gases** need a 'ready-use' store for gas cylinders to be used with anaesthetic machines and ventilators. Consult published official guidance on the storage of gases (e.g. HTM 22) and relevant codes and standards (e.g. BS 1319). It should be easy to identify the type of cylinder and control full and empty cylinders.

• **Blood**: stored blood needs to be held in a refrigerator which is quickly and easily accessible from the operating suites. The staff control base is a convenient place.

Dedicated air compressor

A dedicated air compressor system supplying high-pressure medical air for surgical tools is needed, located outside the department. It may be in the plant room dedicated to ventilating the department.

Cleaners' facilities

There must be sufficient space to park and manoeuvre cleaning machines, and also for its cleansing, the disposal of dirty water and used cleaning materials and for subsequent hand washing.

Equipment servicing room

This space should be adjacent to the main equipment store.

Some user servicing is possible for theatre equipment using manufacturers' manuals. Sometimes this is supplemented by formally agreed local instructions.

There should be space provided to service equipment within the department. It should be large enough to park and manoeuvre the equipment and include a workbench and lockable storage for tools, as well as washing facilities.

A number of engineering services will be required: medical gas outlets for oxygen, nitrous oxide, compressed air and vacuum, together with gas scavenging facilities.

Switch cupboard and battery enclosures

These should be provided, along with a separate enclosure for the emergency lighting batteries and automatic battery charging equipment, which should be directly accessible from a circulation area; away from water surfaces; and lockable. There should be clear and safe access for maintenance staff.

The battery enclosure will require ventilation – this is achieved at the least cost when it is located on an outside wall.

The switch cupboard should preferably be within the department and the battery enclosure should be central to the operating suites. Staff safety should not be compromised by passing traffic or opening doors during maintenance.

Planning a day surgery unit

Day surgery is not a sub-specialty of surgery. (Guidelines for day case surgery – The Royal College of Surgeons, 1992)

A day surgery unit (DSU) should be self-contained and not an adjunct of an operating department. Developments in day surgery will continue to extend the types of procedures which can be carried out within the day. Patients attending the DSU should not need to attend any other department on the day of treatment.

Elective surgery is changing. For instance, the Central Middlesex Hospital is developing the world's first Ambulatory Care and Diagnostic Centre (ACAD). It will be a 'one-stop shop' incorporating consultation and examination suites, radiography, pathology side room, laboratories and overnight stay accommodation. It moves the concept from treatment within the day to treatment within a 24-hour cycle.

A DSU should not be used for:

- surgical procedures on inpatients
- overnight stay of A&E patients
- to provide additional accommodation for inpatients
- a waiting space for patients treated elsewhere.

Carers should be able to accompany children or other special patients as much as possible during their attendance. This has a radical effect on the range of spaces to be provided and the ambience that has to be created: it must be domestic, friendly and as non-clinical as possible. Special arrangements may be necessary for particular groups of patients, e.g. children and people with learning difficulties.

PEOPLE FOCUS

It is generally agreed that hospital patients and visitors are vulnerable groups and that the physical environment can be a source of stress. This stress can impede the ability of patients to recover from their illness. It can also increase hospital costs and decrease the quality of life for patients, visitors and staff. (Carpman, Grant and Simmons, *Design That Cares*)

There are particular issues to be addressed in the DSU.

- **Wayfinding**. The ease with which people can find their way around a building will affect their stress level. Patients and their escorts will not be attending the DSU frequently: not being able to find their way will cause a sense of helplessness and frustration. Signs and artwork can help, but only if they work in conjunction with other parts of a coordinated wayfinding system, such as floor and wall colours and, most importantly, a legible plan. What is simple and obvious probably works best.

- **Physical comfort**. There are two aspects to comfort: the impact of the environment on people, and how easy it is for them to control it. Factors that affect people are temperature, noise levels, smells and lighting. Factors they can control include ventilation and lighting levels and seating arrangements.

- **Privacy and contact**. The tapestry of life does not stop at the door to the DSU. The design must allow for patients and visitors to regulate their contact with others and create opportunities for visual and aural privacy, contact, distraction and solitude. Putting on a hospital gown in particular can make people feel they have lost identity and become an exhibit.

- **Image**. The environment communicates messages as well as providing for physical comfort and enabling clinical procedures. In the DSU environments need to be created which communicate a positive, caring message.

ACCESS

Being able to see the entrance as you approach is more important than the sign which announces the DSU for what it is.

Most patients will come by car or ambulance. Easy access from the approach road to the drop-off area is needed. The drop-off area should be right outside the main entrance and under cover. Access into the building should be barrier free. Ideally staff should be available to help patients from their transport into the unit.

The drop-off area needs to be big enough to allow enough space for collecting patients and visitors as well as dropping them off. Manoeuvring space and space for passing traffic need to be allowed.

Public transport, including taxis, should be able to be reached easily, or alternatively a free phone service may be considered.

Exit signage showing the way back to car parks and public transport is as important as signs to guide people in.

SAFETY AND SECURITY OF ACCESS AND PARKING AREAS

Using car parks at night can make people feel insecure. Lighting levels and obvious video surveillance can provide reassurance. Voice-to-voice call points should be available for help in emergencies.

Parking layouts need to allow ambulance access in case of emergency. Multistorey car parks need to allow ambulance headroom for the same reason. Alternatively, full-size bed lifts are needed to evacuate a patient in distress.

If the DSU is to be in a hospital, then liaison with the car parking manager will be required to ensure that an adequate number of spaces can be reserved for use by patients and escorts as close as possible to the DSU or, if absolutely necessary, away from the DSU.

This is very much a second-best option, as in order to be effective it would have to be policed to ensure that parking spaces designated for the DSU are not abused by people parking on a longer-term basis.

A number of items of legislation address the needs of people with disabilities who have difficulty with mobility or orientation:

- The Building (Disabled People) Regulations 1991 (1992 edition)
- The Disabled Persons (Services Consultation and Representation) Act 1986
- The Chronically Sick and Disabled Persons Amendment Act, 1976
- The Chronically Sick and Disabled Persons Act, 1970.

Design teams should be expected to know the building regulations and other guidance material.

Consultation with local voluntary organizations concerned with caring for disabled people is not recommended, as the level of expertise is extremely variable and can be overspecific to one particular group of people with disabilities. Reliance must be placed on the design team to demonstrate that they have used their best endeavours to adequately meet all foreseeable requirements.

ACCESS FOR DISABLED PERSONS AND PEOPLE WITH YOUNG CHILDREN

People with poor eyesight or with physical disabilities need special design features to help them get around. So do the infirm and the able-bodied with children:

- Footpaths need to be wide enough for two wheelchairs or two pushchairs to pass.
- Footpath surfaces, kerbs and gratings should be designed so that they do not trap heels, sticks or wheels.
- Kerbs should be dropped at road crossings.
- Cues should be provided at road crossings, such as different surfaces, or buzzers.
- Keep all gradients as flat as possible and not exceeding 1 in 20.
- Do not use surface finishes that are inherently bumpy, such as interlocking bricks or paviors.

SEGREGATION OF CHILD PATIENTS AND ADULT PATIENTS

There are four options to consider here, taking account of such factors as the number and case mix of children to be admitted:

- a dedicated children's unit
- a dedicated children's session
- concurrent children's and adults' session
- limited use of the DSU by children.

In a combined unit, providing either dedicated children's spaces or a dedicated session ensures segregation. Areas used by children and their carers need tuning to provide an appropriate environment, and so a dedicated session is not really a satisfactory physical solution.

Ancillary accommodation such as WCs, play spaces and quiet rooms need to be scaled to the child user. Consideration should also be given to providing special waiting and recovery spaces for teenage patients.

NHS guidance suggests that the best compromise may be achieved by limiting the use children make of the DSU. Admitting children to the day-care ward of the children's department and returning them there after surgery for recovery and discharge means that children are in the DSU only for surgery and postanaesthetic recovery.

Such a solution may be imposed by financial constraint but runs contrary to the principle of focusing on the needs of those who use the unit. Moving children from and back to the children's unit increases the opportunities for loss of orientation and feeling undervalued. It underscores the message 'You are being processed', rather than 'We are looking after you'.

CATERING

Patients, escorts and carers should be able to have light refreshments and beverages during the predischarge recovery period. Provision should also be made for staff to relax and to consume snacks and beverages.

The briefing team should consider whether this facility should be shared with the patients, escorts and carers as part of the overall strategy to make the atmosphere of the unit more relaxed.

GENERAL FUNCTIONAL AND DESIGN REQUIREMENTS

Figure 8.8 illustrates overall relationships and access zoning.

The interior decor must help to reassure patients that they are receiving an excellent service.

Facilities must be easy for staff to operate and manage, therefore:

- patients and supplies should be moved forward without unnecessary loops on their journey backwards
- crossover circulation should be avoided
- preoperative and postoperative patients should not meet at any point within a unit
- double handling of patients and supplies should be avoided
- staff travel should be minimized.

Activities occur in the following sequence:

- reception and waiting
- patient assessment
- preoperative preparation
- operative procedure
- postanaesthesia recovery
- predischarge recovery and discharge.

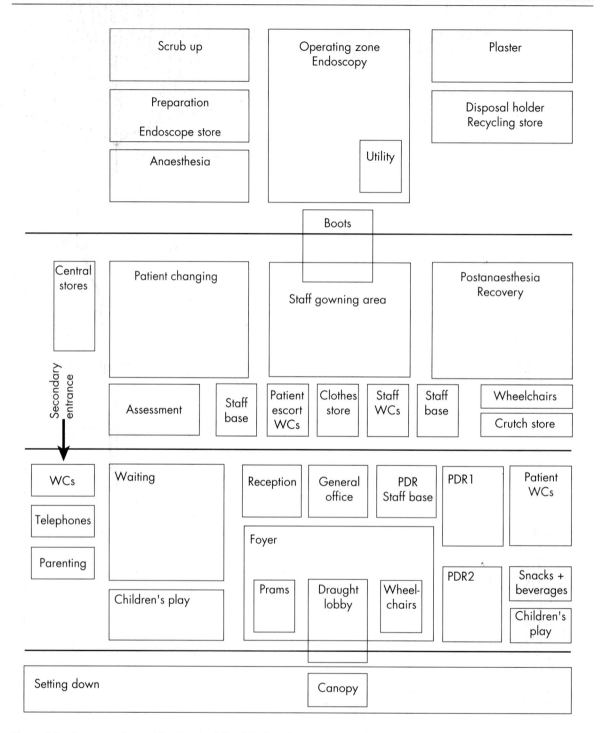

Figure 8.8 Access zoning and functional relationships in a day surgery unit. (Reproduced with permission from NHS Estates 1993 Health Building Note 52.)

Care should be taken to ensure that patients do not feel they are being processed on an assembly line.

Planning separate flow lines for patients and their escorts, staff, supplies and disposal will ensure that clashes between the different types of movement are minimized and the privacy and dignity of patients is maintained. Figure 8.9 shows the key overall flow patterns.

Advise the designers of the planned through-put of patients, the patient management system, the appointments system and the policy for escorts. These decisions will affect not only the overall size of spaces but such things as the number of chairs to provide in the main waiting area.

The section on planning gives guidance on how to calculate the necessary figures.

ENVIRONMENT AND DESIGN

The privacy and dignity of patients should be the main concern. Separate spaces must be provided, with visual and auditory privacy, particularly in patient assessment and postanaesthetic areas. The environment of the DSU should be seen as an extension of daily life rather than a hospital visit. This point should be stressed to the design team.

Separation of men and women waiting for assessment or recovering from anaesthesia is desirable.

COMMUNICATION WITH ESCORTS

While patients are undergoing operations or recovering from anaesthesia their escorts may

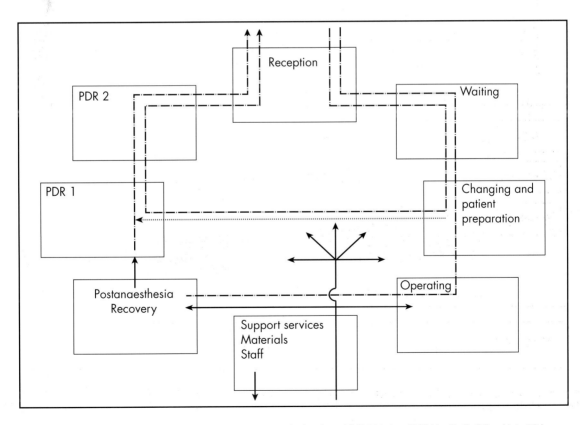

Figure 8.9   General flow patterns. (Reproduced with permission from NHS Estates 1993 Health Building Note 52.)

wish to leave the DSU. They may be provided with a paging device to advise them when it is appropriate to return. Advise the design team if you intend to take up this option.

CLINICAL INVESTIGATION

Day care is being extended to other services, such as endoscopy and medical investigation and treatment. These may be included within the DSU, as shown in Figure 8.7.

LINKS WITH THE OUTPATIENT DEPARTMENT

Conventionally, patients are assessed in the outpatient department to save on making a provision for consulting and examination rooms within the DSU. It is therefore useful to have the two departments close to one another. This allows patients to make their own appointments for day surgery immediately following an attendance at the outpatient department. IT can make this process automatic and relax this requirement.

PARTICULAR SPACES TO CONSIDER

Main entrance canopy

The main entrance canopy can act as a signpost to the entrance of the department. The canopy should be large, to allow sufficient undercover protection both for patients getting out of or entering private vehicles and those being helped out of or into ambulances, which may call from time to time. The canopy should be high enough not to foul aerials or lights on ambulances.

The whole area should be well lit and fully visible from the reception space.

Reception area

This will be continuously occupied during working hours and will therefore need to be protected by a draught lobby with automatic doors.

The foyer can become congested and confusing, especially for elderly people or those with disabilities, and so:

- the doorway should be passable for someone with poor sight or in a wheelchair (or pushing a buggy)
- the doors should open with little applied effort
- the threshold should be flush with indoor and outdoor surfaces
- there should be ample crush space.

There should be sufficient space for people to be able to have their business dealt with by reception staff without encumbering the movement of others.

Secondary entrance

A secondary entrance is needed so that the main entrance can be dedicated to adult patient access and discharge. The secondary entrance can provide access for staff, a delivery point for suppliers, access for children, and, in the reverse direction, access to inpatient accommodation if patients need to be admitted to the hospital. These activities are not fully compatible. In particular, it is probably necessary to segregate access for children from the other activities to avoid accidental trauma.

The secondary entrance needs to be securely controlled and supervised.

Children

Children attending the DSU need to be treated as a separate stream of patients from the adults attending. They may come either direct to the unit or from a children's unit in the adjoining hospital, or even a children's ward.

Children will be escorted either by a member of their family or a nurse, and therefore changing spaces for them must all contain a space for the escort to sit. Separate spaces must also be provided for children to recover prior to their discharge.

Reception point

The reception point should be:

- directly visible from the entrance
- self-evident without signage

- positioned to face the majority of people arriving
- positioned so that queues of people waiting to be attended to do not block the circulation area
- positioned so that they can be attended to in acoustic privacy
- positioned so as to have a clear view over all the waiting areas.

Should a reception counter be provided? A reception counter introduces a separation between those providing care and those about to receive it, which is not appropriate to the atmosphere a DSU should try to create. Cosmetic design to make a reception counter open and friendly is not sufficient. Reception should be welcoming to all users. Consider whether the reception function can be broken down into a series of different spaces and surfaces for greeting people, dealing with their enquiries, reading case histories or preparing files prior to treatment.

Patients may be encouraged to examine and discuss their individual case histories with practitioners. An informal space in which this can be done should be provided. One model for this approach is exemplified by the PLANETREE approach in the USA.

Reception staff may personalize their working space. This helps promote a relaxed atmosphere.

The working spaces should keep out of sight any supplies and equipment not related to the business of receiving people. A separate space is needed for display terminals and to hold a working supply of stationery and office accessories and park a health records trolley.

Work spaces should provide:

- temporary parking space for people's possessions while they are talking to reception staff
- space to sit in a chair or wheelchair while talking to the staff.

Designers should be briefed to consider the visual comfort of those working in reception for extended periods, avoiding very reflective finishes and employing task lighting.

Receptionists will mainly be receiving and registering patients and their escorts as they arrive. They will also be expected to deal with personal enquiries and to remind escorts of arrangements which are being made to collect patients and to pass the patients into the care of nursing staff. A personal carer may be assigned to patients at this point to stay with them for the duration of their stay.

Information on patients and their health records may be provided by document, by IT or by telephone. Discussion of confidential matters relating to patients over the telephone must be discreet.

General office

There should be an office for the general administration of the unit, which also serves as the IT/communication centre.

Main waiting area

The main waiting area should be a place that can support a wide range of activities. It should feel comfortable and safe. It should not feel isolated. Surveys have shown that people in waiting areas like to feel part of what is going on and find watching other people interesting.

Time becomes important, so there should be an easy-to-read clock visible. A calendar helps people to plan future visits to outpatient clinics if required.

Vending machines for beverages and snacks may be included for escorts waiting for patients and for patients prior to their discharge. Tea and coffee making facilities can allow escorts to participate in caring for patients: an important displacement activity psychologically, it can contribute to reducing the patient's anxieties.

Waiting is not just passive: designers should be reminded to provide plenty of space for comings and goings.

There should be secure storage for patients' belongings so they do not have to take them into the unit.

Escorts and patients are likely to want to deposit outerwear; there should be somewhere for it to dry, so a coat room may be more appropriate than coin-return lockers.

Provide a secure parking space for prams and pushchairs, and for wheelchairs.

Maps and way-back directions should be prominently displayed, near bus schedules and taxi phones.

The main waiting area should have a comfortable and relaxing environment with domestic-style finishes and furnishings. Elderly people and young children may require different types of seating, and a check should be made that these have been included by the design team in their proposals. Seating should be informal to allow patients to sit in small groups with their escorts and visitors. There should be space for a patient using walking aids or in a wheelchair to be included unselfconsciously in such groups.

The selection of seating requires special care and ergonomic consideration. People come in a variety of shapes and sizes, with varying degrees of mobility. Professional advice should be sought, but there are two key principles for briefing:

- support of most of the body, from the thighs to the upper back and neck, is needed for long-term sitting.
- getting up out of a chair is the crucial activity.

Brief the design team to provide 'non-institutional' lighting. Surveys have shown that spots are seen as less institutional than strip lights, and tungsten less clinical than fluorescent.

Lighting needs to be intense enough to read but not overbright and glaring.

Think of the waiting area as a series of family-sized territories such as they might occupy on a picnic:

- spaces for families with children, with sound-absorbent finishes, under close supervision by reception
- more remote spaces should be quiet enough for reading
- spaces for people waiting collection and transport
- spaces for snacking
- spaces for telephoning.

Consider audio or visual entertainment systems, as these may help mask any confidential discussions that may be going on.

Play area

There should be a play area off the main waiting area next to the children's waiting area where children can play safely, preferably with an adjacent outdoor play area. The UK's climate means it is likely that the outdoor play area will be used only infrequently, so consider specifying hard but safe surfaces rather than grassed areas.

Children play most safely under the direct supervision of their parents or family. Seating for adults should be provided in the children's play area.

Patient preparation

Patients wait changed in a changing room or a sub-waiting area prior to going to theatre. A base should be provided, overlooking the patient changing rooms and sub-waiting area, for staff managing the preparation of patients before their operations.

Patients' changing rooms

The management of patients' clothes is an important part of the activities of the day centre. Before proceeding to theatre patients need to remove their usual clothes, change into a theatre gown and put their usual clothes into secure storage to be returned to them after the operation. Patients can feel anxiety about clinical procedures and changing into a theatre gown is part of getting prepared psychologically.

Waiting gowned up can be felt to be humiliating or an infringement of modesty, so private cubicles are often preferred. Patients with escorts can be accompanied into the changing area if they so wish.

The space required can be reduced by providing sub-waiting areas for patients to relax and wait once they have changed. Some patients may find it less stressful to be in the company of other patients and escorts rather than in a cubicle by themselves.

Changing cubicles should be placed next to the main waiting area and patient WCs and near the patient preparation staff base. Patients can undress in privacy, staff can carry out some preoperative procedures and confidential discussions may be held. The cubicles should be places where patients can relax and wait prior to being escorted to anaesthetic rooms and therefore should feel as non-clinical as possible.

A cubicle should provide:

- space for undressing, gowning and collecting clothes for storage
- a chair for the patient to sit on while waiting
- space for a wheelchair to be parked or for the patient to be transferred to a wheelchair
- a chair for the escort to sit on or for medical staff to hold confidential discussions
- a stool to lift the foot for shoe tying
- a mirror that can be used by sitting and standing people
- a staff call button.

A window giving on to a pleasant view will help reduce anxiety.

Preclinical checks, such as measurement of blood pressure, may be carried out in the changing cubicles or in the preoperation sub-waiting area once the patients have changed.

The number of changing rooms required will depend on the estimated throughput of the operating theatres. It is preferable for children not to have to use the same changing accommodation as adults. Lockers and seating can be more suitably sized for them in dedicated cubicles.

The NHS suggests that where procedure time is equal to the patient preparation time one changing room should be allowed per operating suite, with one extra to meet the overall demand.

Consulting and examination room

A consulting and examination room should be provided adjacent to and accessible from patient changing and sub-waiting areas, for when medical staff feel that examination and consultation are needed. It requires facilities for patient examination, report writing and clinical hand washing as well as a comfortable arrangement for the doctor and patient to discuss the condition.

Patient ablutions

Adjacent to the main waiting area and to the changing rooms there should be provided:

- toilets for men and women, including bidet facilities in at least one cubicle for each sex
- a wheelchair users' WC cubicle
- a patients' shower, so that patients can take a shower or staff may elect to give a shower before the operation
- a space where babies can be fed and changed in privacy.

In the DSU WCs are required for:

- men, women and children who are disabled, as well as those who are ambulant
- for patients, escorts, staff and visitors, any of whom could be disabled
- for patients and escorts, close to the main waiting area, the patient changing rooms and the predischarge recovery areas.

Single-cubicle WCs complete with hand-washing facilities and a space where a baby can be changed are recommended for use by either men or women.

WCs are usually arranged in groups and each group should include a WC of a standard suitable for use by disabled people and another where seat height and handbasin height are suitable for children.

In the predischarge areas bidets should be included within the WC cubicles.

Operating rooms

General guidelines for operating suites are as set out earlier in the chapter.

Operating rooms in the DSU are subject to a high throughput, and therefore in place of the transfer trolley system used in an operating theatre suite consider using fully adjustable day surgery patient trolleys both in the operating rooms and in postanaesthesia recovery.

Consider including one theatre with an operating theatre table and transfer trolley for more complex procedures.

Anaesthesia may be induced either in an anaesthetic room or in the operating room itself, and the design should permit either option. Patients entering the anaesthetic room will either walk or be brought in a wheelchair or on a trolley. Children will be accompanied by their escort. Most patients will be assisted on to the trolley before preoperative procedures, which are carried out once the patient is comfortable.

Layout considerations for the anaesthetic room were discussed earlier.

Some procedures may require the use of a mobile examination lamp and the rooms should be large enough for such a lamp to be placed.

Postanaesthesia recovery

General requirements for postanaesthesia recovery were set out earlier in the chapter.

Patients requiring supervision by trained staff will be moved after their operations to the postanaesthesia recovery room (PAR). Patients not requiring supervision will move directly to the predischarge stage 1 recovery space (PDR1). Patients are likely to walk from the PAR to the PDR1, which should be as close together as possible.

The number of spaces to be allowed in the PAR will depend on the throughput of the unit and on the need to provide separate recovery spaces for children. It is suggested that the overall number should be equal to the number of operating rooms plus one.

To allow for variations in demand for recovery space in PDR1 those spaces nearest to PDR1 in the PAR should be designed to be used on a swing basis, i.e. to allow recovery either on a trolley or on a semireclining chair.

Predischarge recovery areas (PDR)

PDRs should appear as non-clinical as possible. Separate spaces should be provided for the two stages of PDR, PDR1 and PDR2.

First-stage recovery can take place in a reclining chair in an individual curtained cubicle. Patients who have received a local anaesthetic are likely to walk there from the theatre or to be moved there in a wheelchair or on a trolley. Patients who have recovered in the PDR are likely to move there on foot.

Each first-stage cubicle should have:

- service terminals, including oxygen and medical vacuum, and a staff call button for emergencies
- a reclining chair
- a chair for the patient's escort.

There should be space for the patient to dress in privacy when sufficiently recovered.

The second stage of recovery, PDR2, takes place in an open lounge with informal seating and occasional tables. This space should be close to the main entrance from which patients will leave on discharge. It should be possible for patients and their escorts to provide themselves with refreshments and beverages, i.e. by making tea and coffee and using a microwave oven to heat snacks (in which case there should be storage space for crockery and cutlery and a refrigerator for perishables). Alternatively, a vending machine may be included.

Separate PDR2s should be provided for children, women and men. There should be a play area adjacent to both the adults' and children's PDR2, with design considerations similar to that adjacent to the main waiting area. There should be WCs for men, women and children adjacent to the PDR2s.

Crutches, splints and wheelchair storage

There should be a store for crutches and splints to be issued to patients on discharge, adjacent to the PDR2 areas. Discrete parking areas should also be provided for wheelchairs near the operating theatres and the two PDRs.

PDR staff base

Staff need a base for administrative procedures associated with the discharge of patients, which should be carried out as informally as possible; the design should be open and inclusive, but it should be possible to supervise both PDR1 and PDR2 areas. There should be space for IT activities and shelves for storage of sterile supplies and disposables and for the storage of medical products. There should be facilities for clinical hand washing.

While in the PDR2 patients will be given post-operative instructions and possibly prescribed drugs or medicines. On discharge their records will need to be returned to the DSU general office. Unobtrusive parking space for the records trolley should be provided in this area.

Staff changing

Advise the design team what the policy may be.

Staff may arrive changed from home or from a central uniform exchange, or it may be assumed that staff changing will take place in the unit if hospital uniforms are to be worn.

As part of the intention to make the unit feel as non-clinical as possible, non-theatre staff may wear everyday clothes with their name badges only.

Operating theatre clothing will be issued to staff in the unit. Separate changing areas must be provided for male and female staff in which they can change from their everyday clothes and store their outdoor garments and other personal items. There should be a provision for secure hanging of wet outer clothing and lockers for personal items. Theatre garments will be provided in packs on shelving, and parking spaces should be provided for trolleys to take soiled used theatre clothing.

Returns and disposal holding

Space for the holding of returned items and items for disposal should be provided near the exit from which the collection will be made. Separate spaces need to be provided for:

- Soiled linen, which may be collected from the operating theatre suites and the staff changing area. This will be for short-term holding prior to reprocessing. Theatre garments should be kept in bags colour coded according to Health and Safety Guidelines.
- Soiled returns holding. Space should be provided for SSD trolleys loaded with used instruments and other items for collection and reprocessing.
- Disposal. Items for disposal should be bagged and colour coded in accordance with

Health and Safety Guidelines. Waste may be separated into general non-clinical refuse and clinical waste in separate coloured bags. Alternatively it may be felt that all waste should be treated as clinical waste. Sharps will be in separate containers for disposal.

Incineration of clinical waste may take place on or off site. The briefing group should give careful consideration to the separate processing of non-clinical waste to reduce the overall consumption of energy and reduce atmospheric pollution.

The three areas should be clearly separated and ventilated. A single holding area may be used, but in this case separate enclosed areas for different types of storage should be provided to help to ensure that the different kinds of materials for reprocessing and disposal are not accidentally confused.

The size of the holding facility will be determined in part by the number of operating suites in the unit and the throughput of each suite, and in part by the frequency of collections.

Cleaners' facilities

These were discussed on page 350.

ENGINEERING CONSIDERATIONS
Illuminated signs

Illuminated signs should be discussed with a competent laser/radiation adviser and provided in accordance with recommendations, together with interlocks between doors where radiation or laser is to be used. Relevant technical specification is set out in BSEN0825 *Radiation Safety of Laser Products, Equipment Classification, Requirement and Users' Guide.*

Secondary entrance to DSU

The secondary entrance to a DSU should be linked to reception by an intercom system and interlocked with electromagnetic doors. There should be an internal override for staff to use routinely for entrance and for final exit in the event of fire, but it is recommended that this be monitored at reception to ensure that the door is not abused by being kept permanently open, thereby nullifying its security intent.

Music and TV in the DSU

There may be music outlets in the main waiting area, the patient changing cubicles, theatres and PDR2. TV outlets may be provided in the main waiting area and PDR2.

Staff location and patient call systems

The policy adopted for the hospital in general should be extended to the operating department and DSU. Guidance on systems is contained in HTM 20.

Patient staff call buttons should be provided in the patient changing areas, consultation and examination room and PDR1. Staff to staff call systems should be provided in the postoperative recovery area.

Telephone and data wireways

Standard guidance is contained in the NHS model specification C47. Because of rapidly changing technology briefing teams are recommended to update recommendations on telephone, data links and CCTV links. Requirements should be worked out and specified in detail to the design team.

Information and management technology (IT) now has a central role in health management and health education.

Good communications are of great importance. IT systems selected should be consistent with local and national health service IT strategies. Give detailed consideration to:

- the choice of system
- functions to be included
- location of terminals
- access levels for information.

Functions may include:

- maintaining an appointment system:

  — confirming appointments with patients
  — checking patients intend to attend
  — making appointments with other hospital departments
- running a patient management system:
  — communicating with health record services
  — advising a GP of the results of day care and requesting a follow-up
  — planning visits by district nurse before or after surgery
- managing theatre lists and sessions
- transmitting urgent test results from pathology
- transmitting digital imagery to or from radiography
- managing materials and supplies
- providing clinical audit
- providing management and statistical information, including feedback from patients, GPs and district nurses
- monitoring building security:
  — unauthorized access
  — tampering with secure storage locations
  — fire
- monitoring environmental conditions – link to hospital BMS.

A typical network for a day surgery unit is shown in Figure 8.10.

Fire

The day surgery unit is a high life risk department with highly trained staff available. It is therefore not necessary to have bells, and alarm systems should be designed to avoid causing panic. Visual indicators and buzzers should be called for in preference to bell systems.

Medical gas stores

Briefing teams should refer to the NHS letter WKO(85)1 dated February 1985, *Code of Practice for the Storage of Medical, Pathology and Industrial Gas Cylinders*, especially paragraph 12 which deals with ready to use stores and the requirements therein to prevent the storage of flammable anaesthetic gases.

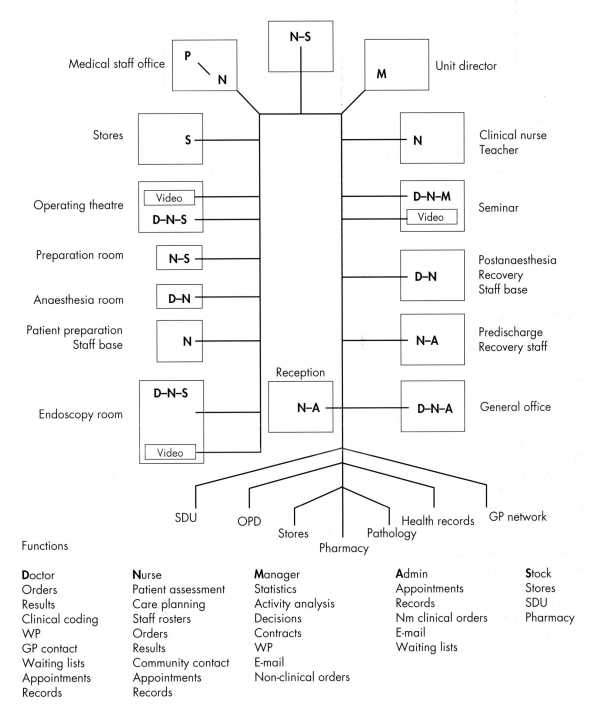

Figure 8.10   IT network diagram for a day surgery unit. (Reproduced with permission from NHS Estates 1993 Health Building Note 52.)

Sizing the facility

The briefing group will have to advise the design team of their requirements in terms of number of spaces or rooms for each activity that will be required. The following method relies on accumulated health management statistics or, in the absence of these, best guesses.

OPERATING THEATRES

Determine for each specialty:

- the number of beds required, using historical data, numbers of beds currently available, demographic trends and local demographic characteristics, N_s
- the average length of stay of patients, T_s
- the bed occupancy factor, which can be current/desired/likely, and should be compared with regional and national factors to calibrate for realism, f_{NS}
- patient throughput per year, Q_s
- average number of cases per theatre session, C_s
- the number of working weeks in the year, W
- the planned preventive maintenance programme: maintenance may take place during working sessions or during the times when theatres are not in use, p
- the number of waiting list patients eventually receiving surgery, f
- the provision of theatres for emergency use, E.

$$
\begin{aligned}
F_s &= \text{average future bed throughput per year} \\
&= f_{Ns} \times 365/T_s & (1) \\
Q_s &= N_s.F_s & (2) \\
&= \text{total bed throughput per year} \\
e_s &= \text{total annual theatre caseload} & (2) \\
&= Q_s.F_s & (3) \\
S_s &= \text{total number of theatre sessions a year for elective surgery} \\
&= e_s/C_s & (4)
\end{aligned}
$$

The total number of sessions required will be the sum of all sessions for all specialties:

$$
\Sigma_n = S_{1-n} \qquad (5)
$$

Provision must be made for emergencies.

Usually one theatre is reserved for emergencies, increasing the total session requirement by 10 sessions a week, assuming two sessions a day, 5 days a week.

$$
\begin{aligned}
E &= 10 \\
A &= \text{number of theatres required} \\
A &= \frac{\Sigma_2 + (W.E)}{W(E-x)} & (6)
\end{aligned}
$$

where x is any reduction from working sessions for planning preventive maintenance.

Round A to the nearest whole number. Rounding up will represent a degree of over-capacity, rounding down undercapacity. Exercise judgement.

DAY CARE

Similar logic may be applied. Determine for each surgical specialty, endoscopy or clinical investigation likely to be required:

- number of cases per year, Q_s;
- average number of cases per working day, C_s;
- length of working week in days, E-x;
- the number of working weeks in the year, W

$$
\begin{aligned}
&= C_s \times W(E-x) & (1) \\
e_s &= \text{total annual capacity for one day theatre} \\
&= Q_s/e_s & (2) \\
S_s &= \text{the total number of theatre sessions required}
\end{aligned}
$$

Again the total number of theatre sessions for all specialties must be summed:

$$
\begin{aligned}
\Sigma_n &= S_{1-n} & (3) \\
A &= \frac{\Sigma_n W}{W(E-x)} & (4) \\
&= \text{the number of theatres required}
\end{aligned}
$$

The number should be rounded as before, with similar implications.

AREA SCHEDULES

The schedule of accommodation and the approximate built area can be derived from Tables 8.1

and 8.2 once the number of theatres is known. The space standards are those recommended by the NHS. Most UK operating departments fall in the range 4–8 theatres and DSUs in the range 2–4 theatres.

Table 8.1 Operating department schedule of accommodation

Space	Unit area m²	4 theatres No.	4 theatres Total area m²	6 theatres No.	6 theatres Total area m²	8 theatres No.	8 theatres Total area m²
Entrance/transfer	49.00	1.0	49.00	1.0	49.00	1.0	49.00
Reception office	11.00	1.0	11.00	1.0	11.00	1.0	11.00
Porters' base	5.50	1.0	5.50	1.0	5.50	1.0	5.50
Staff control base	11.00	1.0	11.00	1.0	11.00	2.0	22.00
Male staff change	20.00	1.0	20.00	1.0	20.00	2.0	40.00
Male staff personal washing	11.50	1.0	11.50	1.0	11.50	2.0	23.00
Female staff change	20.00	1.0	20.00	2.0	40.00	2.0	40.00
Female staff personal washing	14.00	1.0	14.00	2.0	28.00	2.0	28.00
Boot lobby	16.00	1.0	16.00	2.0	32.00	2.0	32.00
Anaesthesia	15.00	4.0	60.00	6.0	90.00	8.0	120.00
Operating theatre	40.00	4.0	160.00	6.0	240.00	8.0	320.00
Scrub-up	10.00	4.0	40.00	6.0	60.00	8.0	80.00
Preparation	12.00	4.0	48.00	6.0	72.00	8.0	96.00
Utility	10.00	4.0	40.00	6.0	60.00	8.0	80.00
Patient exit bay	23.00	2.0	46.00	3.0	69.00	4.0	92.00
Local equipment store	1.00	4.0	4.00	6.0	6.00	8.0	8.00
Recovery		1.0	86.00	1.0	107.00	1.0	164.00
Utility	6.50	1.0	6.50	1.0	6.50	1.0	6.50
Mobile imaging equipment bay	6.00	1.0	6.00	1.0	6.00	2.0	12.00
Staff rest room – 10 places	16.50	1.0	16.50	2.0	33.00	2.0	33.00
Staff rest room – 20 places	30.00	1.0	30.00	1.0	30.00	2.0	60.00
Staff pantry	7.00	1.0	7.00	1.0	13.00	1.0	13.00
Office – theatre manager	11.00	1.0	11.00	1.0	11.00	1.0	11.00
Office – theatre nursing staff	11.00	1.0	11.0	1.0	11.00	1.0	11.00
Office – medical staff	11.00	1.0	11.00	1.0	11.00	1.0	11.00
Cleaners	7.00	1.0	7.00	1.0	7.00	1.0	7.00
Disposal		1.0	8.00	1.0	8.00	1.0	13.00
Endoscope cleaning, etc.	10.00	1.0	10.00	1.0	10.00	1.0	10.00
Central stores		1.0	83.50	1.0	93.00	1.0	137.00
Equipment store		1.0	21.50	1.0	31.50	2.0	43.00
Medical gas store	7.00	1.0	7.00	1.0	7.00	1.0	7.00
Switch room	4.50	1.0	4.50	1.0	4.50	2.0	9.00
Image processing	6.50	1.0	6.50	1.0	6.50	1.0	6.50
Seminar room	20.00					1.0	20.00
Clinical nurse teaching	11.00					1.0	11.00
Net total			889.00		1,201.00		1,631.50
Rounded totals			**1,111.00**		**1,500.00**		**2,040.00**

Essential complementary accommodation

Space	Space area m²	Circulation etc.	Total area m²
Seminar room	22.00	8.00	30.00
Clinical nurse teaching	11.00	2.00	13.00

Table 8.2 Day surgery unit schedule of accommodation

Space	Unit area m²	2 theatres		4 theatres	
		Qty	Total area m²	Qty	Total area m²
Entrance and reception					
Draught lobby	10.50	1.0	10.50	1.0	10.50
Foyer		1.0	27.50	1.0	36.00
Reception		1.0	9.50	1.0	14.50
General office	16.50	1.0	16.50	1.0	16.50
Main waiting		1.0	40.00	1.0	80.00
Play area		1.0	12.00	1.0	18.00
Disabled WC/wash	4.00	1.0	4.00	1.0	4.00
Visitors' WC/wash/parenting	4.00	1.0	4.00	1.0	4.00
Children's WC/wash	2.00	1.0	2.00	1.0	2.00
Patient preparation areas					
Patient preparation staff base/utility		1.0	8.00	1.0	11.50
Patient changing room	6.50	3.0	19.50	5.0	32.50
Consulting/examination & assessment room	14.00	1.0	14.00	1.0	14.00
Colonoscopy preparation room	6.50	1.0	6.50	1.0	6.50
Patient predischarge areas					
Predischarge recovery: stage1		1.0	91.00	1.0	145.50
Predischarge recovery: stage 2		1.0	22.00	1.0	40.00
Predischarge recovery play area		1.0	12.00	1.0	18.00
Predischarge recovery staff base/utility	11.00	1.0	11.00	1.0	11.00
Beverage & snacks	7.50	1.0	7.50	1.0	7.50
Patients' clothing store	4.00	1.0	4.00	1.0	4.00
Wheelchair parking bay	2.50	1.0	2.50	1.0	2.50
Patients sanitary facilities					
Patients' WC/wash	2.00	2.0	4.00	2.0	4.00
Patients' WC/bidet/wash	3.50	1.0	3.50	1.0	3.50
Disabled WC/wash	4.00	1.0	4.00	1.0	4.00
Operating theatre suites					
Anaesthetic room	15.00	2.0	30.00	4.0	60.00
Operating theatre/endoscopy room	40.00	2.0	80.00	4.0	160.00
Scrub-up and gowning	10.00	2.0	20.00	4.0	40.00
Preparation room	12.00	2.0	24.00	4.0	48.00
Utility room	10.00	2.0	20.00	4.0	40.00
Cleansing/disinfecting room	9.50	1.0	9.50	1.0	9.50
Patient exit bay	23.00	1.0	23.00	2.0	46.00
Equipment cupboard	1.00	2.0	2.00	4.0	4.00
Mobile imaging equipment bay	6.00	1.0	6.00	2.0	12.00
Image processing	6.50	1.0	6.50	1.0	6.50
Postanaesthesia recovery room		1.0	48.00	1.0	65.00
Postanaesthesia room staff base/utility	11.00	1.0	11.00	1.0	11.00
Dirty utility		1.0	6.50	1.0	6.50
Male staff change/locker room		1.0	20.00	1.0	30.50
Female staff change/locker room		1.0	23.00	1.0	30.50
Boot lobby	8.00	1.0	8.00	1.0	8.00
Staff WC/wash	2.00	2.0	4.00	4.0	8.00
Staff shower	2.50	2.0	5.00	2.0	5.00
Staff rest room		1.0	16.50	1.0	30.00
Staff pantry	7.00	1.0	7.00	1.0	7.00
Unit director's office	11.00	1.0	11.00	1.0	11.00
Nurse manager's office	11.00	1.0	11.00	1.0	11.00
Medical staff office	11.00	1.0	11.00	1.0	11.00
Central store		1.0	59.00	1.0	83.50
Main equipment store	21.50	1.0	21.50	1.0	21.50
Equipment service room	10.00	1.0	10.00	1.0	10.00
Medical gas cylinder store	7.00	1.0	7.00	1.0	7.00
Cleaners' room	7.00	1.0	7.00	1.0	7.00
Disposal hold		1.0	5.50	1.0	8.00
Switch cupboard		1.0	3.00	1.0	4.50

Table 8.2   Day surgery unit schedule of accommodation (Contd.)

Space	Unit area m²	2 theatres		4 theatres	
		Qty	Total area m²	Qty	Total area m²
Operating theatre suites (cont'd)					
Battery cupboard		1.0	3.00	1.0	4.50
Net total			851.00		1,290.00
Circulation allow 25%			306.50		462.50
Rounded total			**1,060.00**		**1,600.00**

Essential complementary accommodation			
Space	*Unit area m²*	*Circn, etc. m²*	*Total area m²*
Seminar	22.00	8.00	30.00

Optional accommodation and services			
Sub-waiting area (3 persons)	7.50	2.50	10.00
Sub-waiting area (5 persons)	9.50	3.50	13.00
Patients' shower	2.50	1.00	3.50
Children's reception	5.00	2.00	7.00
Plaster room	16.00	6.00	22.00
Clinical nurse teacher	9.50	3.50	13.00
Interview room	6.00	2.00	8.00
Baby feeding and nappy changing room	5.50	2.00	7.50
Crutches and splint store	2.00	.50	2.50

Planning guides

HEALTH BUILDING NOTES

NHS Estates, an executive agency of the UK Department of Health, publish a series of Health Building Notes (HBNs), which are available through HMSO bookshops or by post. HBNs provide advice on the briefing and design implications of departmental operational policies. They are prepared in consultation with representatives of the NHS and appropriate professional bodies. They are probably the best set of documents of this type in the world.

Relevant guides are:

HBN 26   *Operating Department*   (1991)
HBN 52   *Accommodation for daycare*
       Vol. 1 *Day Surgery Unit*   (1993)
       Vol. 2 *Endoscopy Unit*   (1994)
       Vol. 3 *Medical Investigations and*
           Treatment Unit (in preparation)

Related guides published by NHS Estates and others include:

• *Activity Database*: a computerized system for defining the activities which have to be accommodated in spaces within health buildings. *NHS Estates*

• *Design Guides*: complementary to Health Building notes, Design Guides provide advice for planners and designers about subjects not appropriate to the Health Building Notes series. *HMSO*

• *Estatecode*: user manual for managing a health estate. Includes a recommended methodology for property appraisal and provides a basis for integration of the estate into corporate business planning. *HMSO*

• *Capricode*: a framework for the efficient management of capital projects from inception to completion. *HMSO*

- *Concode*: outlines proven methods of selecting contracts and commissioning consultants. Both parts reflect official policy on contract procedures. *HMSO*
- *Works Information Management System*: a computerized information system for estate management tasks, enabling tangible assets to be put into the context of servicing requirements. *NHS Estates*
- *Option Appraisal Guide*: advice during the early stages of evaluating a proposed capital building scheme. Supplementary guidance to *Capricode*. *HMSO*
- *Health Technical Memoranda*: guidance on the design, installation and running of specialized building service systems, and on specialized building components. *HMSO*
- *Health Guidance Notes*: an occasional series of publications which respond to changes in Department of Health policy or reflect changing NHS operational management. Each deals with a specific topic and is complementary to a related Health Technical Memorandum. *HMSO*
- *Encode*: shows how to plan and implement a policy of energy efficiency in a building. *HMSO*
- *Firecode*: for policy, technical guidance and specialist aspects of fire precautions. *HMSO*
- *Nucleus*: standardized briefing and planning system combining appropriate standards of clinical care and service with maximum economy in capital and running costs. *NHS Estates*
- *Concise*: software support for managing the capital programme. Compatible with *Capricode*. *NHS Estates*

Items published by HMSO can be purchased from HMSO bookshops in London (post orders to PO Box 276, SW8 5DT), Edinburgh, Belfast, Manchester, Birmingham and Bristol, or through good booksellers.

ACTIVITY DATA

The Activity DataBase (ADB) is an information system originally developed as part of the 'Nucleus' hospital planning programme and is heavily coloured by the concepts therein. ADB is now software based and updated twice yearly. It comprises three types of information:

- Activity space data sheets (A-sheets)
- Activity unit data sheets (B-sheets)
- A-sheet component listings (D-sheets).

A-sheets record in detail each task or activity performed in a particular activity space, which may be a room, space, corridor or bay, together with recommended environmental conditions and technical data necessary to perform the activities, for example the level of lighting and the power for operating tools to carry out an operation.

B-sheets provide text and scale graphics related to one activity. They show equipment fitted or to be supplied as part of the building and the required engineering services terminals.

D-sheets quantify the total numbers of components extracted from all relevant B-sheets related to an individual A-sheet.

The system has weaknesses:

- It is incomplete: activities tend to be formally planned, whereas a lot of the guidance given here is about informal activities, particularly waiting.
- Formally planned activities tend to be based on preferred British procedures, some of which have as much a cultural overtone as a technical one.
- B-sheets graphics are ageing and reflect the information provided by the manufacturer originally consulted.

Design practices with expertise in healthcare building design are tending to develop their own parallel databases as a result of having to operate in international markets. Anyone briefing a design team should therefore require designers to show evidence of their in-house databases, and should be prepared to depart from national guidance material, such as that published by NHS Estates, wherever the design team's input may be more up to date or where planned practice requires developing unique briefing material.

Where such material is required the ADB presentation provides an excellent pro-forma for establishing the information a design team will require.

Funding building works

GOVERNMENT GUIDANCE

Capital planning requires a strategic approach, asking the three classic questions: Where are we now? Where do we want to be? and How do we get there? In designing a new facility the answer is not always a new building.

In the UK the NHS Executive has published a *Capital Investment Manual* (1994) which should be referred to for public sector projects (Fig. 8.11).

This must also be seen in the context of the Sir Michael Latham's report *Constructing the Team* (HMSO 1994), which is aimed at reducing real construction costs by 30% by the year 2000 by removing from the building procurement process all those factors which add cost but do not add value (such as project managers and CDM supervisors) but which include:

- weak expression of clients' wishes
- poor understanding of the briefing process
- confusion of design responsibility
- unsuitable procurement routes
- wasteful duplication of qualification and pre-qualification procedures
- adversarial contracts
- underuse of standard components and off-site assemblies.

The government intends to become a 'best practice' client and, notably, intends to publish a briefing guide.

RISK MANAGEMENT

The briefing group will be expected to recruit qualified financial advisers to help prepare their business case. This section is a guide to strategic thinking needed when briefing the advisers.

Risk management is part of a strategy which goes back to the 1984 Efficiency Study into Government Purchasing. In 1986 the Central Unit on Procurement was set up within the Treasury to help government departments improve value for money in all aspects of

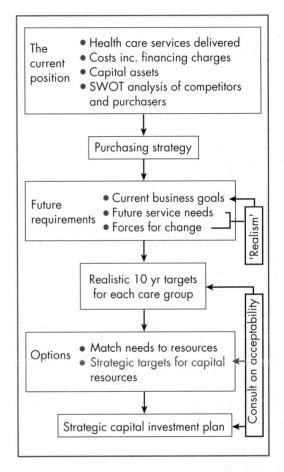

Figure 8.11 A strategic approach to capital investment planning. The test for realism can never be wholly objective as the criteria are best guess estimates, even if tempered by testing against a range of criteria- sensitive analysis. The clear logic of the approach breaks down when the consultation process starts and runs the risk of megaphone decision making by those able to orchestrate and influence opinion. (Reproduced with permission from NHS Estates Concode.)

purchasing goods and services, works projects and project management, by promoting best practice. It is recommended that the briefing group obtain CUP Guidance No. 41, *Managing Risk and Contingency for Works Projects* (1993), which encourages public sector clients to develop a risk management approach to works projects, setting out a strategy and preferred approaches to risk analysis. The process is iterative and contains the following steps:

- **Identification** of what could go wrong so as to identify the risks
- **Assessment**, understanding and quantifying possible impacts on projects
- **Monitoring and control**, to identify options for dealing with unacceptable risks and select risk responses that give better value for money
- **Setting a budget** (contingency), to control expenditure on residual risk after such measures have been taken.

Success means striking a balance between the threat/cost of risk and the opportunity of an outcome that has better value for money. Options might include:

- avoiding risk altogether, by reappraisal of the objectives or organization of the project
- reducing the risk in some way, by further investigation of, say, site constraints, changes to design or building method
- transferring risk to another: the responsibility should only be passed on if another party is better able to control the risk
- sharing the risk, if the risk is beyond the control of any one party and a realistic way of sharing it can be agreed.

Residual risk exposure

CUP guidance calls for an estimate of the most likely time or cost effect of the residual risk, i.e. that which remains after all appropriate risk management steps have been taken, to be provided for when setting the budget.

Risk analysis

Risk analysis of the residual risk should be carried out at key stages of the project:

- to identify all potential risks
- to make a qualitative assessment of them
- to make a quantitative assessment.

The results of any risk analysis should identify:

- the most likely risk scenario with the cost or time provision most likely to be required

- any unusual risk characteristics
- variability of project outturn
- the maximum likely risk estimate.

Benefits

The Treasury has made clear the direction it wishes to see providers take in managing risk on construction projects. It hopes that a risk management approach will lead to an overall reduction in risk exposure and produce better estimates and budgets. Other benefits include:

- more focused, explicit decisions
- clearer definition of risks
- prompter responses to risks that materialize
- full use of project personnel's expertise
- accumulation of knowledge corporately rather than with individuals.

APPROVAL PROCESS

All government departments have delegated authority for projects in the range, typically, of £1–5m. Above those limits projects must go to the Treasury for a three-stage process:

- business case and options appraisal
- approval to take forward planning and design
- final approval for full implementation.

At the final approval the Treasury normally sets out monitoring conditions which contain 'triggers' requiring resubmission of the scheme to its scrutiny. Usually these concern costs, specifically the expenditure of the contingencies sums in the estimate.

Approval budgets

The Treasury wants to see that a project has been well thought out, makes good economic sense and that a positive attitude to risk has been taken. The financial elements of the submission should contain:

- the base estimate of resources, works and other costs, i.e. the total cost or time determined by pricing or programming elements of the project without any provision for residual risk affecting outturn

- a contingency to provide for the most likely cost of the residual risk.

This produces the average risk estimate, i.e the most likely estimate of cost and time to complete the project. This is normally the budget approved by the Treasury.

Sometimes there are projects with a greater degree of residual risk because of complexity, scale, innovation or length of time associated with the development. Such schemes need a tol-erance, or allowance above the budget, to allow for the possibility that further spending may be needed. The tolerance is usually the amount the provider can spend from his own budget without returning to the Treasury for further approval.

Use of contingencies and tolerances should improve the overall accuracy of estimates and help control expenditure on the previous exposure to residual risk.

Health and safety legislation

CDM REGULATIONS

The Construction (Design and Management) Regulations came into force from 31 March 1995. They cover any project where the construction phase is more than 30 days, or where more than 500 man days of work are involved. They cover any of the following types of work:

- construction
- alteration
- conversion
- fitting out
- renovation
- repair
- upkeep
- redecoration
- cleaning
- demolition.

Such works must be notified to the HSE.

Law

- Breach of the Regulations can be a criminal offence (Regulation 21).
- The Regulations represent the law until such time as they are changed, and clients, planning supervisors, designers and principal contractors are obliged to comply with them.
- Not all the Regulations apply to a domestic building for a client user/owner whose habitation it is (see Regulation 5).

- The Regulations apply to certain types of building and certain activities outside the UK (Regulation 20).
- The Regulations do not cover work carried out by a tenant in a client's building; these may require a separate H&S Plan.

What to do

- Consult published guidance (1995): *Approved Code of Practice, Designing for Health and Safety* (Green Book), HSE Books. *Case Study Guidance for Designers*, CIRIA. *RIBA Practice Notes*.
- If in doubt, ask the HSE for guidance and interpretation.
- It is the architect's legal duty to ensure the client is aware of his legal obligations and duties under the Regulations, i.e. to
  - appoint a competent and adequately resourced Health and Safety Planning Supervisor, Designer and Principal Contractor (Regulations 6 and 13)
  - satisfy himself that the Planning Supervisor, Designer and Principal Contractor are competent and have allocated adequate resources for Health and Safety (Regulations 8 and 9)
  - provide the Planning Supervisor with any available information relevant to the Health and Safety of the project (Regulation 11)

— ensure that construction work does not start until a Health and Safety Plan has been prepared (Regulation 10)

— ensure the Health and Safety file is available for inspection by a specified person (Regulation 12).

• This raises interesting issues, such as who can state that a Planning Supervisor is competent and adequately resourced, and how will competence be regulated?

• Suggested checkpoints:

— Does the proposed Planning Supervisor have identified and suitably qualified health and safety staff?

— Does the proposed Planning Supervisor have internal risk assessment procedures?

— Does the proposed Planning Supervisor have any experience of this role under the draft CDM Regulations?

ROLES AND RESPONSIBILITIES

The Planning Supervisor must:

• notify the HSE of the projects (Regulation 7 and Schedule 1)

• ensure designers avoid and control risk

• ensure designers coordinate their work in respect of the health and safety of the project

• prepare the health and safety plan for tender issue

• receive information from the Principal Contractor and Contractors and incorporate this in the health and safety file

• present the H&S file to the client on project completion (Regulation 14).

The Designer must (Regulation 13):

• ensure that considerations of the design for any project to be built include:

— avoidance of reasonably foreseeable risks to the health and safety of anyone constructing the building, cleaning it or working on it or to anyone who may be affected by such a person at work

— combating at source such risks to such persons

— prioritizing measures which protect all such persons rather than those that protect the individual at work

• ensure that the design includes adequate information about foreseeable risks for incorporation in the H&S plan

• cooperate with the Planning Supervisor and any other designer so far as is necessary to allow each of them to comply with the Regulations

• at completion provide the Planning Supervisor with all the information on operation, maintenance and H&S for incorporation in the H&S Plan

• ensure the Regulations make due recognition of 'reasonable' expectations and the practicability of compliance at the time of design.

The Principal Contractor must:

• develop and implement the H&S plan

• ensure the coordination of all contractors

• verify that all contractors and operatives comply with site rules set out in the H&S plan and ensure that operatives are adequately trained (Regulation 17)

• obtain from contractors their risk assessment methodology so that he can comply with his duties under the regulations (Regulation 19.1)

• display notices and exclude unauthorized persons

• ensure the views and advice concerning H&S of persons at work on a project or of their representatives are received, discussed and coordinated (Regulation 18)

• pass information to the Planning Supervisor for the H&S file (Regulation 16.1).

APPOINTMENTS

• The appointment of a qualified competent and adequately resourced Planning Supervisor should be a separate appointment with a distinct fee.

• The duties of the architect in applying the Regulations should be subject to a separate agreement and fee.

• The architect must not enter into a collateral warranty which imposes on him, unwillingly, the function of Planning Supervisor.

• The architect (or any other person) should be qualified to act as Planning Supervisor. If wishing to offer his services in this capacity he should be able to demonstrate evidence of his competence and of professional indemnity insurance to cover this function.

COMMENTARY

The principles of risk management usually involve an appraisal of the costs and benefits of different options, typically avoiding the risk altogether, reducing the risk in some way, and transferring the risk to another party. However, the object of transferring risk is to pass responsibility to someone able to control it better. The CDM Regulations have transferred H&S risks to the client, etc. Are these persons best able to control it?

The H&S file provided for under the Regulations notably fails to include works carried out by tenants in a building. Coordination will be a major issue.

In making a cost–benefit appraisal of H&S risks, clients should be aware that actual risk reduction can perhaps be best achieved by an incentive scheme rather than reliance on legislative provisions. Custom and practice on site is the key.

In the absence of recognized criteria for qualification, and until such time as these are available, clients should scrutinize the representations made to them by others offering services in accordance with the Regulations, applying the test of reasonableness.

Look for evidence that knowledge has been organized corporately rather than lying in the experience of individuals.

Appendices

CONTENTS

Appendix 1

Day surgery nurse assessment clinic

PURPOSE

To assess patient suitability for day-case surgery. This will be done in the form of a preadmission interview between nurse and patient. Physical, psychological and social aspects will be discussed. Specific information for pre- and postoperative care will be given, both verbally and in a printed document. There will be a contact telephone number of the day-case unit should the patient need further advice. The patient and their carers will be asked to read their instructions prior to hospital admission. It is hoped that this will help in planning for a safe early discharge.

The assessment should ideally be carried out 2–8 weeks prior to surgery.

INVESTIGATIONS

Patients will have their blood pressure, pulse and weight checked. They will be asked to complete a questionnaire on their medical condition; depending on the results, further tests such as ECG, LFTs, U&Es, FBC and sickle test will be initiated. The results of these will be assessed by a consultant anaesthetist and recommendations given.

INFORMATION

The length of time needed for recovery, length of time needed off work, level of assistance required and level of incapacity should be discussed. This should be particularly borne in mind for patients with a manual occupation having a hernia repair.

It must be emphasized that a patient must be taken home in a car and have a fit responsible adult to care for them for 24 hours. The journey should be no more than 1 hour's drive from the hospital. Adults taking a child home are advised to have another adult driving.

Good home support and conditions are essential, so it must be ascertained that patients have access to a toilet and a telephone.

Adult patients who do not have a level of understanding that would enable them to comply with treatment should be excluded.

No upper age limit is set, as physical and social conditions should be considered more important than chronological age.

If the assessing nurse is in any doubt about the patient's suitability for day-case surgery they should discuss the case with the anaesthetist.

MEDICAL CRITERIA FOR ACCEPTANCE OF DAY-CASE SURGERY.
(Using recommendations from the Royal College of Surgeons and ASA I & II)

Inclusions

Patients that:

- are free from disease
- have a disease that is controlled
- are asthmatic but not requiring steroid therapy
- are hypertensive with a diastolic pressure below 100 mmHg (with treatment)
- have diet-controlled diabetes but do not have glycosuria.

Exclusions

Patients with:

- heart disease, heart murmurs or having had heart surgery
- chest disease, chronic respiratory disorders or severe asthma
- insulin-dependent diabetes
- epilepsy, who have had a fit in the last 3 years
- severe rheumatoid arthritis
- symptomatic hiatus hernia
- chronic neurological disease
- renal failure
- uncontrolled hypertension
- necessity to take steroid therapy or anticoagulant therapy
- severe psychiatric illness
- uncontrolled thyroid disorders
- a body mass index index greater than 34%
- known previous adverse anaesthetic reactions (or who have had a relative who has had an adverse anaesthetic reaction).

All patients over 60 should have an ECG.

NURSE ASSESSMENT CLINIC

Date of assessment: Assessing nurse:

Name:
Date of birth:
Address:

BP: Pulse: Weight:

MEDICAL HISTORY

Heart disease ....Yes/No
Chest disease (asthma) ....Yes/No
Hypertension ....Yes/No
Diabetes ....Yes/No
Thyroid problems ....Yes/No
Rheumatoid arthritis ....Yes/No
Renal problems ....Yes/No
Bleeding disorders ....Yes/No
Gastric problems (including hiatus hernia) ....Yes/No
Psychiatric illness ....Yes/No
Anticoagulant therapy ....Yes/No
Steroid therapy ....Yes/No
Current medication (please list) ....Yes/No

No. of units of alcohol consumed weekly
No. of cigarettes smoked daily

SOCIAL HISTORY

Do you live within 1 hour's drive? ....Yes/No
Do you have access to a telephone? ....Yes/No
Do you have a fit responsible adult to care for you for 24 hrs? ....Yes/No
Will you be able to organize for someone to drive you home? ....Yes/No
If you have any small children will you be able to organize
assistance for a few days if mobility is reduced? ....Yes/No

Appendix 2
Health and safety audit tool

HEALTH AND SAFETY AUDIT

LOCATION: _____

NAME OF AUDITOR: _____ **DATE OF INSPECTION:** _____

1.	Policy	Yes	No	Remarks	Action	Date & signature
1.1.	Does the department have a copy of the facility's health & safety policy?					
1.2.	Does the department have its own health & safety policy?					
1.3.	Are copies available for the staff to read?					
1.4.	Are records maintained of staff having read the policies?					
1.5.	Are the department's policies reviewed regularly? Give date of last review.					
1.6.	Have all amendments been brought to the attention of all staff?					
2.	Management	Yes	No	Remarks	Action	Date & signature
2.1.	Is the responsibility for health and safety clearly identified?					
2.2.	Is there an identified safety representative?					
2.3.	Are departmental audits carried out? If yes state frequency.					
2.4.	Does the responsible person carry out: Staff training; Health and safety audits; Check safe working practices, ensure personal protective equipment is utilized, etc.; Ensure emergency equipment is working and maintained correctly?					

2.	Management (cont'd)	Yes	No	Remarks	Action	Date & signature
2.5.	Are the following names clearly displayed in the department: First aider Safety adviser?					
2.6.	If a first aid box provided is it checked regularly?					

3.	Audits	Yes	No	Remarks	Action	Date & signature
3.1.	Are documented audits carried out regularly (minimum annually)?					
3.2.	Do supervisors accompany safety personnel during audits?					
3.3.	Have previous audits been reviewed to ensure appropriate action was taken?					
3.4.	Are all hazards in the work area detailed and checked during audit?					
3.5.	Date of last audit?					
3.6.	Have copies of audits been sent to the facility's health & safety officer?					

4.	Accident reporting and investigation	Yes	No	Remarks	Action	Date & signature
4.1.	Is an accident/incident form always completed?					
4.2.	Are all accidents/incidents investigated?					
4.3.	Is an analysis of accident/incidents occurring over time carried out?					
4.4.	Are results of the analysis used in staff training?					
4.5.	Following investigation and analysis are recommendations made to prevent recurrences?					
4.6.	Is there an effective follow-up procedure to ensure that recommendations are carried out?					

5.	Fire safety	Yes	No	Remarks	Action	Date & signature
5.1.	Are fire procedures clearly displayed?					

5.	Fire safety (cont'd)	Yes	No	Remarks	Action	Date & signature
5.2.	Are fire exits clearly marked with appropriate signs?					
5.3.	Are fire exits kept clear at all times?					
5.4.	Can the fire alarm be heard in all parts of the area being audited?					
5.5.	Date of the last fire alarm test?					
5.6.	Date of the last fire evacuation practice?					
5.7.	Are the fire appliances appropriate for the types of fire in this area?					
5.8.	Is there any storage in front of the fire appliances?					
5.9.	Do staff know the location of the fire appliances, exits and assembly point?					
5.10.	Is there a record kept of the staff training and annual up-dating?					
5.11.	Date of the last emergency lighting test?					
6.	**Access, egress and environment**	**Yes**	**No**	**Remarks**	**Action**	**Date & signature**
6.1.	Is there adequate access and egress from all working areas of the department?					
6.2.	Are traffic routes blocked at any time?					
6.3.	Are doorways blocked at any time?					
6.4.	Are all floors free from holes, slopes, pitting, unevenness, etc?					
6.5.	Are floors free from water?					
6.6.	Are drains flush with the floor?					
6.7.	Are drains free from blockage?					
6.8.	During working hours is the temperature maintained at or above 16°C					

6.	Access, egress and environment (cont'd)	Yes	No	Remarks	Action	Date & signature
6.9.	Are suitable thermometers available to determine workplace temperatures?					
6.10.	Is there suitable and sufficient lighting in all work areas?					
6.11.	Is emergency lighting provided where necessary?					
6.12.	Are doors provided with panels to provide visibility if necessary?					
6.13.	Are there sufficient safeguards to prevent injury to people from falling or falling objects?					
6.14.	Is there restricted access to potentially dangerous areas?					
6.15.	Are procedures in place to protect those who enter dangerous areas?					
6.16.	Have staff working in dangerous areas been given adequate instructions regarding the risks and safety measures?					
6.17.	Is there sufficient space in each work area for the tasks to be undertaken?					
6.18.	Is there a restriction on the maximum number of staff and/or visitors in any work area?					
6.19.	Is this restriction complied with?					
6.20.	Do any furnishings, machinery, equipment, etc. impinge on the workspace?					
6.21.	Are staff trained in the risks of equipment, etc. in the work-space?					
6.22.	Is there suitable ventilation in all work areas?					
6.23.	Are there adequate lockers and changing facilities for the staff and visitors?					
6.24.	Are there adequate toilet and washing facilities available for staff and visitors?					

6.	Access, egress and environment (cont'd)	Yes	No	Remarks	Action	Date & signature
6.25.	Are rest rooms and eating facilities adequate for the staff?					
6.26.	Is drinking water available within the department?					
6.27.	Are all areas cleaned daily?					
6.28.	If there are windows are these cleaned regularly?					
6.29.	Are all light fittings and switches in good repair?					
6.30.	Are all leads and plugs in good repair?					
6.31.	Are there sufficient sockets?					
6.32.	Are there any adaptors in use?					
6.33.	Is all electrical equipment checked at least once per year and the checks recorded?					
6.34.	Is the work area clear of trailing leads?					
6.35.	Does the safety supervisor check for unsafe behaviour: Safety devices or equipment not being used? Reaching into machinery when in use? Horseplay? Are there any reasons which create a poor safety attitude?					
6.36.	Do staff understand written instructions, abbreviations, technical information?					
6.37.	Is there training where deficiencies are identified?					
6.38.	Are the individuals physically suited to the tasks to be undertaken?					
7.	Handling and storage of materials	Yes	No	Remarks	Actions	Date & signature
7.1.	Are there written procedures in place for the handling, use and storage of substances?					

7.	Handling and storage of materials (cont'd)	Yes	No	Remarks	Actions	Date & signature
7.2.	Are procedures in place in the event of spillage and/or staff contamination (e.g. cytotoxics)					
7.3.	Are there suitable storage facilities for volatile/inflammable liquids and materials?					
7.4.	Is there adequate storage for substances and/or materials?					
7.5.	Have substances been assessed as required by the Control of Substances Hazardous to Health Regulations (COSHH)? Are the assessments up to date?					
7.6.	Have staff been trained in the use of risk substances?					
7.7.	Are there training records?					
7.8.	Are warning notices displayed where necessary?					
7.9.	Is suitable personal protective equipment available?					
7.10.	Are suitable engineering controls in place where necessary?					
7.11.	Are all portable gas cylinders properly stored, restrained and secured?					
7.12.	Are all storage areas adequately ventilated?					
7.13.	Are all storage areas free from combustible materials?					
7.14.	Are all storage areas secured and of non-combustible construction?					
7.15.	Has environmental/testing monitoring been undertaken, such as: Noise Solvents Fumes (explain)					
7.16.	Are systems exhausted to a safe point external to the workplace?					

7.	Handling and storage of materials (cont'd)	Yes	No	Remarks	Actions	Date & signature
7.17.	Are fume cupboards tested regularly?					
7.18.	Are local exhaust ventilation systems tested as per statutory requirements?					
7.19.	Is there a system for recording testing and problems with ventilation systems?					

8.	Waste collection and disposal	Yes	No	Remarks	Action	Date & signature
8.1.	Is there a departmental waste disposal policy?					
8.2.	Do staff understand and comply with the policy?					
8.3.	Is waste collected in appropriately coloured bags?					
8.4.	Are bags sealed before collection?					
8.5.	Are all waste containers labelled as to their source?					
8.6.	Is there a sharps disposal policy?					
8.7.	Do staff understand and comply with the policy?					
8.8.	Are all sharps injuries reported as per the policy?					
8.9.	Are all sharps injuries dealt with as per the bloodborne diseases policy?					
8.10.	Have relevant vaccinations/ immunizations been offered to staff?					

9.	Equipment and machinery	Yes	No	Remarks	Action	Date & signature
9.1.	Is machinery/equipment suitable by design, construction or adaptation for the purpose intended? If no, explain.					
9.2.	Is there a planned preventative maintenance programme for all equipment?					
9.3.	Is a maintenance log kept?					

9.	Equipment and machinery (cont'd)	Yes	No	Remarks	Action	Date & signature
9.4.	Are information and instructions provided for all equipment and machinery?					
9.5.	Are all appropriate staff trained in the use of departmental equipment before they are required to use it?					
9.6.	Is the training documented?					
9.7.	Can equipment/machinery be isolated from sources of energy if necessary?					
9.8.	Are control systems of work equipment safe?					
10.	**Personal protective equipment (PPE)**	**Yes**	**No**	**Remarks**	**Action**	**Date & signature**
10.1.	Is suitable protective clothing provided for staff?					
10.2.	Is suitable protective equipment provided for staff?					
10.3.	Is PPE provided as a last resort where other controls cannot be implemented?					
10.4.	Does PPE comply with UK legislation and carry the 'CE' mark?					
10.5.	If wearing more than one type of PPE has compatibility been considered?					
10.6.	Has an assessment of need and suitability been carried out and documented?					
10.7.	Is equipment checked regularly for efficiency and effectiveness and examination recorded?					
10.8.	Are all relevant staff trained in equipment function and use?					
10.9.	Is training recorded?					

10. Personal protective equipment (cont'd)	Yes	No	Remarks	Action	Date & signature
10.10. Which of the following PPE are provided: Head protection, Face protection, Eye protection, Ear protection, Respiratory protection, dust, fumes, gases, solvents, etc., Overalls/coveralls, Disposable clothing, Gloves, Footwear, Describe others					
10.11. Are staff monitored in PPE use?					
10.12. Is this monitoring documented?					
10.13. Are there adequate emergency: eye wash stations, showers, first aid boxes					

11. Staff health	Yes	No	Remarks	Action	Date & signature
11.1. Is there a full occupational health service?					
11.2. Is pre-employment screening undertaken?					
11.3. Are health surveillance programmes available for those staff requiring them?					
11.4. Are staff referred to occupational health when a problem arises?					

12. Purchasing controls	Yes	No	Remarks	Action	Date & signature
12.1. Is there a policy on purchasing?					
12.2. Are occupational health, environmental and infection control issues and advice considered when purchasing supplies?					
12.3. Are specifications prepared for suppliers on above issues?					

13.	General issues	Yes	No	Remarks	Action	Date & signature
13.1.	Is the health and safety law poster displayed?					
13.2.	Have health and safety leaflets been given to all staff?					
13.3.	Where applicable, are relevant posters displayed in the work area?					
	Other issues, comments, general assessments in this department.					

14.	Display screen equipment	Yes	No	Remarks	Action	Date & signature
14.1.	Has an inventory of display screen equipment and workstations been undertaken?					
14.2.	Have display screen users been identified?					
14.3.	If necessary have workstation layouts been assessed?					
14.4.	If necessary has the working environment been assessed?					
14.5.	Have findings been reviewed and appropriate action taken?					

15.	Manual handling operations	Yes	No	Remarks	Actions	Date & signature
15.1.	Do manual handling operations involve a significant risk?					
15.2.	Can operations be avoided/mechanized					

Appendix 3
Nursing care plan for a major surgical operation

Activity of living	Usual routines What patient can do independently	Patient's problem (P) Potential problem	Goals
Maintaining a safe environment	Normally independent in all activities of living	Patient unable to regulate position of his body when anaesthetized, possibility of pressure sores	To prevent formulation of pressure sores caused by position on theatre table
		p) Possibility of electrical burns from electrosurgery unit	To prevent electrical burns from electrosurgery unit
		p) Possibility of wrong operation, or wrong side opened	Correct operation on correct side, performed on correct patient
		p) Possibility of swab, needle or instrument left inside wound	No swabs or instruments left inside wound
		p) Shock due to haemorrhage	Minimal shock due to blood loss. Fluids and electrolytes within normal parameters
		p) Injury when being transferred to and from theatre table, and when being positioned	No injury while in theatre
		p) Damage to eyes due to foreign bodies causing corneal abrasions	Patient's eyes will remain undamaged while unconscious
Communication	Normally independent. Pleasant, easy to talk to and interested	p) Unable to express anxiety preoperatively	Allowed to express fears and anxieties. Opportunity to ask questions given, in order to reduce anxiety postoperatively
		Unable to communicate while undergoing anaesthetic	Nurse to act as patient's advocate

Nursing intervention	Rationale	Evaluation
Ripple mattress on table, bony prominences protected with foam pads	Pressure sores can develop due to external pressures, such as hard surfaces. The concentration of body weight on a hard surface is on bony prominences[1,2]	Pressure areas and bony prominences checked when leaving theatre, no skin damage or colour change
Check all jewellery is removed. Safe placement of electrosurgery pad. Protection of skin from metal. Use quiver for blade	The size, shape and placement of the electrosurgery pad is important to prevent burns. Points of contact between patient and metal can cause burns[3]	No burns when leaving theatre
Check patient on arrival – use nameband, notes, consent form and op-list. Check verbally with patient	[2,4]	Patient checked by theatre practitioners, anaesthetist and surgeon. Correct operation performed
Scrub person to count all swabs, needles and instruments with another theatre practitioner before operation begins and just before wound is ready to be closed, and again before skin closure	[2,4,5]	At end of operation all swab, needle and instrument counts correct
Blood loss in theatre monitored. Intravenous infusion in left hand commenced. Blood available if required	The theatre nurse should monitor the patient's blood loss and keep the anaesthetist informed. Blood should be adequately replaced, to prevent shock and hypovolaemia[5]	Minimal blood loss in theatre. Intravenous infusion in progress. Blood transfusion not required
Correct lifting technique used. Adequate number of people to lift patient. Limbs supported at all times	[4]	No injury received while in theatre
Close patient's eyes carefully following induction of anaesthesia. Tape horizontally with hypoallergenic tape: avoid inversion of lashes	Guard eyes against foreign bodies and exposure[4]	Eyes free of foreign body at end of surgery
Preoperative visit by theatre nurse to discuss any fears regarding surgery. Opportunities to ask questions given. Information about postoperative care and analgesia given. Stay with patient until asleep	[6–8]	Patient's questions answered preoperatively. Not unduly anxious. No problems in anaesthetic room
Theatre practitioners should make representations on the patient's behalf as he/she would make themselves if able. Theatre practitioners must be sure that the interests of the patient are promoted	Advocacy for patients essential feature of accountability[5,9,10]	Patient's wellbeing safeguarded.

Activity of living	Usual routines What patient can do independently	Patient's problem (P) Potential problem	Goals
Breathing	Normally independent, does not smoke	Will require intubation with minimal difficulties	To intubate patient quickly and easily causing minimal harm
		Will require ventilation during surgery due to action of muscle relaxant needed for surgery	To ventilate the patient during surgery
		p) Possible chest infection postoperatively	To prevent chest infection postoperatively
Eating and drinking	Normally independent	p) Patient may vomit during induction or postoperatively if food is in stomach	To prevent vomiting during induction and postoperatively
		p) Dehydration due to being 'nil by mouth' pre- and postoperatively	To prevent dehydration and electrolyte imbalance postoperatively
Eliminating	Normally independent	p) Temporary retention of urine due to anaesthetic drugs	Patient will pass urine within 8 hours post-operation
Personal cleansing and dressing	Normally independent	Appropriate clothing needed for day of surgery	To be appropriately bathed and gowned for day of surgery
		p) Possibility of wound infection	To prevent wound infection
Controlling body temperature		p) Possibility of becoming cold during long operation	To keep patient's temperature within normal range during operation
Mobilizing	Normally independent	Patient unable to regulate position of his body when anaesthetized – possibility of nerve damage to cranial/peripheral nerves	To position patient safely, causing no nerve damage

Nursing intervention	Rationale	Evaluation
Check preoperatively if patient has any crowns/loose teeth. Ensure anaesthetic room is fully prepared, assist with intubation	5,10	Patient has a loose crown. Intubation performed quickly and easily, no trauma to crown
Check ventilator is properly prepared, assist with commencing ventilation	10	Patient ventilated throughout surgery, no problems occurred
Intubate with clean endotracheal tube. Explain postoperative deep breathing and coughing preoperatively	5,11,12	Clean endotracheal tube is used. Patient is able to deep breathe and cough. Sputum clear 1 day postoperatively
In anaesthetic room check patient has been 'nil by mouth' 6 hours preoperatively. Give prescribed antiemetics postoperatively	13,14	Checked on arrival in anaesthetic room, has been 'nil by mouth' for 6 hours
Ensure intravenous infusion is commenced and continued in recovery	Body fluids lost during surgery. Intravenous fluid given to maintain fluid and electrolyte balance[5,10,15]	Intravenous infusion commenced preoperatively and continued in recovery
Fluid balance monitored during surgery. Pain relief and privacy provided postoperatively	All anaesthetic agents depress renal haemodynamics and interfere with renal function[16]	Patient passed urine 3 hours postoperatively
Give patient gown to wear to theatre, help to bath preoperatively	17	Patient bathed and dressed in theatre gown
Ensure theatre is clean and instruments sterile. Trolleys and patient's skin prepared aseptically by scrub staff	All patients who undergo surgery have the potential to acquire an infection. The nurse should perform activities to produce a controlled aseptic environment[2,18]	Aseptic environment maintained. No signs of wound infection observed postoperatively
Warmed ripple mattress on theatre table, space blanket to cover patient, temperature monitored during operation	General anaesthetic, skin preparation, preoperative drugs and low ambient theatre temperature contribute to intra-operative hypothermia. Shivering postoperatively may increase pain[15,19]	Patient's temperature remained stable, no shivering postoperatively
Correct transfer from trolley to theatre table, supporting limbs at all times. Protect peripheral nerves with padding	Pressure on peripheral nerves may impair nerve function, resulting in a sensory and/or motor loss. Nerve damage is most likely to occur in areas exposed to hard surfaces[1,4]	Patients safely transferred to table and protected with padding. No nerve damage observed 2 days later

Activity of living	Usual routines What patient can do independently	Patient's problem Potential problem	Goals
Working and playing	Copes with full time job. Leisure mostly involves family	Patient wishes to return to work and normal life as soon as possible	To enable patient to return to normal life as soon as possible
Expressing sexuality	Normally able to express sexuality	p) Concerned about being exposed on the operating table	Patient's dignity will be maintained during surgery
Sleeping	No problems sleeping	p) Physiological changes due to anaesthetic may lead to cardiac or respiratory changes	Patient to experience a safe administration and maintenance of anaesthetic with satisfactory recovery
Dying	Says he does not think of death. Copes with illness and looks forward to a good recovery	p) Minimal risk of death intraoperatively for all patients undergoing surgery	To guard against the minimal risk of intraoperative death

Nursing intervention	Rationale	Evaluation
To prepare patient fully preoperatively both physically and psychologically	Patients who are fully prepared recover more quickly and with fewer complications[7,8]	Patient was prepared both physically and psychologically
No unnecessary exposure of patient during surgery, patient reassurance to be gained	Patients are modest about nudity and feel they have no control over privacy[20]	
Induction and intubation equipment available. Cardiac monitoring to be used	Anaesthetist should check equipment is available and working and have a competent assistant[21]	
Ensure all staff are aware of cardiac arrest, difficult intubation and other emergency procedures	Cardiac arrest or respiratory arrest can occur at any moment in the intraoperative period.[22] Malignant hyperpyrexia can be triggered by anaesthetic	Patient's operation and anaesthetic went well. Emergency procedures not required

REFERENCES

1. Foster C 1987 Positioning the patient. In: Kneedler J, Dodge G (eds) Peri-operative patient care, 2nd edn. Blackwell Scientific Publications, Boston, Chapter 22
2. NATN 1983 Codes of practice, 3rd edn. National Association of Theatre Nurses, Harrogate
3. Elliott C, Pfister JI 1987 The patient is free from harm. In: Kneedler J, Dodge G (eds) Peri-operative patient care, 2nd edn. Blackwell Scientific Publications, Boston, Chapter 11
4. Medical Defence Union 1988 Theatre safeguards. Medical Protection Society, Medical Defence Union of Scotland, National Association of Theatre Nurses, Royal College of Nursing, London
5. Harris L 1980 The specialised role of the neurosurgical operating room nurse. Journal of Neurosurgical Nursing 12: 128–133
6. Wicker P 1987 The role of the nurse in theatre. Senior Nurse 17: 19–21
7. Hayward J 1975 Information, a prescription against pain. Royal College of Nursing, London
8. Boore J 1978 Prescription for recovery. Royal College of Nursing, London
9. UKCC 1989 Exercising accountability. United Kingdom Central Council for Nursing, Midwifery and Health Visiting, London
10. Carrie L, Simpson P 1982 Understanding anaesthesia. Heinemann, London
11. Bernard H 1977 The control of infection. In: Kinney J et al (eds) Manual of surgical intensive care. W.B. Saunders, Philadelphia, Chapter 15
12. Rie M, Pontoppiden H 1987 Ventilatory complications: prevention and treatment. In: Kinney J et al 1977 Manual of surgical intensive care. W.B. Saunders, Philadelphia, Chapter 16
13. Hamilton-Smith S 1972 Nil by mouth? Royal College of Nursing, London
14. Thomas E 1987 Pre-operative fasting – a question of routine? Nursing Times 83: 46–47
15. Rice M 1987 Maintenance of fluid and electrolyte balance. In: Kneedler J, Dodge G (eds) Peri-operative patient care, 2nd edn. Blackwell Scientific Publications, Boston, Chapter 10
16. Hunt P 1985 Post-operative sequelae. In: Smith G, Aitkenhead A (eds) Textbook of Anaesthesia. Churchill Livingstone, Edinburgh, Chapter 21
17. Grundemann B, Huth Meeker K 1987 Alexander's care of the patient in surgery, 8th edn. C.V. Mosby, USA
18. Garner JS, Schultz JK 1987 Absence of infection. In: Kneedler J, Dodge G (eds) Peri-operative patient care, 2nd edn. Blackwell Scientific Publications, Boston, Chapter 13
19. Armstrong M 1980 Current concepts in pain. AORN Journal 32: 383–399
20. Alexander C, Pearson A 1987 Collecting psychological data. In: Kneedler J, Dodge G (eds) Peri-operative patient care, 2nd edn. Blackwell Scientific Publications, Boston, Chapter 5
21. Fell D 1985 The practical conduct of anaesthesia. In: Smith G, Aitkenhead A (eds) Textbook of anaesthesia. Churchill Livingstone, Edinburgh, Chapter 17
22. Persson J 1987 Instruments and equipment. In: Kneedler J, Dodge G (eds) Peri-operative patient care, 2nd edn. Blackwell Scientific Publications, Boston, Chapter 20

Appendix 4
Theatre care plan

PRE-OPERATIVE CARE

Pre-op Visit Performed   Yes/No

PATIENT'S GENERAL DETAILS

1. **ACTIVITY Breathing**	Allergies	
Premedication	YES/NO	
	Time	
Other comments		

2. **Circulation** Pre-op B.P.		Pulse	Temp.
Height	Weight	Other	

3.   **Neurological level/communication**

Pre-operative awareness of operation suggested.

Action required

4.   **Patient comfort/skin**

Difficulties in positioning the patient.

T.E.D.	YES/NO
Isolation requirements	YES/NO

Relevant medication

Relevant blood results

Correct position on canvas

5.   **Specific issues relating to operation**

Time of last nutrition/fluid

Opsite marked

Identity bracelet

Removal of prosthesis	Consent	YES/NO
	Notes and X-rays	YES/NO

WARD NURSE Signature	PRINT
THEATRE RECEIVING PERSONNEL	PRINT

PRE-OPERATIVE VISIT

Date of visit	Time
Patient's preferred name	
Are relatives aware? YES/NO	
Next of kin Tel. No.	
Patient expressed worries or specific wishes	
Any other relevant information	
Signature of visiting/ward nurse	PRINT

ANAESTHETIC ROOM CARE

1.	**ACTIVITY Breathing**		
Type of anaesthesia: General YES/NO		Local YES/NO	
Intubation YES/NO	Mask YES/NO	Laryngeal mask	YES/NO
Packs: Throat YES/NO		Nasogastric tube	YES/NO
Others – state			

2.	**Circulation**	Peripheral line YES/NO	Site
Neck line	YES/NO	Site	
Arterial line	YES/NO	Site	
TOURNIQUET	time on	pressure	position

3.	**Patient comfort**	Warming blanket YES/NO
Other comments		
Personal belongings – state/stored		

OPERATIVE CARE

Hand over given to: NAME	

Safety issues communicated

Patient identity	YES/NO
Consent	YES/NO
Allergies	YES/NO
Difficulties in positioning	YES/NO

1. ACTIVITY Breathing   Specific complications. State:

2. Circulation   Blood loss volume

Diathermy   mono   site   Bipolar   YES/NO

Tourniquet time off

3. Comfort/pressure area care   Appropriate care taken   YES/NO

Pack in situ	YES/NO	
Drains in situ	YES/NO	
Urinary catheter	YES/NO	Size
Type of dressing		

4. Specific issues   Incision site

Skin closure type clips   YES/NO   Absorb   YES/NO   Non absorb   YES/NO

Skin prep used   Irrigation/washout fluid

STATE IF ACTION TAKEN

SWABS correct	YES/NO
SHARP correct	YES/NO
INSTRUMENTS correct	YES/NO
SPECIMENS SENT	YES/NO

MICROBIOLOGY	PATHOLOGY
HISTOLOGY	CYTOLOGY
HAEMATOLOGY	OTHER

SCRUB NURSE Signature   PRINT

CIRCULATING NURSE Signature   PRINT

ACTIVITY	INTERVENTION	INITIAL ASSESSMENT
1. Breathing **GOAL** Maintains adequate ventilation	Maintain airway, check spontaneous breathing. Place patient in optimum position for recovery. Give prescribed O_2. Report to anaesthetist and take necessary action if patient is not breathing.	
2. Circulation Maintains haemodynamic stability. Detection of bleeding. Maintain body fluid and nutritional needs.	Monitor pulse, BP and Sa O_2. Recognise and report significant changes. Maintain accurate fluid balance charts and analyse losses from drains and dressings. Report as required. Observe dressing sites.	
3. Neurological level communication Ensure safe return to pre-operative state.	Remain with unconscious patient, monitor and report changes in pupil reaction and responses to verbal and tactile stimulation.	
4. Comfort and pain relief Alleviate pain and discomfort. Prevent the formation of pressure sores. Access skin for adverse reaction. Offer support to patient and relatives.	Correctly position limbs as per postoperative instruction. Give analgesia as prescribed. Check patient's skin regularly. Recognise the needs of the patient and relatives.	
5. Hygiene and dressing Maintenance of asepsis. Maintenance of dignity.	Check dressing sites and cannulation sites. Ensure patient is afforded privacy.	
6. Specific to operation		

RECOVERY CARE

OPERATION PERFORMED.
BRIEF EVALUATION BEFORE DISCHARGE TO THE WARD

1.	**ACTIVITY Breathing**

2.	**Circulation**

3.	**Neurological level and communication**

4.	**Comfort and pain relief**

5.	**Hygiene and dressings**

6.	**Specific issues relating to operating**

POST-OP INSTRUCTIONS

Personal belongings returned

State

NOTES   YES/NO   X-ray   YES/NO

RECOVERY NURSE   PRINT
Signature

HANDOVER GIVEN TO   PRINT
Signature

Appendix 5

Patient-controlled analgesia protocols

The following protocols are samples and for reference purposes only.

SAMPLE 1

Core intravenous PCA regimen

Drug of choice: morphine
Concentration: 1 mg/ml
Mode: continuous plus PCA
Loading dose: as required
Dose each PCA demand: 1 mg
Lockout period: 5–10 min
Background infusion rate: 1–3 mg/h

General guidelines

Infusion bags will be prepared by: anaesthetist
100 ml saline plus
100 mg morphine

When appropriate, PCA will be set up by: anaesthetist in recovery room

Bags should only be prepared for immediate use

Sets and bags will be stored: in theatres

Key to lock box should be kept with the controlled drugs keys and can be located in: ward using the pump

Maximum duration of
PCA: 48 hours

All patients should be
counselled preoperatively

Specific guidelines

In addition to standard postoperative observations, the following should also be recorded:

- pain scores
- sedation scores
- respiratory rate
- pulse
- blood pressure.

Once the patient is stable the frequency of these observations should be:

- HALF-hourly for 2 hours
- HOURLY for 2 hours
- TWO-hourly thereafter.

Special instructions

If the respiratory rate falls to less than 10 per minute, *STOP PCA* and call the anaesthetist.

If the patient is receiving inadequate analgesia, you believe they understand how to receive doses when in pain and the history button confirms they are demanding and receiving analgesia, call the duty anaesthetist to reassess therapy.

Prescription and dose administration records

Required documents:

- PCA prescription sheet

- ward record sheet
- hospital inpatient prescription chart.

The PCA prescription should be written clearly on the prescription sheet by the prescribing anaesthetist.

Under PRN section of hospital inpatient prescription chart should be written 'Pain relief, see PCA prescription sheet'.

The morphine should be logged in the recovery room's controlled drugs record book.

Additional analgesics should also be prescribed here, or as a STAT dose with very clear prescribing indications. Generally no additional analgesics should be prescribed, and should only be given upon clear instructions.

Loading doses should be recorded clearly in the hospital inpatient prescription chart as a STAT dose and in bold print on the PCA prescription sheet.

If PCA therapy is discontinued before the infusion bag is empty, the contents must be destroyed and this witnessed by two nurses and/or pharmacists; the amount destroyed must be recorded in the ward record sheet.

Upon completion of therapy the duration of therapy and the total amount of drug administered should be recorded on the PCA prescription sheet.

Dose administration records need to be kept:

- when PCA is first set up
- when PCA is discontinued.

SAMPLE 2

Ward: _____

Hospital: _____

_____

_____

_____

Core regimen

Drug of choice: _____

Concentration: _____

Mode: _____

Loading dose: _____

Lockout period: _____

4-hour limit: _____

Background infusion rate: _____

General guidelines _____

Bags will be prepared by: _____

    Daytime: _____

Bags will be changed by: Nocte: _____

PCA will be set up by: _____

Sets and bags will be
stored: _____

A loading dose will be
given: _____

Antiemetics and night sedation will be prescribed on a PRN basis:
_____

Keys to PCA pumps should be kept with the controlled drug keys and can be located in:

_____

All patients should be counselled preoperatively.

Specific guidelines
In addition to standard postoperative observations the following should also be recorded:

Pain scores
Sedation scores
Respiratory rate

Once the patient is stable the frequency of these
observations should be:
_____ hourly for _____ hours
_____ hourly for _____ hours
_____ hourly thereafter.

Special instructions
If the respiratory rate falls to _____ /minute
remove patient pendant.

If the respiratory rate falls to _____ /minute STOP
PCA and call

_____ .

If the patient is receiving inadequate analgesia,
you believe they understand how to receive
doses when in pain and the history button
confirms they are demanding and receiving
analgesia, call _____ to reassess therapy.

Prescription and dose administration records
The PCA prescription should be written clearly
on _____ by the prescribing anaesthetist.

The _____ should be logged in the
controlled drugs record book as per usual.

The bag contents, drug and mg/ml concentration should be entered as given in the nursing
Kardex, with the date and time of set-up.

Under PRN section of standard prescription
sheet should be written 'Pain relief, see PCA prescription sheet'.

Additional analgesics should also be prescribed here, or as a STAT dose with very clear prescribing indications. As a rule no additional analgesics should be prescribed, and are to be given only upon clear instruction.

Loading doses given independently of the infuser should be recorded clearly in the Kardex, as a STAT dose and in bold print on the PCA prescription sheet, as this dose will not be included in the cumulative dose displayed on the front panel of the infuser.

If PCA therapy is discontinued mid-syringe/bag the contents must be destroyed and witnessed by two nurses and/or pharmacists, and the amount destroyed should be recorded in the controlled drug book, Kardex and prescription charts.

Upon completion of therapy the duration of therapy and total amount of drug administered should be recorded.

Dose administration records need to be kept:

- when PCA is first set up
- at each syringe/bag change
- when PCA is discontinued.

Collation of evidence

Upon completion of therapy the patient is invited to fill in the Patient Evaluation of PCA.

The nurse should complete her evaluation independently of the patient in order that realistic comparisons between actual and perceived efficacy of therapy may be judged.

Index

Prongs, nasal 312
Propanolol 328
Propofol 134
Prostheses 99
Protamine sulphate 328
Protocols, wound management 199
Providers
    and day surgery 24–25
    role in contracting 8
Provision and Use of Work Equipment
        Regulation 1992, 63
Pulse oximetry 127–128
Puncture, gloves 191
Purchasers
    and contracts 8, 11
    and day surgery 24–25
Purchasing, information technology 22
Purpose, defining departments' 5–6
Pyrogens, and gloves 190

Q

Quality
    in contracts 9, 11
    definition 10
Quality assurance 13
    benefits 14
    definition 10
    electrosurgery 237
Quantiflex flowmeters 104
Questionnaires
    day surgery 31
    satisfaction 13

R

Radiation Protection Advisor 79
Radiation Protection Supervisor 79
Radiology
    facilities 341–342
    and safety 79–80
REACT score 316
Real–time data entry systems 18
Reassurance, in anaesthetic room
        95–96
Rebreathing bags 107
Reception, of patients 98–100
Reception area, day surgery unit,
        design 356–357
Receptionists 357
Records
    errors 48
    and information technology 15
    legislation 48
    patients' access 36, 42–43
    for theatre 98
Recovery
    area design 347–348
    in day surgery units 25, 26, 360
    drugs 308
    equipment 308–309
    from endoscopy 220

gases in 347–348
    observations 310–314
    patient care 309–310
Reflexes, vagal 133
Refusal, of treatment 41
Regional anaesthesia 100–101, 117–121,
        143
Regulations, health and safety 63,
        74–78
Religious needs, in anaesthetic room
        96
Remifentanil 140
Reporting
    incidents 83
    and information technology 18–19
Reservoir bags 107
Resources, scheduling 16
Respiratory system, and position 293
Respirometer 128–129
Rest, in recovery 314
Rest rooms, design 349
Results, for theatre 98
Resuscitation
    equipment 117
    procedure 320
Retraction, by sutures 163
Retractors 157
Reverse Trendelenburg position 289
Rhys–Davies exsanguinator
        247–248
Rights, patients' 40–43
Ringer's solutions 144
Risk, definition 59
Risk estimate 371
Risk management 59–60, 61, 66
    audit 66
    benefits 370
    and buildings projects 369–370
    and design 66–68
    infection control 64–65, 70–73
Robertshaw laryngoscopes 113
Rocuronium 135
Roper, Logan and Tierney's model of
        nursing 271–273
Roy's model of nursing 269, 271

S

Safety
    see also hazards, infection control,
        risk management, fire safety
    and access 66
    audits 62, 380–389
    checklists for theatre 98–100
    chemicals 74–76, 205, 206
    correct operation 299–302
    and day surgery units 352
    during anaesthesia 97–98, 141, 143
    electrical 78
    and electrosurgery 235–237
    endoscopy 215–217
    environmental 66–70
    instruments 161

lasers 80–81, 226–227
    needlestick injuries 191
    policy 62
    positioning 286–287, 295–296
    and radiology 79–80
    regulations 63, 74–78
    reporting staff 45
    training 62, 64
Salbutamol 328
Satisfaction, questionnaires 13
Saws 239–241
Scabs, formation 195
Scavenging 109
Schedules, and information
        technology 16
Scope of Professional Practice 37–38
Scopolamine 133
Screening
    and exposure to infection 65
    staff 71
Scrub area
    design 346–347
    supplies for 149
Scrub practitioners
    duties 186, 209, 258–260
    and infection control 71, 252
Scrub room 252
Scrubbing, surgical, procedure 252–253
Seating, day surgery units 358
Secretions, reduction 132
Security 335
    and access 66
    data 20
    and day surgery units 352
    information technology 19–20
Sedation 132–133
    Castle Hill Conscious Sedation Scale
        220
    endoscopy 218–219
Semiclosed systems 109
Seminar rooms, design 349–350
Seroma 207
Services
    care services 8
    trends 334
Servicing, equipment 350–351
Servoflurane 139
Seward laryngoscopes 113
Sharps
    categories 153
    disposal 70, 259
    injuries 191
Shear, and pressure sore development
        276
Shelanski test 191
Shelves, infection risk 148
Shock 318
Signs 351–352
    day surgery units 361
Silicone implants 193
Sinks 346
Sizing
    day surgery units 364
    theatres 67, 364–367